PREGNANCY AND BIRTH
IN EARLY MODERN FRANCE

The Other Voice in Early Modern Europe:
The Toronto Series, 23

The Other Voice in
Early Modern Europe:
The Toronto Series

SERIES EDITORS Margaret L. King *and* Albert Rabil, Jr.
SERIES EDITOR, ENGLISH TEXTS Elizabeth H. Hageman

Previous Publications in the Series

MADRE MARÍA ROSA
Journey of Five Capuchin Nuns
Edited and translated by Sarah E.
Owens
2009

GIOVAN BATTISTA ANDREINI
Love in the Mirror: A Bilingual Edition
Edited and translated by Jon R. Snyder
2009

RAYMOND DE SABANAC AND SIMONE
ZANACCHI
Two Women of the Great Schism: The
Revelations *of Constance de Rabastens
by Raymond de Sabanac and* Life of
the Blessed Ursulina of Parma *by
Simone Zanacchi*
Edited and translated by Renate
Blumenfeld-Kosinski and Bruce L.
Venarde
2010

OLIVA SABUCO DE NANTES BARRERA
The True Medicine
Edited and translated by Gianna
Pomata
2010

LOUISE-GENEVIÈVE GILLOT DE
SAINCTONGE
Dramatizing Dido, Circe, and Griselda
Edited and translated by Janet Levarie
Smarr
2010

PERNETTE DU GUILLET
Complete Poems: A Bilingual Edition
Edited by Karen Simroth James
Translated by Marta Rijn Finch
2010

ANTONIA PULCI
*Saints' Lives and Bible Stories for the
Stage: A Bilingual Edition*
Edited by Elissa B. Weaver
Translated by James Wyatt Cook
2010

VALERIA MIANI
*Celinda, A Tragedy: A Bilingual
Edition*
Edited by Valeria Finucci
Translated by Julia Kisacky
Annotated by Valeria Finucci and Julia
Kisacky
2010

The Other Voice in
Early Modern Europe:
The Toronto Series

SERIES EDITORS Margaret L. King *and* Albert Rabil, Jr.
SERIES EDITOR, ENGLISH TEXTS Elizabeth H. Hageman

Previous Publications in the Series

Enchanted Eloquence: Fairy Tales by Seventeenth-Century French Women Writers
Edited and translated by Lewis C. Seifert and Domna C. Stanton
2010

Leibniz and the Two Sophies: The Philosophical Correspondence
Edited and translated by Lloyd Strickland
2011

In Dialogue with the Other Voice in Sixteenth-Century Italy: Literary and Social Contexts for Women's Writing
Edited by Julie D. Campbell and Maria Galli Stampino
2011

Sister Giustina Niccolini
The Chronicle of Le Murate
Edited and translated by Saundra Weddle
2011

Liubov Krichevskaya
No Good without Reward: Selected Writings: A Bilingual Edition
Edited and translated by Brian James Baer
2011

Elizabeth Cooke Hoby Russell
The Writings of an English Sappho
Edited by Patricia Phillippy
With translations by Jaime Goodrich
2011

Lucrezia Marinella
Exhortations to Women and to Others if They Please
Edited and translated by Laura Benedetti
2012

Margherita Datini
Letters to Francesco Datini
Translated by Carolyn James and Antonio Pagliaro
2012

The Other Voice in
Early Modern Europe:
The Toronto Series

SERIES EDITORS Margaret L. King *and* Albert Rabil, Jr.
SERIES EDITOR, ENGLISH TEXTS Elizabeth H. Hageman

Previous Publications in the Series

Delarivier Manley & Mary Pix
English Women Staging Islam,
1696–1707
Edited and translated by Bernadette
Andrea
2012

Cecilia Del Nacimiento
Journeys of a Mystic Soul in Poetry and
Prose
Introduction and prose translations by
Kevin Donnelly
Poetry translations by Sandra Sider
2012

Lady Margaret Douglas and
Others
The Devonshire Manuscript: A
Women's Book of Courtly Poetry
Edited and introduced by Elizabeth
Heale
2012

Arcangela Tarabotti
Letters Familiar and Formal
Edited and translated by Meredith K.
Ray and Lynn Lara Westwater
2012

Three Spanish Querelle *Texts:* Grisel
and Mirabella, The Slander against
Women, *and* The Defense of Ladies
against Slanderers
Edited and translated by Emily C.
Francomano
2013

Barbara Torelli Benedetti
Partenia, a Pastoral Play: A Bilingual
Edition
Edited and translated by Lisa Sampson
and Barbara Burgess-Van Aken
2013

Pregnancy and Birth in Early Modern France

Treatises by Caring Physicians
and Surgeons (1581–1625)

FRANÇOIS ROUSSET, JEAN LIEBAULT,
JACQUES GUILLEMEAU, JACQUES DUVAL
AND LOUIS DE SERRES

Edited and Translated by

VALERIE WORTH-STYLIANOU

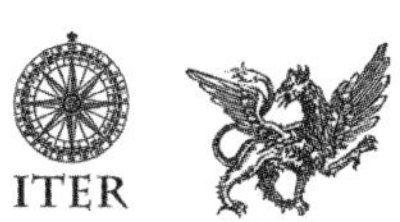

Iter Inc.
Centre for Reformation and Renaissance Studies
Toronto
2013

Iter: Gateway to the Middle Ages and Renaissance
Tel: 416/978–7074   Email: iter@utoronto.ca
Fax: 416/978–1668   Web: www.itergateway.org

Centre for Reformation and Renaissance Studies
Victoria University in the University of Toronto
Tel: 416/585–4465   Email: crrs.publications@utoronto.ca
Fax: 416/585–4430   Web: www.crrs.ca

Iter and the Centre for Reformation and Renaissance Studies gratefully acknowledge the generous support of James E. Rabil, in memory of Scottie W. Rabil, toward the publication of this book.

Library and Archives Canada Cataloguing in Publication

Pregnancy and birth in early modern France : treatises by caring physicians and surgeons (1581–1625), François Rousset, Jean Liebault, Jacques Guillemeau, Jacques Duval and Louis de Serres / edited and translated by Valerie Worth-Stylianou.

(Other voice in early modern Europe. Toronto series ; 23)
Translated from the French.
Includes bibliographical references and index.
Contents: New treatise on hysterotomotoky, or childbirth by Cesarean (1581) / François Rousset -- Three books dealing with the infirmities and illnesses of women (1582) / Jean Liebault -- On the safe delivery of women (1609) / Jacques Guillemeau -- On hermaphrodites, deliveries of women (1612) / Jacques Duval -- Treatise on sterility among women (1625) / Louis de Serres.
Issued in print and electronic formats.
Co-published by: Iter Inc.
ISBN 978-0-7727-2138-9 (pbk.).--ISBN 978-0-7727-2139-6 (pdf)

1. Pregnancy--France--Early works to 1800. 2. Childbirth--France--Early works to 1800. 3. Birth customs--France--Early works to 1800. 4. Women--Health and hygiene--France--Early works to 1800. 5. Obstetrics--France--Early works to 1800. 6. Physicians--France--Early works to 1800. 7. Surgeons--France--Early works to 1800. I. Worth-Stylianou, Valerie, editor of compilation, translator II. Guillemeau, Jacques, 1550–1613? De l'heureux accouchement des femmes. English. III. Liébault, Jean, approximately 1535–1596. Trois livres appartenant aux infirmitez et maladies des femmes. English. IV. Duval, Jacques, 1555?–1615? Hermaphrodits, accouchements des femmes, et traitements qui est requis pour les relever en santé, et bien élever leurs enfants. English. V. Serres, Louys de, active 1625. Discours de la nature, causes, signes et curation des empeschemens de la conception, et de la stérilité des femme. English. VI. Rousset, François, 1535?–1590?. Traité nouveau de l'hysterotomotokie, ou enfantement caesarien. English. VII. Victoria University (Toronto, Ont.). Centre for Reformation and Renaissance Studies VIII. Iter Inc IX. Series: Other voice in early modern Europe. Toronto series ; 23

RG518.F8P74 2013   618.20094409'031   C2013-902924-9
                                                     C2013-902925-7

Cover illustration:
Birthing chair in use. Midwife delivers the mother, while another woman supports the mother from behind. 16th-century woodcut from Eucharius Rösslin *The Garden of Roses*. / Universal History Archive / UIG / The Bridgeman Art Library UIG 527516.

Cover design:
Maureen Morin, Information Technology Services, University of Toronto Libraries.

Typesetting:
Julian Littlewood, Oxford

Production:
Iter Inc.

Table of Contents

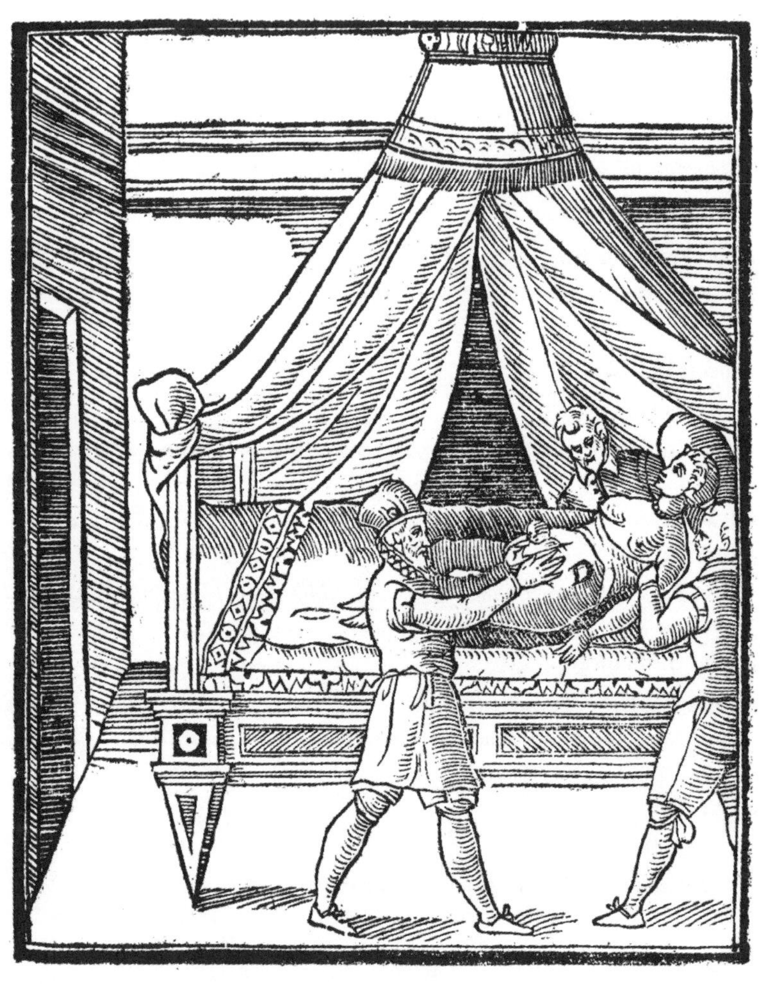

1) Cesarean section on a living woman

Scipio Mercurio, *La Commare*, Venice, 1601
(Wellcome Library, London)

Table of Illustrations

Acknowledgments

This book has been some six years in gestation, and over that period I have been fortunate to work with outstanding colleagues and students, first at Exeter University, and now at Trinity College Oxford. My warmest thanks go to all those — in Exeter, Oxford and elsewhere — who have helped and encouraged me. Among colleagues who have generously shared their knowledge with me on points large and small, I am particularly indebted to: Peter Brown, Jonathan Downing, Lisa Downing, Michael Inwood, Joy Littlewood, Ian Maclean, Emma Percy, Hugh Roberts and Brenda Stones. I must also pay a special tribute to the friendship of Robbie Hyland, Isabel Lough and Annabel Ownsworth in the Academic Office and Ulli Parkinson in the President's Office, and to the Fellowship of Trinity College Oxford, which, since 2009, has provided the ideal environment for academic discussions.

While undertaking the research, I have benefited greatly from discussions and collaborations with colleagues working on diverse aspects of early modern science and women's reproductive health. This book would have been far poorer without the scholarly insights (and friendship) of Janette Allotey, Violaine Giacomotto-Charra, Philip Ford, Monica Green, Elaine Hobby, Helen King, Alison Klairmont Lingo, Stephanie O'Hara, Jacqueline Vons and Adrian Wilson. My thanks also to all the delegates who attended the interdisciplinary conference on 'Retelling Familiar Tales of Pregnancy and Birth' in Oxford in 2012, and shared in two days of lively discussions on this subject!

Even in the digital era, early modern scholarship requires frequent access to libraries, and it is a pleasure to acknowledge here the unfailingly generous help of all the librarians I consulted (in the UK, France and the US), and especially Sharon Cure (Trinity College Oxford), and the librarians of the Taylor Insitution and the Bodleian Library, Oxford, and of the Royal College of Obstetricians and Gynaecologists, London. I was equally fortunate to be supported in IT matters by Jamie Aylward at Exeter (who set up my research website, www.birthingtales.org) and by Alastair Johnson at Trinity College Oxford.

As the book came close to its final shape, far more debts were incurred. Alison Klairmont Lingo very generously shared with me the draft of her magisterial introduction and notes, which will appear shortly in this series, accompanying Stephanie O'Hara's fine translation of the works of the midwife Louise Bourgeois. It has been invaluable to exchange ideas and questions with Alison over the past few years, and she, Stephanie and I see our two volumes as complementary sides of a coin.

The external reader of my manuscript, Gianna Pomata, provided welcome encouragement and some extremely helpful new insights into my texts, which I have been pleased to acknowledge in the footnotes. I could not have asked for a wiser or kinder Series Editor than Al Rabil, who has supported this project every step of the way, and provided invaluable academic and practical guidance. My copy editor, Cherry Mosteshar, tamed lengthy sentences, inserted commas in the right places and clarified my English expression with a secure yet light touch. Martin Sanders (of MapArt) produced two maps that illustrate concisely Rousset's travels. The typesetting of the volume bears testimony to Julian Littlewood's superb professional skills, and I am ever grateful for his good humour while translating the author's wishes into material form. Finally, thank you to Margaret English-Haskin and Anabela Carneiro for their great care in designing the front cover and seeing the volume through the press at Iter.

I am indebted to the British Academy and the National Endowment for the Humanities Board for the grants they awarded me, which provided vital financial support for various stages of this project. The NEH's award has, in particular, funded the reproduction of images for this volume, and I am also grateful to all the libraries and museums which have kindly allowed me to reproduce these.

Finally, my special thanks to my family, Nick, Anastasia and Christopher (and our cats). To my husband for his generous encouragement, unfailing and stimulating interest in things early modern, and for sharing his wealth of classical scholarship with me. To our children for their tolerant curiosity about my project, and for asking some very searching questions! And to our cats for distracting me regularly from over-serious thoughts…

All errors of fact and judgment remain my own.

Conventions

Where proper names or medical terms are essential to the understanding of the immediate context, I use footnotes. For other key references to people, medical terms and herbs or medicines, the reader should consult the Glossaries (349-371).

Titles of works originally published in a language other than English, but of which well-known English translations exist (e.g. works by Galen, Hippocrates, Aristotle) are given in the standard English form only. In the case of works first published in languages other than English for which there is not a well-known translation — or sometimes no translation at all — I provide my own English translation of the title, followed in square brackets by the title of the original text: e.g. *On Betrothals* [*De sponsalibus*].

In citing any early modern text in a sixteenth or seventeenth-century edition, I retain the original spelling, but resolve i/j and u/v and any contractions.

Spelling of proper names in early modern texts is often irregular, sometimes even within one text. For simplicity, I have adopted one standard spelling of each proper name throughout, indicating any significant variant forms in a footnote on the first occurrence. Capitalization in early modern texts is also often irregular, and generally reflects the practice of an individual printer rather than the author. I have standardized it in accordance with modern conventions, except in the translation of title pages where I reproduce the original capitalization. Similarly, except in the case of title pages, I have not retained the original use of fonts (e.g. italic versus Roman), with the one exception of Pena's additions to Liebault's texts (see 69), where the italic characters in the seventeenth-century editions of the text invited the reader to distinguish the writings of Pena from Liebault's original text.

GENERAL INTRODUCTION

*Conception, Pregnancy and Childbirth
in Early Modern France*

Medical Treatises in French, c. 1550–1650

> … so that women of all stations may receive […] good support, and so that their cruellest mortal sufferings may be reduced, alleviated and ended; their illnesses cured; their lives saved and preserved; and their children, who would otherwise perish at birth, may be delivered more easily and safely while they enjoy good health and recovery.[1]

The sixteenth and earlier seventeenth centuries in western Europe are marked by the rising number of volumes circulating in both Latin and, increasingly, in vernacular languages on the subject of women's health in general, and on conception, pregnancy and childbirth in particular. France was at the forefront of the growth in such vernacular medical treatises: some twenty works were published in French between 1530 and 1630, and over seventy editions of these have been documented to date.[2] For this reason alone, the French treatises merit attention, but in addition a number of them were also translated into other languages, including English and even Latin, which remained the international language of medicine well into the seventeenth century,[3]

---

1. Jacques Duval, *On Hermaphrodites and Deliveries of Women* (1612): see 232.

2. I provide full bibliographical details of these French works in my volume *Les Traités d'obstétrique en langue française au seuil de la modernité: bibliographie critique des 'Divers Travaulx d'Euchaire Rösslin' (1536) à l'Apologie De Louyse Bourgeois sage femme' (1627)*, (Droz: Geneva, 2007). I draw on the pioneering study of the treatment of women in French Renaissance medicine by E. Berriot-Salvadore, *Un corps, un destin: la femme dans la médecine de la Renaissance* (Paris: Champion, 1993), and on the analysis of scholarly Renaissance debates and beliefs (in Latin and vernacular texts) about the female body and procreation in I. Maclean, *The Renaissance Notion of Woman. A study in the fortunes of scholasticism and medical science in European intellectual life* (Cambridge: Cambridge University Press, 1980). For other medical texts published in French, it is still useful to consult the census by H. Stone, 'The French Language in Renaissance Medicine', *Bibliothèque d'Humanisme et Renaissance* XV (1953), 315–343.

3. I. Maclean provides an analysis of trends in the composition, publishing and circulation of Latin medical works in the Renaissance in his chapter, 'The diffusion of learned medicine in the sixteenth century through the printed book', in eds. W. Bracke and H. Deumens, *Medical Latin from the Late Middle Ages to the Eighteenth Century* (Brussels, 2000), 93–114. He demonstrates (100–101) a particularly sharp increase in the production of medical works in Latin across Western Europe between 1570 and 1630.

and so their significance is extensive. The number of vernacular medical works published in French was significantly higher than that for other languages, a fact that admits no simple explanation.[4] We may conjecture that, in part, the success of the first treatises probably encouraged other French medical writers to follow suit.[5] Equally, the international reputation of the medical faculties in Montpellier and Paris attracted students from France and beyond who were eager to learn under leading physicians and anatomists, and the interest in conception, pregnancy and delivery shown by such distinguished figures as Ambroise Paré, André Du Laurens and Jean Riolan the younger undoubtedly fueled the energy of those who studied under them.

Who were the authors of these French vernacular treatises, and what do we know of their envisaged and actual readerships? All but one of the works were written by men, most often by physicians, and in a few cases by surgeons; the one exception was the royal midwife, Louise Bourgeois, who recorded her *Observations* based on her care and delivery of some 2,000 women in a series of three volumes appearing in 1609, 1617 and 1626.[6] These *Observations* apart, the

---

4. See *Les Traités d'obstétrique au seuil de la modernité*, p. 46. The treatment of women's health, pregnancy and childbirth in French medical texts also encouraged writers of fiction and poetry to take up some of these themes, as explored by H. Tucker in *Pregnant Fictions: Childbirth and the Fairy Tale in Early Modern France* (Detroit: Wayne State University Press, 2003), and by K. Read in *Birthing Bodies in Early Modern France: Stories of Gender and Reproduction* (Farnham: Ashgate, 2011).

5. See the number of French editions between 1536 and 1632 of Eucharius Rösslin's midwifery treatise (*A Rosegarden for Pregnant Women and Midwives*); and from 1549–1685 of Ambroise Paré's works concerning pregnancy and birth; and the run-away success from 1578–1608 of Laurent Joubert's *Popular Errors* [*Erreurs populaires*], largely concerned with women's sexual and reproductive health (*Les Traités d'obstétrique*, 96–117, 123–142, 194–233).

6. Bourgeois was ahead of her counterparts in other European countries: see *Diverse Observations on Sterility, Miscarriage, Fertility, Childbirth, and the Diseases of Women and Newborn Children (1626)*, O'Hara, and Klairmont Lingo. (Toronto: Toronto University Press, forthcoming). In her introduction, Klairmont Lingo draws attention to Bourgeois's 'commanding style with an assured rhetoric that underlines her right to contribute to medical knowledge'. For an earlier study of Bourgeois's career, see W. Perkins, *Midwifery and Medicine in Early Modern France: Louise Bourgeois* (Exeter: University of Exeter Press, 1996). The first treatise published by a midwife in England was Jane Sharp's *The Midwives Book* of 1671, and in Germany Justine Siegemundin's *The Court Midwife* of 1690.

medical treatises offer only a masculine, professional perspective on the uniquely female activity of bearing children.[7] However, the male authors are often aware that they are addressing a mixed audience, comprising professionals and lay readers, the latter including men and women. Some of the treatises are clearly directed at fellow practitioners, sometimes physicians and often surgeons (who, as a group, could not be expected to have the physicians' ability to read Latin fluently). Occasionally they are directed at apothecaries, or midwives — an exclusively female group, which ranged from skilled, trained, literate women at the highest end (especially in major cities) to unskilled, untrained and illiterate practitioners, the least reputable of whom were typical figures of satirical humor.[8] Other texts are either primarily or partly directed at lay readers, especially literate women of childbearing age.

In most respects, historians of medicine would argue that the theoretical understanding and practical care of pregnancy and childbirth does not change markedly between the Middle Ages and the mid- to late-seventeenth century. Abraham Bosse's etching of a family scene of childbirth in 1633, and the accompanying (anonymous) verses, shown opposite, are representative of this continuum.[9] However, other areas of women's medicine — what today would be termed gynecology — did evolve. In particular, Monica Green has convincingly argued that 'the gendering of gynecology took a different path from that of obstetrics', so that, by the turn of the sixteenth century, 'while care of uncomplicated births remained in the hands of women, gynecological care (as well as certain aspects of emergency obstetrical care) had passed into the hands of men.'[10] It

7. Even literate women of this period do not often record in writing intimate details of their experiences of pregnancy and giving birth, judging by the various letters and journals I have perused without finding the autobiographical information a modern perspective might lead us to anticipate.

8. See for example the incompetent, avaricious midwives who swarm to attend Gargamelle in Rabelais's *Gargantua* (1534), ch. VI.

9. I would observe that it was unlikely a father would often be present at the birth; this is probably a rhetorical rather than realistic aspect of the representation, whereas most other details of the picture appear a very close reflection of contemporary social reality. On reading Bosse's image see: C. Goldstein, *Print Culture in Early Modern France. Abraham Bosse and the purposes of print* (Cambridge: Cambridge University Press, 2012), 59–68.

10. *Making Women's Medicine Masculine. The rise of male authority in pre-modern gynaecology* (Oxford: Oxford University Press, 2008), x.

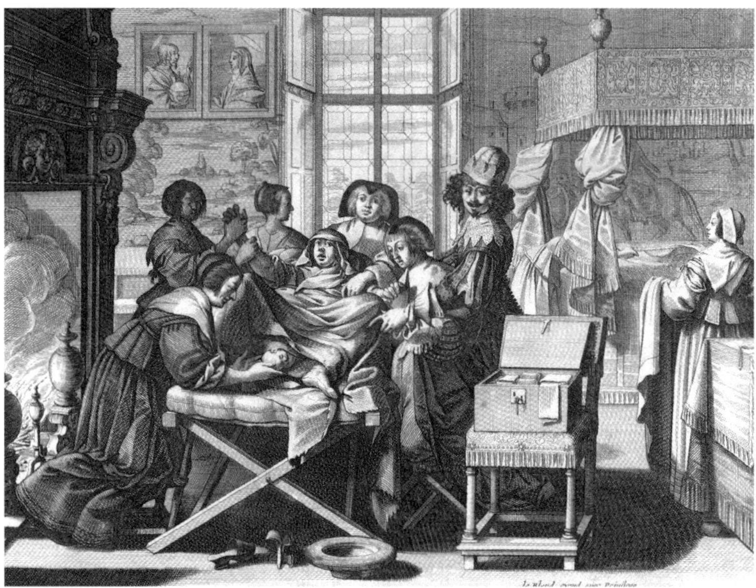

2) Family scene of childbirth

Abraham Bosse, *L'Accouchement* (etching), Paris, 1633
(The Metropolitan Museum of Art, Harris Brisbane Dick Fund, 1926. 26.49.40 Image)

Alas! I can bear it no longer: the suffering
which grips me
Weakens me completely;
My body is dying and there is no cure
For the pains I feel.
THE MOTHER IN LABOR[11]

Madam, be patient,
Do not cry out in this way;
It's finished, and I swear
You are giving birth to a fine Boy.
THE MIDWIFE[12]

This news brings me relief,
Now all my grief is wiped away,
Come, my dear, be brave,
Your suffering will soon be over.
THE HUSBAND[13]

In this painful labor, to which no other
torment
Can be compared;
Deliver her, Lord, and keep her safe
In giving birth.
THE WOMAN PRAYING[14]

11. I have given an English translation of the four short (anonymous) poems which Bosse had printed beneath the etching. The French original reads: 'Hélas! Je n'en puis plus: le mal qui me possede / Affoiblit tous mes sens; / Mon corps s'en va mourant et n'est point de remede / Aux peines que je sens.' L'ACCOUCHÉE

12. 'Madame prenez patience, / Sans crier de ceste façon; / C'en-est faict, en ma conscience / Vous accouchez d'un beau Garçon.' LA SAGE FEMME. (In French, the lines spoken by the midwife and husband are markedly shorter than those of the mother or woman praying.)

13. 'Cette nouvelle me soulage, / Voylà tout mon dueil effacé, / Sus, mon coeur, ayez bon courage, / Vostre mal est tantost passé.' LE MARY

14. 'Dans ce penible effort, à qui n'est comparable / Aucun autre tourment; / Delivrez-la, Seigneur, et soyez secourable / A son enfantement.' LA DEVOTE

was not, however, until 1650–1700 that the rise of the male-midwife or obstetric surgeon began to challenge the midwife's traditional role as the medical attendant at normal, uncomplicated births.[15] Similarly, it was not until the development of the microscope in the late seventeenth century that such fundamental discoveries as the existence of the ova and of the spermatozoa were made, which would gradually change key assumptions about the nature of generation. These significant developments lie beyond the temporal scope of the present volume,[16] but the preceding period leaves us with a different question. If the medical treatises in French on pregnancy and childbirth from the mid-sixteenth to the mid-seventeenth centuries were written by male authors, to what extent do they nonetheless find space for 'the other voice', that voice of protest raised in favor of women?

The 'Other Voice' in Male-Authored Treatises

The history of the emergence of the male surgeon specialized in childbirth, whose advent was often to reduce the laboring mother to a literally supine role, came to be traditionally presented as the heroic triumph of male skill over nature.[17] In such narratives, the woman risked being anonymized and relegated to the passive role of the vehicle from which the expert surgeon would seek to extract the child. It is true that authors of such accounts, including the most celebrated French obstetrician of the later seventeenth century, François Mauriceau, might express compassion for the women they treated,[18]

15. On the rise of the male-midwife or specialist surgeon in England, see the study by A. Wilson, *The Making of Man-Midwifery: childbirth in England 1660–1770* (London: UCL Press, 1995). For the same phenomenon in France, see J. Gélis, *La Sage-femme ou le médecin. Une nouvelle conception de la vie* (Paris: Fayard, 1988).

16. I do, however, highlight several early indications — well before 1650 — of male surgeons or physicians attending normal births without any apparent controversy. (See 143.)

17. L. McTavish offers a full account of this development over the mid-seventeenth to early-eighteenth centuries in France in *Childbirth and the Display of Authority in Early Modern France* (Aldershot: Ashgate, 2005).

18. Notably the moving account of the death of his own sister in childbirth, recorded in his *Treatise on the Diseases of Pregnancy and Childbirth* [*Traité des maladies des femmes grosses et de celles qui sont accouchées*], first published in 1668. See the analysis of this episode by L. McTavish: *Childbirth and the Display of Authority in Early Modern France*, 155–157.

but this was frequently counterbalanced, or outweighed, by the desire to promote their own achievements. A similar tension between professional male pride and pity for women's physical suffering is also present in many of the earlier birthing treatises, but I would suggest that prior to the rise to prominence of the male midwife (known in French as the *accoucheur*), French treatises more easily afforded space to what I shall identify as the 'other voice'.

In this volume, I have translated substantial sections of the works of five French authors, all of whom can be considered to merit the title 'caring' physicians or surgeons. In the introductions preceding each translation, I offer a more detailed overview of the authors in question, and of the works and their distinctive contribution to 'the other voice'. Here, I wish to draw attention to some of the most important common threads.

All five authors write because they are strongly motivated by a desire to save women from some of the worst horrors of pregnancy and childbirth, whether through their advocacy of particular techniques or operations, or through explanations of the principles of good care. François Rousset, physician to the Duke of Savoy and a lone voice in defending the viability of cesareans on living women, ascribes his desire to publish his work in 1581 to the need to change what he has witnessed:

> Above all, I have been led to do this by the pitiful sight
> of the agonies, helplessness, prayers and pitiful looks of
> those poor creatures who are so tortured, and cry murder,
> as they appeal only to us, begging with clasped hands for
> such help as we may be able to give them.[19]

Jacques Duval, a physician in Rouen, published a work in 1612 that combined a sensational report of his involvement in a case of transsexual identity with a treatise on generation, pregnancy and birth. Like Rousset, he affirms that one of his main reasons for writing was to prevent the agonies and deaths of mothers and newborn infants. His resolve sprang partly from his personal experience of losing his

19. See 23.

first wife after an obstructed labor,[20] and partly from his conviction that poorly instructed midwives in Rouen were responsible for the deaths of some 500 newborns a year.[21] Jacques Guillemeau, the only surgeon in the company of the four physicians translated here, specifically entitles his volume of 1609 *On the Safe Delivery of Women*, and his treatise advises both on how to avert the causes of mortal danger to mother or infant (such as untreated hemorrhage in labor), but also, in a fascinatingly modern approach, on the benefits of medical attendants heeding the individual mother's temperament and the powers of nature.[22]

By devoting volumes to the medical health of women, the authors I have translated had cause to reflect more broadly on the nature of women. Rousset's and Guillemeau's comments are mainly confined to women's roles during pregnancy and childbirth, with both authors expressing sympathy and sometimes admiration for the parturient mother, and giving a nuanced evaluation of midwives according to their individual skills (a position shared by all these authors). Duval's work is distinctive in treating procreation in at least as much detail as pregnancy and childbirth. He praises both male and female sexual anatomy (chapter 2), but has distinctly more to say about women (chapters 7–15) than about men (chapters 5–6). However, the treatises by the slightly earlier Parisian physician, Jean Liebault, and his continuer (Lazare Pena), and by the last author I present, a seventeenth-century physician from Lyons, Louis de Serres, contain significant sections of praise for women which go beyond the immediate subject of childbearing. Both Liebault's *Three Books*

---

20. See 287.

21. See 248. On the training of midwives in this period, see Klairmont Lingo's analysis in her introduction to Bourgeois's *Observations* (Klairmont Lingo and O'Hara), which gives a very full overview of developments in Paris from the Middle Ages to the mid-seventeenth century. However, other urban centers, such as Rouen, lagged behind the capital in terms of their organization. The broader context of women's roles in all fields of medical work in this period is the subject of S. Broomhall's monograph *Women's Medical Work in Early Modern France* (Manchester: Manchester University Press, 2004). On the development of male (as well as female) medical roles over this same period, see also L. Brockliss and C. Jones, *The Medical World of Early Modern France* (Oxford: Clarendon Press, 1997).

22. It is tempting, even if only partly accurate, to see Guillemeau as an early advocate of some of the 'gentle birth' or 'natural birth' philosophies and practices of the later-twentieth century, such as those pioneered by Michel Odent.

Dealing with the Infirmities and Illnesses of Women (1582, revised and expanded by Pena in 1609) and de Serres's *Treatise on the Nature, Causes, Signs and Remedies concerning Failures to Conceive, and Sterility among Women* (1625) are indebted to the Italian neoplatonic tradition, which celebrated woman's dignity and civilizing influence. Silently drawing on one key Italian source, the humanist physician Marinelli,[23] Liebault praises the distinctive nature of the female sexual anatomy, while Pena goes much further in his praise of women's beauty and their power to allure men, concluding:

> All these wonders together teach us that woman is one of the great miracles of Nature, and a subject in which philosophy finds more to study than in all the other things in creation.[24]

Louis de Serres's defence of women appears initially to be rooted in a more practical concern, the consolation and encouragement of women not yet able to bear an heir. Yet in chapter III of his work, which purports to discuss 'whether women who bear only daughters should be called sterile?', he engages in a familiar but extraordinarily wide-ranging *pro et contra* debate on the equality of women, including their ability to hold temporal power, their part in the Christian mysteries of creation and redemption, and the Christian doctrine on their nature in the afterlife. His clear affirmation that to bear female children is in no way to be considered a form of sterility is one of the most resounding and unexpected examples of how early modern birthing treatises in French afforded space to the 'other voice'.

We should, nonetheless, not be overly surprised that medical texts make a contribution to the later-sixteenth-century reworking of the *'querelle des femmes'*. If the commonplaces and general ramifications of the debate had been explored, above all in works of

23. For a detailed discussion of Liebault's use of Marinelli, see 67-68. It should be noted that Giovanni Marinelli's daughter, Lucrezia Marinella, was herself an influential advocate of women's standing in her treatise *Nobiltà e eccellenza delle donne, coi difetti et mancamenti degli uomoni*, published in Venice in 1600 (translated into English and edited by A. Dunhill, with an introduction by L. Panizza: *The Nobility and Excellence of Women and the Defects and Vices of Men*, Chicago: Chicago University Press, 1999).

24. See 87.

literature and treatises such as Agrippa's seminal *Declamation on the Preeminence and Nobility of the Female Sex* (1529)[25] in the earlier part of the century, the increasing acceptance of a number of anatomical discoveries and revised theories affecting the medical perception of the female sex meant that by 1600, as Maclean concludes, 'many doctors are convinced that the notion of woman has changed, and that by the removal of the taint of imperfection she has attained a new dignity.'[26] Most critically, woman is rarely still held to be a monster or mistake of nature, an imperfect man; instead, she is believed to be equally perfect in her own sex. It follows that by the end of the century, female discharges, notably the menses, are thus conceived — when regular — as a harmless excrement rather than inherently noxious; and the existence and efficacy of female 'seed' are now rarely doubted.

Hence we can agree with Maclean's assertion that it is 'possible to argue that there is a feminist movement in the medical spheres, where in theology there is little evidence of one'.[27] However, he rightly reminds us of the twists and turns these debates took, and particularly of the general reluctance among most physicians to accept women as equal to men in the workings of the mind and passions. Precisely because of the specificity of their bodily organs (notably the uterus) and the balance of their humoral temperament, they were still often depicted as intellectually inferior, their minds subject to the forces of the emotions and the imagination.[28] Although none of the five authors presented in this volume radically challenges conventional views of male/female difference in the way Pomata has shown the Spanish author Oliva Sabuco to do in *The True Medicine* of 1587,[29] Liebault (and his continuer, Pena) and de Serres argue explicitly

25. See the translation and critical edition by A. Rabil, *Henricus Cornelius Agrippa: Declamation on the Preeminence and Nobility of the Female Sex* (Chicago: University of Chicago Press, 1996).

26. *The Renaissance Notion of Woman*, 44.

27. *The Renaissance Notion of Woman*, 29.

28. Note, however, that in the section of her introduction to Bourgeois's *Observations* treating 'Bourgeois and the Querelle des femmes', Klairmont Lingo argues convincingly that Bourgeois makes the case for women being able to control their emotional state through the exercise of their mental faculties.

29. Pomata argues that Oliva Sabuco (or the author writing under Oliva Sabuco's name) 'put deeply into question the axiom that was the cornerstone of woman's inferiority — the

against misogynist stereotypes. Their celebration of women's physical and mental powers provides significant examples of the 'other voice' being raised in defence of women in a medical context.

I have found no evidence that the five authors translated in this volume were personally acquainted with each other, although it is possible that Liebault's and Guillemeau's activities overlapped in Paris. However, there is evidence that they had some familiarity with each other's writings.[30] In addition, they can be seen to share a commitment to the general principle of defending and improving the medical care of women and infants in childbirth through the circulation of knowledge in the vernacular. In this, they are indeed representative of a professional, masculine 'other voice', which should be read alongside the exceptional contribution by the one professional woman writer, the midwife Louise Bourgeois.[31] On many key aspects of obstetrical care, the five authors are readily in agreement, such as the importance of diet and regimen throughout pregnancy to prepare the mother for an easier labor, or the need for the medical attendants to encourage the mother and offer psychological as well as physical support throughout the delivery. Yet there are some differences, indicative both of evolving medical debates and of the writers' individual commitments to continue to search for the best practices.[32] I shall conclude this general introduction with comments on the significance of two such divergences.

First, as indicated above, there is a very sharp dissension between advocates and opponents of cesareans on living women. Rousset and Duval fall into the former camp, whereas Guillemeau refuses to subscribe to their arguments.[33] That Rousset and Duval ultimately won the day, in the light of subsequent medical history, is less important

---

centrality of blood and of innate heat' (*The True Medicine*, 63), thus undercutting the conventional measure by which women could be judged inferior to men.

30. In the material in this volume, for example, Liebault cites Rousset (74), Guillemeau alludes to him (214), and Duval cites Liebault (251) and draws extensively on him.

31. On Bourgeois's subtle presentation of midwives as at once needing to learn from surgeons and physicians, yet on occasion more skilful than inept or arrogant male practitioners, see Klairmont Lingo's section 'Authorizing the Text' in her introduction to Bourgeois's *Observations* (Klairmont Lingo and O'Hara).

32. See the Table (xxviii) detailing the treatment of key subjects by the five authors.

33. See 214 and 287.

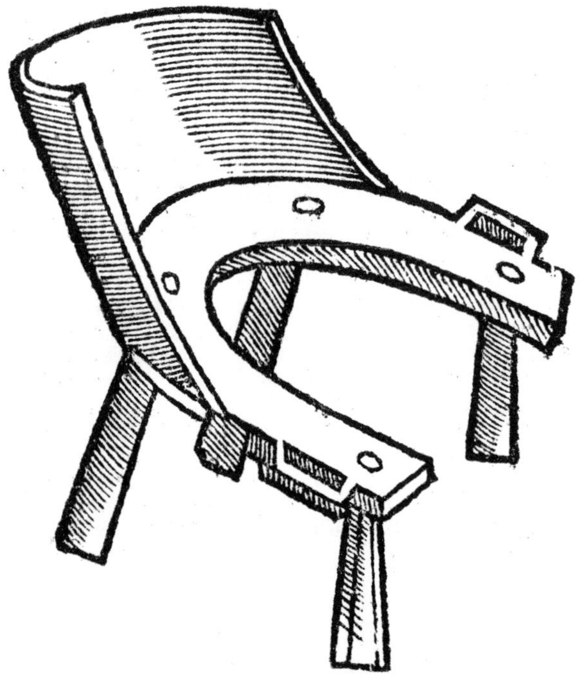

3) Birthing chair

Eucharius Rösslin, *Des divers travaulx et enfantemens des femmes*, Paris, 1539
(Library of Royal College of Obstetricians and Gynaecologists, London)

than the fact that both sides vigorously defend the positions they espouse because of their deep-rooted concern to recommend the best care for a woman struggling to deliver her child.

Less immediately divisive, yet suggestive of fierce debates to follow, are the comments of three of the authors concerning the best position for an unobstructed delivery. Liebault inclines, in 1582, for the traditional birthing chair because, as a physician with a keen interest in anatomy, he believes it favors easier dilation; nonetheless, he permits the woman to choose to deliver lying on a bed if she will 'be more at [her] ease'.[34] Guillemeau, writing in 1609, is equally liberal in recording that the woman should have a choice of positions, enumerating standing, sitting, kneeling or lying, before he

34. See 118.

expresses his own preference: 'But the best and safest way for them to give birth is in bed (this is what I advise).'[35] We might assume that this recommendation was in part explained by the fact that he had obtained most of his professional experience as a surgeon summoned to difficult deliveries, were it not for the fact that it closely accords with the advice of the midwife Louise Bourgeois. Bourgeois also allows the woman to move around and adopt the position of her choice, but concludes that for uncomplicated labors, which do not last too long, the woman will be more comfortable in bed. Only in the case of difficult protracted labors does she recommend that the woman would be aided by adopting a standing or sitting position so that the weight of the child (i.e. gravity) aids the delivery.[36] Duval's advice, three years later in 1612, is far closer to Liebault's, again based on anatomical observations: a preference for a standing or seated position, with some use of kneeling to encourage the woman to bear down through contractions. He reserves delivery on a bed for cases when 'a woman is so weak that she cannot remain in a sitting position'.[37]

These divergences were to be at the center of major changes in childbirth in France over the course of the next century, yet Liebault, Guillemeau and Duval, while advocating different practices, still respect the need to suit the physician's or surgeon's preferences to the wishes and physical state of each mother. The expression of concern for women as individuals is as central to the distinctive 'other voice' of these caring physicians and surgeon as it is to that of the midwife Bourgeois.

---

35. See 195.

36. See *Diverse Observations*, O'Hara and Klairmont Lingo, I. 10.

37. See 272.

Table of Key Subjects Treated by the Five Authors

The following table highlights the chapters translated in this volume that deal in detail with the key stages of pregnancy and delivery. Its purpose is to facilitate comparisons between the different authors.[38] In addition, I indicate in square brackets some chapters from the works which are not translated in this volume, but which may be of further interest.

	ROUSSET	LIEBAULT	GUILLEMEAU	DUVAL	SERRES
Conception and early miscarriage	VI	[I. 25, II. 2, 5, 7, 41]	[I. 1, 20]	XV	3, 10, 14
Regimen in pregnancy		III. 20, 32	I. 5–7	XV, XVIII	
Regimen in preparation for delivery		III. 45	I. 6	XVIII	
Choice of midwife		III. 45	II. 3	XIX	
Normal delivery		III. 45	II. 1,5–7	XIX	
Difficult, obstructed labor	I	III. 45–46	[II. 10–15]	XX	14
Assisted delivery		III. 46	II. 16	XXII-XXIII	
Foetal death in utero	IV	[III. 49]	II. 16	XXII	14
Cesarean delivery	I	[III. 49]	II. 28	XXII	
Care after delivery		[III. 50]	II. 9, III. 1	[XXV]	

38. For a detailed list of all subjects treated by each author, see the Index.

A Note on the Translations

In general, I have sought to balance the need for an intelligible English translation with the desire to provide a fairly close rendering of the source texts. While I have aimed to reflect something of the sentence structure of each of the original texts, in the interests of clarity, I have frequently subdivided some of the longer, hypotactic sentences common in later-sixteenth and early-seventeenth-century French prose, and have followed modern conventions of punctuation. I have also avoided the French practice of starting many sentences with 'And' ('*Et*') or 'But' ('*Mais*'). Where appropriate, I have introduced additional paragraph divisions, following modern usage, to break up very lengthy blocks of text.

The figure of reduplication — the use of two almost or fully synonymous words to express a single concept — is a common characteristic of early modern French style. Although I have retained it on some occasions, in part to give a period flavor, the repeated use of the figure can become awkward, so I have more often translated it by a single word in English.

The translation of medical terms raises a particular issue, given that the early modern understanding of the human body, and especially of female physiology and anatomy, is sometimes radically different from that of modern medicine. In order to avoid anachronistic renderings, I have, in particular, retained the literal translation 'mouth of the womb' (for '*bouche matricale*' or '*bouche de la matrice*'), rather than employing the modern term 'cervix'. Similarly, I have avoided introducing the modern distinction between the vulva and vagina. In place of the more technical modern term 'genitalia', I have generally used 'lower parts' or 'lower regions' to translate a range of early modern French terms (including '*la partie honteuse*', literally 'the shameful part'). However, where authors such as Jacques Duval have used the adjective '*genital*' in French (generally in the sense 'procreative'), I have adopted the cognate form in English. Finally, early modern writers often use the term '*vaisseaux spermatiques*' (literally, 'spermatic vessels') to designate the Fallopian tubes, reflecting the assumption that women's seed might be analogous to men's; I translate this by 'seed-bearing vessels'.

FRANÇOIS ROUSSET

New Treatise on Hysterotomotoky,
or Childbirth by Cesarean
(1581)

TRAITTE
NOVVEAV DE
l'Hysterotomotokie,
O V
Enfantement Cæsarien.

QVI EST

*Extraction de l'enfant par incision laterale du
vẽtre, & matrice de la femme grosse ne pou-
uant autrement accoucher. Et ce sans preiu-
dicier à la vie de l'vn, ny de l'autre; ny em-
pescher la fæcondité maternelle par aprés.*

PAR
Françoys Rousset Medecin.

A PARIS,

Chez Denys du Val, au cheual volant,
rue S. Iean de Beauuais.

M. D. LXXXI.

Auec priuilege du Roy.

4) Title page: François Rousset, *Traitté nouveau de l'hysterotomotokie,*
Paris, 1581

INTRODUCTION

TRANSLATION OF EXCERPTS FROM *NEW TREATISE ON HYSTEROTOMOTOKY, OR CHILDBIRTH BY CESAREAN* (1581)

INTRODUCTION

The first of these five authors to publish a complete work in French treating women's reproductive health and childbirth was the physician to the Duke of Savoy, François Rousset (1535–1590), whose treatise promoting cesarean operations on living women created enormous interest and controversy in France and beyond.

Life and Works of François Rousset

The life of Rousset is relatively uncharted, and but for his *New Treatise on Hysterotomotoky,* he would probably have passed into the annals of medical history almost unknown. From contemporary bibliographers, we glean that he was a friend of Ambroise Paré, a French surgeon to the royal court, and had studied medicine at Montpellier, under two of the great professors, Houllier and Rondelet, before returning to take up residence in his hometown of Pithiviers, some 100 km south of Paris.[1] The evidence of the *New Treatise on Hysterotomotoky* suggests that Rousset was an intellectually curious practitioner, well grounded in classical theories of medicine,[2] but equally alert to the new lessons of contemporary practice. His advocacy of the use of cesarean operations in the most desperate cases of obstructed labor relies above all on the authority of case histories, which he has been able to verify, either personally or through trustworthy intermediaries.

Thus, we build up a picture of a Renaissance physician who studies cases that come to his personal attention, corresponds with colleagues in other regions, and travels eagerly around the country, notebook in hand, to interview physicians, surgeons — sometimes mere barber surgeons — and patients and their relatives or neighbors. In this respect, Rousset provides a very interesting example of the increasing phenomenon of practitioners — mainly physicians, but also some surgeons — in the second half of the sixteenth century keeping

---

1. See the entry on Rousset in François de La Croix Du Maine, *Les Bibliothèques françoises de La Croix Du Maine et de Du Verdier, sieur de Vauprivas,* 6 vols, ed. M. Rigoley de Juvigny (Paris: Taillant and Nyons, 1772; first edn, 1584), vol. I, 237.

2. See for example his scholarly discussion of a disputed locus in Galen's commentary on an aphorism of Hippocrates, 61-62.

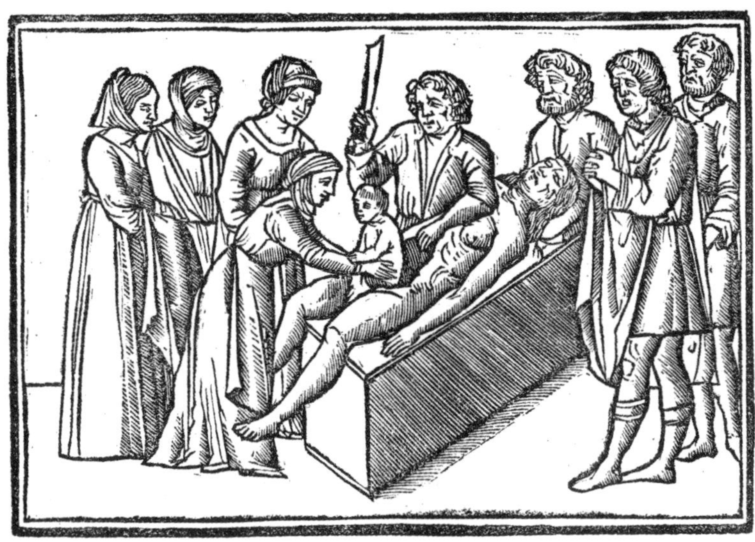

5) Cesarean section performed on a dead woman

Suetonius, *Vitae Caesarum*, Venice, 1506
(Wellcome Library, London)

detailed records of their cases. Some collections were published, in Latin, under the title *Observationes,* a new epistemic medical genre that combined the writer's personal authority, as detailed professional observer, with the desire to share cases among the wider medical fraternity.[3] Occasionally, Rousset includes references to events in his own life which affected his task, such as the time he was seriously ill and could not personally attend the delivery of a woman who needed a surgeon to deliver her by cesarean,[4] or the intrusion of the civil wars that prevented him from following up one contact as he would have liked.[5] Most frequently, however, Rousset relies on a blend of what he defines as 'verified experience, appropriate reasoning and convincing

3. The rise and significance of the genre of *Observationes* is identified and charted by G. Pomata in 'Sharing Cases: the *Observationes* in early modern medicine', *Early Science and Medicine* 15 (2010), 193–236. On the preference, some 20 to 30 years later, for case histories above ancient textual knowledge, see Klairmont Lingo's 'The Superiority of Practice over Ancient Wisdom' in her general introduction to Louise Bourgeois's *Diverse Observations* (edited and translated by Klairmont Lingo and O'Hara).

4. See 40.

5. See ibid.

authority'[6] to press his case. The balance is weighted, however, towards contemporary experience rather than the authority of classical written sources, since, as Rousset explains at the outset of his treatise,[7] no Greek or Latin author had discussed the possibility of carrying out cesareans on living women, although cesareans on women who had died were customary in order to deliver a foetus.

Unlike the other authors in this volume, Rousset does not appear to have written treatises on any other area of medicine. The subject of cesareans prompted his only known incursions into print, first the *New Treatise*, and then, a decade later, a dialogue[8] and a final short response[9] in Latin defending his views against critics of his treatise – notably Jacques Marchant, a Parisian surgeon considered an expert on deliveries.[10]

In the prefatory letter to the reader of the *New Treatise*, Rousset gives the impression that he took up his pen only because of his passion for this single issue. Furthermore, he indicates that the project took shape slowly. Initially, he intended to produce a simple account in French, then drafted a longer, unpublished treatise in Latin, from which he extracted an abridged version to publish in French, in Paris in 1581. Although this French edition was not reprinted, we can assume it circulated quite widely, to judge by the number of copies surviving in libraries across Europe and beyond, and by direct and oblique reference to Rousset in works published subsequently in French.[11]

6. See 34.

7. See ibid.

8. *Dialogue in Defence of Cesarean Delivery* [*Dialogus apologeticus pro caesareo partu*, Paris: Denis Duval, 1590]. In this, Rousset gives a spirited defence of the broader principle of courageous innovation in medicine.

9. *Response to the Declamation of Jacques Marchant* [*Responsio ad Jacobi Marchant declamationem*, Paris, n.d. ?1590].

10. Jacques Marchant (or Marchand) was the son-in-law of Jacques Guillemeau, and sometimes worked with him. In her *Observations*, Bourgeois praised his skill in deliveries: *Diverse Observations on Sterility*, O'Hara and Klairmont Lingo, I. XXXIX. In the 1590s, Marchant published a series of increasingly vitriolic attacks on Rousset's advocacy of cesareans, in the form of several poems and two prose works, *Declamation against François Rousset's Apologia* [*In Fr. Rosseti apologiam, declamatio*, Paris: Nicolas Delouvain, 1598], and *Third Declamation against François Rousset* [*Declamatio III in Fr. Rosseti*, n.d]. A summary of this exchange is provided by R. Blumenfeld-Kosinski, *Not of Woman Born. Representations of caesarean birth in medieval and Renaissance culture* (Ithaca and London: Cornell University Press, 1990), 43–45.

11. For example, Guillemeau's criticism that points to, but does not name, Rousset (214).

However, the most important indication of Rousset's significance is the fact that Caspar Bauhin (1560–1624), a leading Swiss physician and anatomist, undertook a translation of the *New Treatise on Hysterotomotoky* into Latin for inclusion in the second (1586) edition of the renowned Latin compendium of medical writings on women's health, the *Books on the Diseases of Women* [*Gynaeciorum libri*]. This meant that the international community of scholarly readers, whether physicians or laymen, now had access to Rousset's text, to which Bauhin appended further case histories he had collected to support the viability of cesareans on living women.[12] Rather surprisingly, in 1590 there appeared a separate edition of another Latin version of Rousset's work,[13] far longer than Bauhin's translation for the *Gynaeciorum libri*. In all probability, Rousset had himself belatedly decided to publish his original Latin treatise, which ran to more than 500 pages. Its appearance coincides with his responses to his critics, and suggests that his defence of cesareans had moved to a new stage. However, this time the debate was played out on a far more acrimonious and personal level between medical professionals writing in Latin, rather than in the wider and more civil public arena of the vernacular.

Circulation and Afterlife of the 'New Treatise on Hysterotomotoky'

Thus, the significance of the *New Treatise* as a contribution to women's medicine and to evolving debates on medical ethics far outstrips the single French edition of the work. Alongside the number of copies in circulation in the vernacular, the treatise reached a broad international audience through the Latin texts. The co-existence of the French and Latin versions means that we need to be aware that the text was potentially read by quite different groups of readers: learned humanist physicians in many countries, French-speaking surgeons, and also the burgeoning class of lay-readers of books in the vernacular treating

12. On the composition and contents of the *Gynaeciorum libri*, see H. King's masterly study: *Midwifery, Obstetrics and the Rise of Gynaecology. The uses of a sixteenth-century French compendium* (Aldershot: Ashgate, 2007), 1–8.
13. *Hysterotomotokias, id est Caesarei partus assertio historologica* (Paris: Denis Duval, 1590).

women's health and, more generally, topics linked to generation and sexuality.[14]

Rousset makes it clear throughout the 1581 French treatise — on which my analysis will focus — that he is writing primarily for surgeons, because it is they who could be called upon to perform the cesarean. Ultimately, the surgeon must feel confident that he can carry out this rare operation, and persuade the patient and her family to trust him to do so. Hence, the liminary sonnet is headed 'Sonnet by the Author to the Reader who is a Surgeon', and the preface speaks of 'some of our French surgeons, having little or no reading knowledge of Latin, [who] have been urging me to share [my treatise] with them'.[15] Equally, most of the case histories recounted by Rousset report the work of surgeons or barber surgeons, and not infrequently he includes comments designed to assist any inexperienced surgeon who — in Rousset's view — should not hesitate to conduct the operation as a last resort to save a laboring mother's life.[16]

Yet the issue was, of course, one that required physicians and surgeons to make an ethical choice, for in cases of difficult labor — when a midwife recognized that she could proceed no further alone — either a surgeon or a physician would be summoned. The choice as to which would depend in part on the family's station and wealth, and on geographical factors: the small villages cited by Rousset in the first section had local barbers or surgeons, whereas a physician would often reside in a nearby town. However, it would also depend on any local surgeon's reputation for assisting in childbirth. If a physician was summoned, he might then advise that a surgeon should also be called, as in the case of Bernarde Arnoul,[17] when Rousset himself recommended a surgeon to deliver the woman by cesarean. Thus the physician would bear some of the moral responsibility for the cesarean. For this reason, physicians and surgeons hotly debated Rousset's proposals. The majority of the reactions recorded in print

---

14. Compare the immediate success of Laurent Joubert's *Popular Errors* [*Erreurs populaires*], first published in 1578: at least 19 French editions appeared by 1608 (see Worth-Stylianou, *Les Traités d'obstétrique*, 187–233). The attraction of the volume was due, in no small measure, to its direct engagement with questions about sexual and reproductive health.

15. See 23.

16. See his advice on suturing, for example, 42.

17. See 40-41.

appear to have been sceptical or hostile, but a small minority were won over by Rousset — some largely by his treatise, as in the case of the Italian doctor Scipione Mercurio,[18] or others, like Jacques Duval,[19] because the treatise confirmed their own experience.

Unlike some other French medical treatises of this period,[20] there is no evidence that either the French or Latin versions of Rousset's treatise were translated into any other vernaculars in the century following their appearance. However, Helen King has established that the Latin text of the *Gynaeciorum libri* compendium continued to be widely owned as a '"must have" in the medical libraries of individuals and institutions, into the Victorian era',[21] and cites the example of a bibliography of forensic medicine in 1819 that refers to the Latin edition of the *Hysterotomotokias*.[22] It is also worth noting that an English translation of the third section of Rousset's text was included in William Cheselden's *A Treatise on the High Operation of the Stone* in 1723. While this version was confined to Rousset's discussion of operations to extract stones from the bladder rather than the sections on women's health, it provides further proof that the treatise continued to circulate and to be read closely long after it was first published.

In 2010, a modern English translation of the whole of Rousset's *New Treatise* appeared, translated by Ronald Cyr and edited by Thomas Baskett.[23] Since a present-day medical practitioner undertook the translation, it contains some very informative medical insights, but there are some inaccuracies or anachronisms, with the style leaning towards modern terminology,[24] and the notes do not always engage in detail with early modern thought. My translations of extracts from Rousset offer a more historically-based version, and my

18. *The Midwife* [*La commare o raccoglitrice*, Venice: G. B. Ciotti, 1601], II. 28.

19. See Jacques Duval's account of the death in childbirth of his first wife. As a physician who had witnessed successful cesareans conducted under his father's orders, he had wanted to call a surgeon to perform the operation, but was overruled by the wife's parents (287).

20. For a discussion of the English translation of Guillemeau's work, see 146.

21. *Midwifery, Obstetrics and the Rise of Gynaecology*, 6–7.

22. *Midwifery, Obstetrics and the Rise of Gynaecology*, 45.

23. *Caesarean Birth. The work of François Rousset in Renaissance France. A new treatise on Hysterotomotokie or caesarien childbirth* (London: RCOG Press, 2010).

24. Particularly in the medical sphere, but sometimes in the translator's use of social or political terminology.

footnotes compare and contrast him with other contemporary writers, demonstrating his unusual contribution to the 'other voice'.

Structure of the 'New Treatise on Hysterotomotoky' and Selection of Sections for Translation

Rousset divides his French treatise into six sections. The first outlines the reasons why a cesarean may prove necessary and furnishes a series of case histories of successful cesareans. The next two sections provide technical discussions of anatomical and physiological difficulties in conducting the operation and how the surgeon should overcome these (second section), followed by an extended comparison between cesareans and standard operations to remove stones from the bladder (third section). The fourth section continues to look at comparable dangerous but beneficial operations and records cases of other operations conducted on women's reproductive organs. In the fifth section, Rousset returns to more theoretical and technical arguments about cesareans, before finally addressing two distinct subjects in the sixth section — whether cesareans render women infertile (he believes they do not), and the separate topic of uterine pessaries.

My translation reproduces the first and fourth sections in their entirety. They not only exemplify Rousset's position on cesareans but also his wider attitude towards the care of women's health. These sections are among the most accessible to lay readers. In contrast, I have not translated the second, third and fifth sections, which consist substantially of technical descriptions and of discussions of operations, and are addressed to practicing surgeons or physicians. Readers wishing to pursue these should consult Cyr's and Baskett's version. I conclude my translation with the final part of the sixth section in which Rousset's discussion of uterine pessaries demonstrates again his particularly sympathetic attitude towards women's medical problems.

Rousset's Arguments and Style

The most striking aspect of Rousseau's treatise, when compared with most other contemporary medical treatises in French, is, as

Blumenfeld-Kosinski has remarked,[25] the passionate tone that permeates it. On occasion, he makes blatantly emotional appeals, notably in the preface 'To the Reader', where he paints a harrowing picture of the suffering of women in obstructed labor who call out to physicians and surgeons:

> Just the report of such a pitiful scene is horrifying to the most barbarous heart in the world, even when one is not present.

Frequently, however, in the sections expounding his arguments, he relies upon logical persuasion rather than pathos, skilfully using traditional devices such as irony, rhetorical questions and accumulation,[26] while in the case histories he adopts a deliberately neutral, factual tone, so that the reader is more likely to trust the veracity of his reports.

These different persuasive techniques are all designed to support the one argument of which Rousset most wants to persuade his reader — that, as a last resort, cesareans can, and should, be safely carried out on living women. He was writing in an age and culture that approved the use of cesareans to excise a living child from the womb of a dead mother,[27] but in which performing the operation on living women was considered impossible because it was assumed it must result in the death of the mother. Hence, the subtitle of Rousset's thesis proclaims his unlikely case: he will argue that the operation can be undertaken 'without endangering the life of either (mother or child), nor preventing the woman from bearing other children hereafter'. Throughout the treatise he can thereby avoid the vexed

---

25. *Not of Woman Born*, 43.

26. A particularly striking example of what could be termed Asiatic rhetoric occurs in the Epilogue concluding the fourth section (54).

27. French law followed the requirement of Roman law under the *rex legia*, and confirmed by Justinian in his sixth-century digest of legal texts, that a pregnant woman should not be buried before the foetus had been cut out, to avoid the possibility of a living child perishing. By the later-sixteenth century, concern for the survival of the child was, in Catholic theology, associated with the imperative of baptizing any living child, even if it would not survive for long, to ensure the salvation of its soul.

ethical question that troubles other writers — whether priority should be given, in extreme cases, to saving the mother or the child.[28]

The reference in the subtitle to preserving a woman's fertility, even if a cesarean is undertaken, is an interesting indication of his respect for women's anxiety not to compromise their marital relations by losing their ability to bear children or to satisfy their husbands.[29] Thus, in his reports on the uses of uterine pessaries, he makes a point of not citing the names of those women he had interviewed who prefer their husbands to remain ignorant of their recourse to such a device.[30] In other ways, too, Rousset shows sensitivity towards women's conventional reticence in matters pertaining to their sexual health, even if this might sometimes stand in the way of a physician carrying out his duty. At a number of points, for example, he acknowledges uncritically the habitual modesty that forbids women to uncover themselves before a male doctor or physician.[31]

Alongside this understanding of women's personal and moral responses to the role enjoined upon them by social conventions, Rousset also praises those exceptional women who defy received wisdom by themselves seeking cesarean operations as a means of delivery. Thus in the case history of Bernarde Arnoul, he reports collusion between the woman and himself, against the husband:

> She got her husband to send for me in order to seek some urgent advice on how she could be saved, and was brave enough — in defiance of her husband's wishes — to allow herself to be opened.[32]

He is far more critical when the men standing in the way of a woman's brave resolve to undergo a cesarean are the surgeons

28. E.g. Guillemeau acknowledges this dilemma and comes down in favor of saving the mother (see 211).

29. In this respect, his attitude is quite close to that of Joubert who, in his *Popular Errors* three years earlier, had shown concern for the good sexual relations of married couples, and a positive attitude towards sexuality in itself, rather than only as a means to procreation. In both cases, these attitudes might be associated with Protestant beliefs.

30. See 57.

31. E.g. 60.

32. See 40.

themselves, as in the case of Agnes Boyer, who lost her life as a result of such reticence:

> And so, of her own accord, she asked to have an incision performed as before, but beg as she might she could not prevail upon the two new, young surgeons who had been sent to attend her from Neufville where they had taken over after Philippot had died of the plague. As a result, she and her unborn child both died pitifully because of their lack of resolve — unless it was weaknesses or some other regrettable reason which prevented them from acting.[33]

For Rousset, it is the practitioners above all who must lead the way in promoting this innovative means of saving women's lives, and he considers them deserving of censure if they show any hesitation. Yet this does not, as it might have done, lead to an arrogant celebration of the surgeon's powers; his frame of reference is always defined by how far the physician and surgeon have fulfilled their duty towards God, allowing the proper workings of Nature to triumph. Indeed, in the absence of classical written sources on the operation, he effectively sets God in the position of authority, affirming in the closing pages of the treatise that on the one hand the surgeon or physician has a duty to use the knowledge revealed to him:

> … nonetheless it would be a dereliction of our duty to allow any good thing to be wasted when God reveals it by such means and ministers as please Him, whenever this may chance to occur.

On the other hand, he attributes to God this timely revelation of an innovative procedure:

> Being the daughter of time, truth has learned from her father not to produce everything at once, but whenever it may come, we must accept it like every other good thing, receiving it with a grateful hand when it offers itself to us

33. See 43.

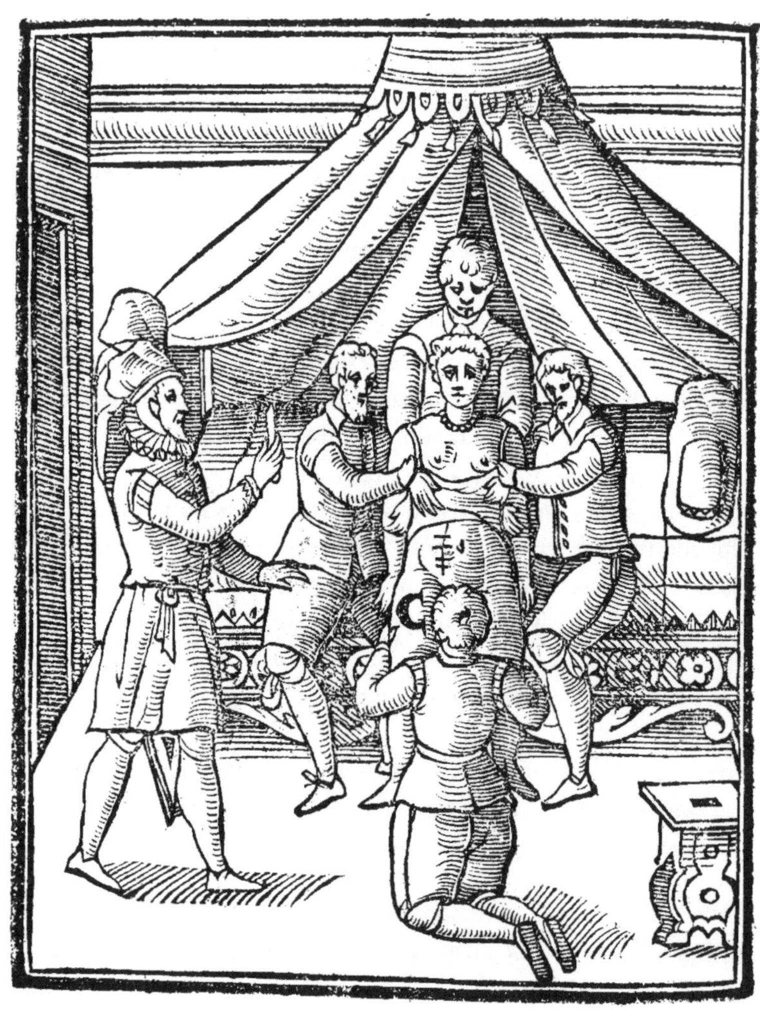

6) Preparation for cesarean section on a living woman

Scipio Mercurio, *La Commare*, Venice, 1601
(Wellcome Library, London)

> in the fullness of time, in such ways, and by such means,
> as it pleases God, the ancient of days and Father of ages, to
> send it to us.

This final appeal to a higher authority mirrors Rousset's dedication of his project at the start of the volume to earthly sponsors, the Duke of Savoy and the late Duchess of Ferrara. Presenting himself as a God-fearing physician and a dutiful subject, concerned only for the good health of women, he has placed a firm shield against his critics.

What, finally, is Rousset's attitude to women not as patients but as medical practitioners? Like all the authors presented in this volume, he worked alongside midwives, and his attitude seems to reflect the diversity of good and bad practice he met. Thus, there are some moments of harsh criticism for what he perceives as midwives' incompetence, on the grounds of the suffering they cause laboring women. Agnes Boyer is said to have 'had her body quite broken for four days by the incompetence of the midwives, all to no avail',[34] while in the case of Jeanne Michel, the midwives fail to deliver a woman so that the foetus dies and its limbs putrefy.[35] Yet in other cases, it is a midwife who correctly diagnoses a pregnancy when the physicians fail to,[36] and he is not slow to report the skills of Madame Preignon 'who is much sought after by the great households because of her long experience and her skill at her craft'.[37] In short, his appraisal of midwives, like that of their male counterparts, whether surgeons or physicians, depends entirely on how well they perform their task. He is as willing to praise a good midwife as a good barber surgeon — or to castigate either if they cause suffering to the parturient mother, who alone is never criticized.

34. See 42-43.
35. See 44-45.
36. See 48.
37. See 57.

TITLE PAGE [1581]

NEW TREATISE ON *Hysterotomotoky*,[38]
OR
Childbirth by cesarean.

THAT IS

Extraction of the child by means of a lateral incision of the abdomen and womb of the pregnant woman unable to give birth by other means. And without endangering the life of either, nor preventing the woman from bearing other children hereafter.[39]

BY

Françoys Rousset, Physician.

IN PARIS,

From the press of Denys du Val,[40]
at the sign of the flying horse,
in the rue Saint Jean de Beauvais.

M.D.LXXXI.

With the King's Privilege.

---

38. From the Greek, literally 'womb-cutting'. I have compared my translation with the version recently published by Cyr and Baskett. In the places where I have gained specific insights from their translation and notes, this is indicated in the footnotes. Equally, I point out occasions where I disagree significantly with details of their version or notes.

39. In the subtitle, Rousset already responds to two of the chief criticisms levelled by his opponents: that the operation would kill mother or child (or both), and that even if she survived, the woman would never be able to bear other children.

40. More commonly written as Denis Duval (c. 1553–1614): Paris printer and bookseller, who took over from Chrétien Wéchel.

SONNET BY THE AUTHOR TO THE
READER WHO IS A SURGEON

If any man in the past could undo the Gordian Knot,[41]
Unravelling it completely, the Oracle claimed
That he would easily possess the whole of Asia;
But if he could not, never should he hope so to do.

Alexander[42] seeing (as he dreamed of this subject)
That, if he persisted in trying, he would labor in vain,
Come what may, resolved that he would make
His plan rest upon the knife (a bloody portent).

Friend, the birth which is presented here
Is a Gordian Knot; and Alexander, in his assistance
Is human, not cruel; he desires no ill.

To this great hero Asia never brought as much glory
As the happiness of those born by cesarians[43] will give you
    in the world;
Their mothers and they will owe their lives to you.

41. According to legend, Alexander the Great solved the problem of undoing the Gordian Knot by slicing it with his sword. Some of his biographers recorded that he thereby fulfilled an oracle's prediction that the person who undid the knot would be ruler of Asia.

42. The sonnet reworks the standard comparison of the achievements of Alexander the Great and Julius Caesar (see for example Plutarch's *Parallel Lives*), but compares instead Alexander's slicing of the Gordian Knot with the surgeon's use of the cesarean operation.

43. According to legend, Julius Caesar had been delivered by cesarean. Since his mother, Aurelia, did not die in the birth, the episode supports the claims Rousset makes in his treatise.

TO THE MOST ILLUSTRIOUS PRINCE, JACQUES OF SAVOY, DUKE OF GENOA AND NEMOURS.

Sir,

I observe that in both small and great matters you practice what you most praise in a Prince,[44] which is to add to his natural goodness the imitation, in words and deeds, of that which has been most particularly prized in all those on whom virtue has bestowed both high rank and praise: namely, that they have shown themselves humane and accessible to those around them. I am therefore emboldened not to be fearful of offering you this gift on account of my low rank. It is a small book, born from my studies, entitled 'Childbirth by cesarean'. I hope that you will look favorably upon it, like the Great King of Persia who did not scorn the apple that one of his peasants gave him; or like Jupiter who loved the small quantity of incense burned by the common people, or even little cakes left in place of incense, as much as the extravagant sacrifices of the richest people. Or like God himself, who in the Gospel did not consider the mite of the poor widow any less valuable than the substantial offering of the great Pharisees, who gave only what they did not need from their riches.[45]

Indeed, I see every day that if one of your gardeners brings you some fruit he has grown which seems to be new or out of season, and which is thought to be pleasing, even though it is not one of the most excellent; or if someone brings you some medicinal minerals[46] or an unusual crystal, even though it is not one of the finest, you desire both of those people to be allowed to see you. I, therefore, must hope for no less, as your humble servant and Ordinary Physician, as I bring you this small gift, which, however, if I may say, is not as small as it may first appear. Thus I hope that when you have looked at it more closely, you will find it to be a good fruit, even though in truth it

---

44. Jacques of Savoy (1531–1585), by whom Rousset was employed, became the second Duke of Nemours in 1533. He was married to Anne d'Este, daughter of Duke Ercole II of Ferrara and Renée of France. For a fuller account of his life, see Cyr and Baskett, 120–123.

45. Mark 12. 41–44; Luke 21. 1–4.

46. The French uses the term 'terre', literally 'earth' or 'soil', referring to the practice of travelers bringing back samples of foreign soils thought to contain valuable minerals.

is not quite ripe and may still have a slightly uncultivated taste. Yet, it is of good quality and of no less repute than the finest fruit from your trees, even though they were once the true bezoars of the ancient Medes, who gave them their name.[47] I trust that one day you will hold in no lesser esteem the finest medicinal minerals of your own Savoy,[48] even though this work is at present only a crude mass, not yet refined, and you will come to prefer it to the most precious stones sent to us from the East, since it suffices better to pay the ransom for the life of a princess, queen or empress and their most illustrious descendants (in case of need) than a whole mine of gold or silver could do.

However, I do not doubt that it would be ridiculously arrogant of me to praise this gift so highly, with splendid words, to you who are so perceptive, were the gift not indeed equal to my praise. I should also be ungrateful in the sight of God and men, and a traitor to my own profession if, having uncovered with His help, over a very long period and with great effort, the value of this new gift which will be useful to all humanity, I did not reveal it, and principally to yourself, who can keep it from perishing if you once accept it as your own.

It is true that its novelty and unfamiliarity, qualities France esteems too greatly, might for a while commend its subject. However, it is to be feared that the fact of its being home-grown (something which is held in low esteem among our countrymen) rather than foreign, together with the very lowly regard for its little-known author, may immediately suffice to condemn it in the eyes of our fellow Frenchmen, who nowadays set the least store by what their own country produces.[49] We see this with this excellent French clay, which they value so little that it is profaned by intelligent people who use it only to clean bonnets in Paris.[50] Yet, if one considers it

47. A bezoar is a mass trapped in the stomach, believed by classical physicians to be a universal antidote.

48. I.e. Rousset's present work.

49. Like many contemporary writers (e.g. Henri Estienne or François de La Noue), Rousset laments the growing taste in France in the later sixteenth century for importing expensive, exotic products from abroad. Cyr and Baskett misrepresent this sentence slightly, since 'nom' in sixteenth-century French means 'reputation' rather than 'name'.

50. Cyr and Basket (23, n. 25) provide a good rationale for the translation 'clay', explaining that its 'strong, absorptive powers' were used to remove stains from clothing.

dispassionately and without prejudice, in all its qualities and effects it is infinitely better than the finest red earth of Lemnos and other such strange soils, which are sold to us for more than the price of gold. And this is all because it was praised by those from that region — notably the Greek author Galen, who had never seen our soils. This is despite the fact that the earth is now taken from a different place from that which he described, and that one lot is almost never the same as the next in the same year, whether it appears to bear an authentic stamp or a false one — both from the same pasha. This shows the great deception of something that should not be reckoned a worthy subject of deception even if it were entirely genuine. I do not want to enter here into a discussion of an infinite number of other abuses which involve foreign impostors coming from far away to take advantage of our credulity: let it just be mentioned in passing in respect of this small gift.

For my part, as the bearer of it, I thought I should follow the advice of the Greek lord who held that the wise and useful advice of a private citizen, having been found good (as it was), should be made public through the mouth of a great magistrate, or some other person of standing. In this way, he taught lesser people to obtain a sponsor in order to protect the results of their good industries. Resolved to apply this, after handing this little work to the gentlemen of the Faculty of Medicine in Paris,[51] and seeing that it was accepted and approved by them, I thought I could obtain no better protection for it to dwell safely in this kingdom, nor any stronger escort to leave it in safety,[52] than the safe-conduct of your name, which it greatly needs. Otherwise it risks an unfavorable reception by some, since it seems to promise something new, which has rarely been heard of, never written down, scarcely credible even to people who see it. Consequently, until now, it has been held to be impossible, even by the most learned and experienced physicians and surgeons from the most

51. Following a decree issued by the Paris Parlement on 3rd May 1535, all works on medicine required the prior approval of the Paris Faculty of Medicine. See the Approval (29), which originally appeared at the end of the treatise.

52. Rousset envisages at the outset that his work may be of interest outside France, as proved to be the case when it circulated in Latin in the collection *Books on the Diseases of Women* [*Gynaeciorum libri*]. See 7.

famous universities in the world.[53] Now since this is a matter of great significance, not only for the acceptance of this new method that I am recommending (if it be considered useful and sometimes necessary, as it is), but also because it could wrongly be banned if it were to be carried out without due care and with unfortunate consequences, it is quite reasonable to hold me responsible, as I am before God, yourself and all men, as to the absolute truth of all the circumstances which I record having heard, read about or seen, and I submit myself willingly to any penalties appropriate if the contrary were shown to be the case.

I ask God, my Lord, to grant you and your family long life, good health, and His holy grace at all times,

Your most humble servant and faithful physician,

Fr. Rousset.

53. Compare Guillemeau's report of Ambroise Paré's later opposition to cesareans on living women (214).

TO THE READER

I had not originally intended, dear Reader, to do more than record in writing a simple account and several small and amicable debates which Monsieur Paré[54] and myself had previously had on the subject of the delivery which I called Cesarean. These conversations were in French, the language Monsieur Paré uses most readily in his lectures and writings.[55] But, after the sight of my testimony had shown him the truth of the facts recorded, and the likelihood of my arguments seemed to have persuaded him of what he had held to be impossible, I decided not to write down anything at all of this. However, some learned persons of high reputation, having taken his place and gained the opportunity to contradict me more strongly than before, forced me to resume my defence of the subject (so that such a useful matter did not perish through fear or lack of effort), and to develop further some subjects related to it.

Because of this, I drafted a longer treatise than before, this time in Latin, at the command of my excellent mistress, the late Madame Renée of France, Duchess of Ferrara, so that I did justice to her rank.[56] Shortly before her death, she asked me to undertake this so that it should be accessible to foreign nations (and especially, among the Italians, her own people of Ferrara). I believe that by the private circulation of it, I have already, on an individual level, satisfied most of my opponents. I intend shortly to publish it, since it is a most important matter, not only for surgery and medicine, but also for the whole commonwealth.[57]

54. Ambroise Paré (?1509–1590), the most famous surgeon of the French Renaissance, and surgeon to four successive kings of France.

55. Many editions of Paré's collected works were published in French from 1575. See J. Doe, *A Bibliography of the Works of Ambroise Paré* (Chicago: University of Chicago Press, 1957). The Latin translation of his works appeared in 1582, produced by an anonymous translator, but overseen by Jacques Guillemeau.

56. Renée of France (1510–1575), the second daughter of Louis XII and Anne of Brittany, married Hercule, Duke of Ferrara, in 1540, converting to Protestantism the same year. Her court was a center of Renaissance culture and also an asylum for Protestants fleeing from persecution.

57. On the publishing history of the French and Latin versions of the treatise, see 6-7.

However, the delay in introducing this operation, which the fuller Latin treatise describes (but it has not yet wanted to leave my hands), may be harmful to a large number of poor pregnant women in France, who die because they do not have the opportunity to be saved in this way that we hope to provide. And also, some of our French surgeons, having little or no reading knowledge of Latin,[58] have been urging me to share it with them, and I wish to satisfy their request without delaying such an essential, urgent means of saving the lives of women who are left, once all other solutions have been attempted in vain, with only this last option. So, I have included in this shorter French version a good number of the main points of the longer treatise which, like this French one, I wish to declare that I undertook not out of idle curiosity or vain ambition, but because of the important nature of its subject. Principally I did so seeing that none of those who could have expressed it better than myself accepted, as they should have done, when I invited them to do so — rather they refused as though it were an absurd or impossible undertaking.

Above all, I have been led to do this by the pitiful sight of the agonies, helplessness, prayers and pitiful looks of those poor creatures who are so tortured, and cry murder, as they appeal only to us, begging with clasped hands for such help as we may be able to give them. For it is in this more than in any other calamity that the greatest women suffer everything.[59] Thus, let us for our part, when all other means have failed, and having wiped the tears from our eyes, take courage, trusting in God's help, and acting with due care, so that we may use the only means left to us to save the lives of the mother and the child from the tomb into which they would shortly be consigned. Just the report of such a pitiful scene is horrifying to the most barbarous heart in the world, even when one is not present.

---

58. Rousset's comment fits with the general picture provided by sixteenth-century surgical treatises. Unlike physicians, surgeons were not required to know Latin, and so their ability to read it was very variable indeed. Hence French translations of works on surgery constituted a lucrative market for printers and booksellers.

59. Rousset is discretely arguing that childbirth — like death — is the greatest social leveller among women, since even the highest born may suffer or die.

Thus I promise you, for these reasons, to write more about this soon, dear Reader, if I find that this short account pleases you, since I guarantee that it is entirely true, and that I give it to you in all good faith. May you use it in the name of God, whoever you may be, either applying it with great care and patience (as befits such a serious matter), if there is need in your household or among your friends, or carrying it out for someone else, as a wise and careful surgeon, without undue haste. You will do so not for gain or vain glory — for these would bring you misfortune and shame — but acting out of compassion and Christian charity and for the glory of God. To whom be honor and thanksgiving, through Jesus Christ His Son, Our Lord. Amen.

TABLE OF THE MAIN POINTS AND MOST REMARKABLE THINGS CONTAINED IN THIS BOOK

Of the risk of hernia as a result of the incision of this part.

Of uterine hemorrhage, which is not substantial.

Of the site where blood from the uterus will pool.

That there is not a risk of spasms when cutting through this section of the womb.

Third section (p. 51)

Third sort of proof, based on authorities.[60]

Of epigastric muscles, from the authority of reports.

Of the peritoneum, from authorities.

Of the womb, from authorities.

Comparison of the incised womb with the incision of the bladder in case of stones.

Discussion on the related topic of the extraction of stones from the hypogastrium or lower abdomen.

Example of a history on the subject of this new advice.

Response to common objections against the incision of the bladder in its membranous part through the epigaster.

Further confirmatory example.

Fourth section (p. 100)

Citing, in place of authorities, other dangers to this same afflicted part which are worse than a cesarean section.

First part, containing three histories.

First history.

Second history.

Third history.

Second part.

Aliboux[61] to Rousset, greetings.

Second history on a similar subject from the same Aliboux.

---

60. We might expect Rousset here to follow the standard practice of looking to classical authors (Galen, Hippocrates, etc.) to support his arguments, but in the absence of any classical accounts of cesareans on living women, he has to draw on the authority of respected physicians and surgeons of his own century.

61. Jean Ailleboust: see 38.

Two other histories on a similar subject from Nicolas
de Villeneufve.[62]
Another history from him.

Third part.
First history.
Second history.
Third history.
Proof of the incredible nature of the history related above.
Fourth history on this same subject.
Fifth history.
Sixth history.

Fourth part.
History.
Another history.
Another history.
Other histories.
Another new history.

Fifth part.
First history.
Second history.
Epilogue to the preceding histories.

Fifth section (p. 150)
Other less learned proofs.
Another unlearned proof.
Of some dangers, which may be alleged to result from this
cesarean section.
That the pain from the incision of the womb cannot provoke
a spasm, and that at the place of the incision there is very
little sensitivity.
History.

62. On de Villeneuve, see 50.

Sixth section (p. 165)

Of fertility that remains after the cesarean section.

As to the scar, that it does not impede fertility.

Another proof that the scar does not impede fertility: by argument from the strongest to the weakest, consisting in the assertion of a new paradox proved to be true by experience and medical reasoning.

Of the invention of the pessary, and of its various forms.

Histories about this subject.

Paradox concerning conception, while still wearing this pessary in the womb.

Confirmation of what is said above, through arguments that answer several objections against it.

Answer, by means of a corollary, of another dispute, over what is predicted concerning the opening of the mouth of the womb in pregnant women.

Histories concerning these matters.

That the pessary does not prevent the seed being fully received and securely lodged in the womb.

Answer to several other objections, and that the use of this pessary is not new, although the assertion of conceiving while wearing it is a new observation.

Small warning to the reader on the use of this cesarean operation.

APPROVAL BY THE FACULTY OF
MEDICINE OF PARIS[63]

I have read this book, the teachings of which on what is called cesarean childbirth seemed to me so well founded on reason and experience that I thought it worthy of being published. Yet the reader should be advised only to use it in the cases specified, and with great caution. Henry de Monanthueil,[64] the King's Professor of Mathematics and Dean of the Faculty of Medicine at the University of Paris.

I confirm as above,

A. Paré[65]
J. Viard

63. This appears at the end of the 1581 treatise, without a title.

64. Dean of the Faculty of Medicine, 1578–1580 (Cyr and Baskett, 113).

65. On Paré's later rejection of cesareans on living women because of the likelihood of maternal death, see Guillemeau's coments (214).

FIRST SECTION

Definition of Cesarean Childbirth

By the term cesarean birth, we mean the swift extraction of the child from the mother's side if she cannot give birth in any way other than by an incision of both the epigaster (or outer abdomen) and the body of the uterus.[66] This is to be done, nonetheless, without risk to the life of either mother or child (unless they suffer for some other reason), and even without the mother thereby losing her ability to bear a child hereafter. This applies to a child that is still alive in the mother's womb.

The term also covers the similar extraction of a child that has already died inside the mother, when it is impossible to remove it by means of any other help from the midwife,[67] or other simpler, safer and more common medical or surgical means, and when it is seen that otherwise it will cause the mother's death. This happens daily to women of every status, after having been uselessly ripped apart and pitifully injured.

As for the extraction of children that are still alive in the womb of a mother who has already died (who could have been saved by this expedient), given that it has already been discussed by both classical and modern writers in greater detail than necessary, and that it requires no great skill, I do not intend to treat it here, even though such an incision gave his name to the first of the Caesars, Scipio Africanus,[68] who came into the world in this way. It is after him that this incision was also named a 'cesarean' by us. However, we hope that (with God's grace) it will be carried out with greater success, that is to say without causing the death of the mother, which did not happen in Scipio's case, as is recorded by the Latin poet Silius Italicus.[69]

66. Translated into modern medical English by Cyr and Baskett (29) as 'incision performed in the mother's anterior abdominal wall and uterus'.

67. Cyr and Baskett's translation (29) omits the mention of the midwife and medical and surgical means.

68. Scipio the Elder (Publius Cornelius Scipio Africanus, 236–183 BC), a statesman of the Roman Republic and general, who defeated Hannibal at the end of the Second Punic War.

69. Tiberius Catius Silius Italicus (25–101), Latin epic poet and author of the 17 books of the *Punica*. The death in childbirth of Pomponia, mother of Scipio Africanus, is recorded in *Punica* XIII. 615–646, although Silius does not explicitly claim that Scipio Africanus was delivered by cesarean.

Of the Usefulness and Necessity of This Cesarean Section

Regarding not only the usefulness, but also the necessity of this operation, it must be noted that if it happens that children, dead or alive, strong or weak, cannot be delivered by any other means, for the reasons that we shall explain hereafter, it is necessary to have recourse to it. Otherwise the children and their mothers will both inevitably die, even if the mothers are still strong. And even more so if the mothers are already weak and close to death; in such cases it is absolutely imperative to open them.

The benefit is twofold, because then the child escapes with its life, instead of dying as a suffocated prisoner, and not only does the mother not die, as she would have done — I mean provided she is opened in a good and timely fashion, while she is still strong — but also she will be no less healthy than before, even still being able to bear children. If she should be already weak, and her life despaired of at this stage, she will still have some hope of escape if, after it has been explained, she is skillfully cut open. For this is better, even though uncertain, than absolute despair.

This operation not only contributes to sustaining marriages, alliances and other such arrangements that involve private individuals, but also serves commonwealths and institutions on this earth. By this means it ensures the survival of those whose races depend on the succession from father to son, or from one relative to another, for the inheritance of belongings, titles, realms and empires, which often change hands in the absence of this expedient, damaging states and causing great regret among subjects. It was for less cause than this that Hippocrates wrote his 59th aphorism in the fifth book, starting, 'If a woman does not conceive', etc. ['*Si mulier non concipit…*'].[70] We can see this from Galen's commentary on this locus.

---

70. Hippocrates's aphorism (V. 59) reads, 'If a woman does not conceive and wishes to establish whether she can conceive, after she has been wrapped in blankets, fumigate her below, and if it seems that the scent passes through the body to the nostrils and mouth, it is clear that in herself she is not sterile.'

Causes of the Impossibility of Natural Delivery, Which Give Rise to the Need for This Operation

The causes which prevent any other delivery and that may, on occasion, render this operation necessary are varied. Some come from the child, others from the mother. As far as the child is concerned, it may be that it is unusually heavy or large; or it may be one of twins or a multiple pregnancy, with one child preventing another's delivery; or there may be a fleshy mole;[71] or it may be deformed or monstrous; or, if it is wrongly positioned, it may be unable to right itself or be assisted into a position allowing a better delivery. Or if it is already dead, it can no longer play a part in its birth as it should.[72] Or it may be so swollen that it cannot pass through the normal passage.

As for the mother, she may be too narrow, which occurs in diverse manners: as a result of her natural build, some women being more constricted than others, just as all men do not have their genital parts of identical size; or because of the tender age of girls who are married too young, and are still only partly open;[73] or those who are too old and already hardened, especially when they married very late; or others who have had several pregnancies which did not reach full term, the long interruption causing them to become more closed up as a result of the hardening due to their age. Because of this, the pubic bone that usually moves in labor, although some say it does not,[74] has more difficulty opening.

71. Renaissance physicians write extensively about moles, even though modern statistics suggest a hydatidiform mole (placental tissue that develops in the absence of a viable foetus) is a rare condition, affecting only 1 in c.1500 pregnancies in Western society. On the Renaissance fascination with uterine moles, see H. King, *Midwifery, Obstetrics and the Rise of Gynaecology*, 59–64.

72. A comment reminding us that Renaissance physicians assumed it was the foetus's active efforts to be born which ensured its delivery.

73. Like many other physicians and moralists, Rousset opposes early marriages because they may damage the pubescent female body.

74. There was a vigorous debate over whether the pubic bone actually opened in labor. Modern medicine confirms that the pubic bones do ease apart, partly due to softening of the pelvic joints, which during a normal pregnancy loosen the usually small gap between the two pelvic bones (4–5mm) by a further 2–3mm. See also Liebault's and Guillemeau's comments on this topic: 119, 187.

For some women, this happens accidentally when (contrary to the normal conformation of other women), since birth[75] they have had a defect at the entrance, or in the middle, or deep inside the uterus. This acts like a barrier which means they are shielded or suffer an obstruction and the seed is hardly able to enter; then, having grown for nine whole months to the size of a child, the baby cannot be delivered from this enclosure. By longstanding defect, I also mean any obstacle that has developed since the birth of the woman, whether she has been affected in this area by an ulcer, the scar of which has healed over and hardened making these parts very narrow; or whether because of previous births; or the badly accomplished extraction of a stone; or bitter discharges which have damaged these parts; or because of an abscess which started and developed there.

Such malformations, generally known by the Greeks as φιμωσεις (or phimosis), and commonly called obstructions, are described by Celsus, Aegineta,[76] and other surgeons, both ancient and modern, who hold a good many of these obstructions to be incurable even if they are known, and the modesty of ladies does not easily allow them to be. Furthermore, even though some of these may be cured in women who are not pregnant, if they were willing to reveal them in good time, still pregnancy — during which the area cannot be touched — puts them, like the first group, beyond hope of a cure, and consequently beyond hope of the women giving birth.[77]

In all these cases, which often arise and affect many women, cesarean section is not only desirable, but also absolutely necessary. The failure to recognize these malformations, and in the absence of any other assistance to carry out this section — for it is the only remedy — means that every day an infinite number of wretched women die, both poor women and princesses, and the greatest regret

---

75. Cyr and Baskett's version of this sentence is misleading, implying that the defect has been present only 'from the beginning of pregnancy' (p. 31), and that what grows is a uterine tumor, not the foetus.

76. See Celsus, *On Medicine*, trans. by G. F. Collier, VII.28, and Paulus Aegineta, *The Medical Works*, trans. by F. Adams, VI.72.

77. Compare (288-291) the use some exceptionally skilled surgeons made of the speculum [*speculum matricis*] to widen obstructed vaginal and cervical passages in the early seventeenth century.

the loss of their lineage. And their subjects, as said above, regret the loss of the natural line of their ancient princes.

I would readily group together with these causes an infinite number of temporary tumors, inflammations, prolapses, abscesses, schirruses,[78] tumors and other hard swellings. These can, and in these places usually do, as elsewhere, obstruct the passages and towards the end of pregnancy prevent women from giving birth, since they are unable to wait for these tumors to burst or be cured because of the urgency of the impending delivery, and yet the delivery, because of the tumor, cannot be accomplished.

Three Sorts of Proof of This Matter

Now since this matter has never been treated by any ancient or modern author, and since it is still only very rarely practiced by a few rural barbers,[79] and, moreover, since it is held to be false and impossible even by the physicians and surgeons whose knowledge and experience is the most renowned — and by whom the practice should be promoted in order for it to become accepted, gain recognition and be used — it is necessary to employ all the means of persuasion which can be found. Of these, there are commonly three: verified experience, appropriate reasoning and convincing authority, if such can be found. As for the first, it will be demonstrated through histories which have been confirmed; the second, through medical debates; we lack the third since no one has ever written anything on it as far as we have seen. But in place of this, we shall proceed by analogy or by reference to similar or more dangerous operations on these same parts and others near them — indeed to some more major and thus more crucial ones, yet which have enjoyed good success, and consequently promise even better success for this operation. I myself have had some of them performed, and I have drawn the others in part from the practice of famous doctors who are still alive, and in part from the writings of various authors, both ancient and modern.

78. A type of hard tumor.
79. I.e. barber surgeons.

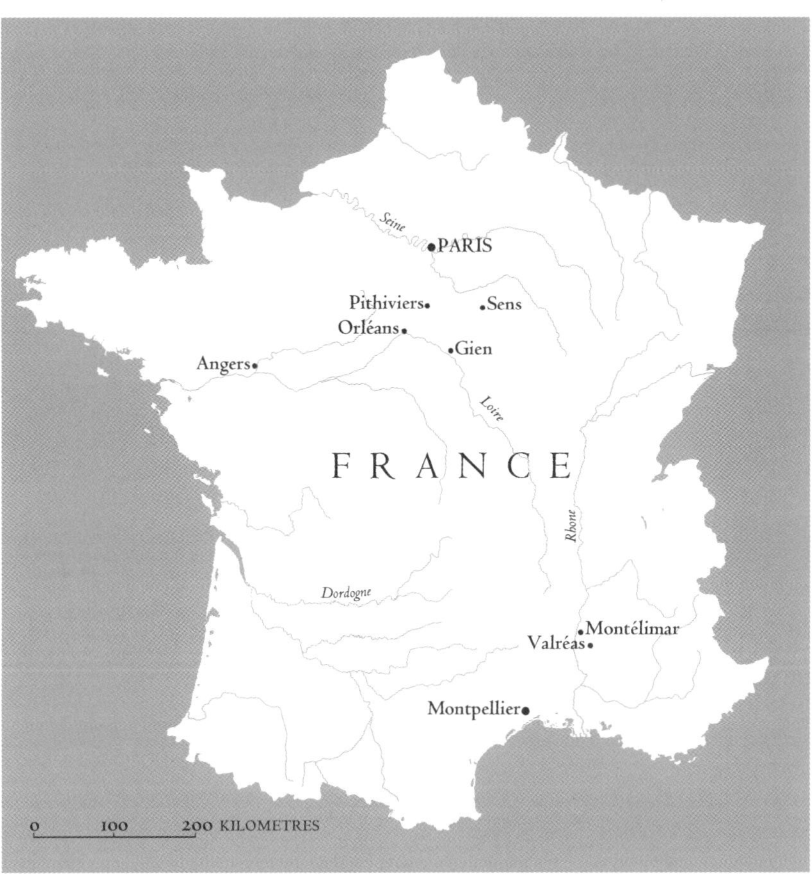

7) Map of France showing towns cited by François Rousset

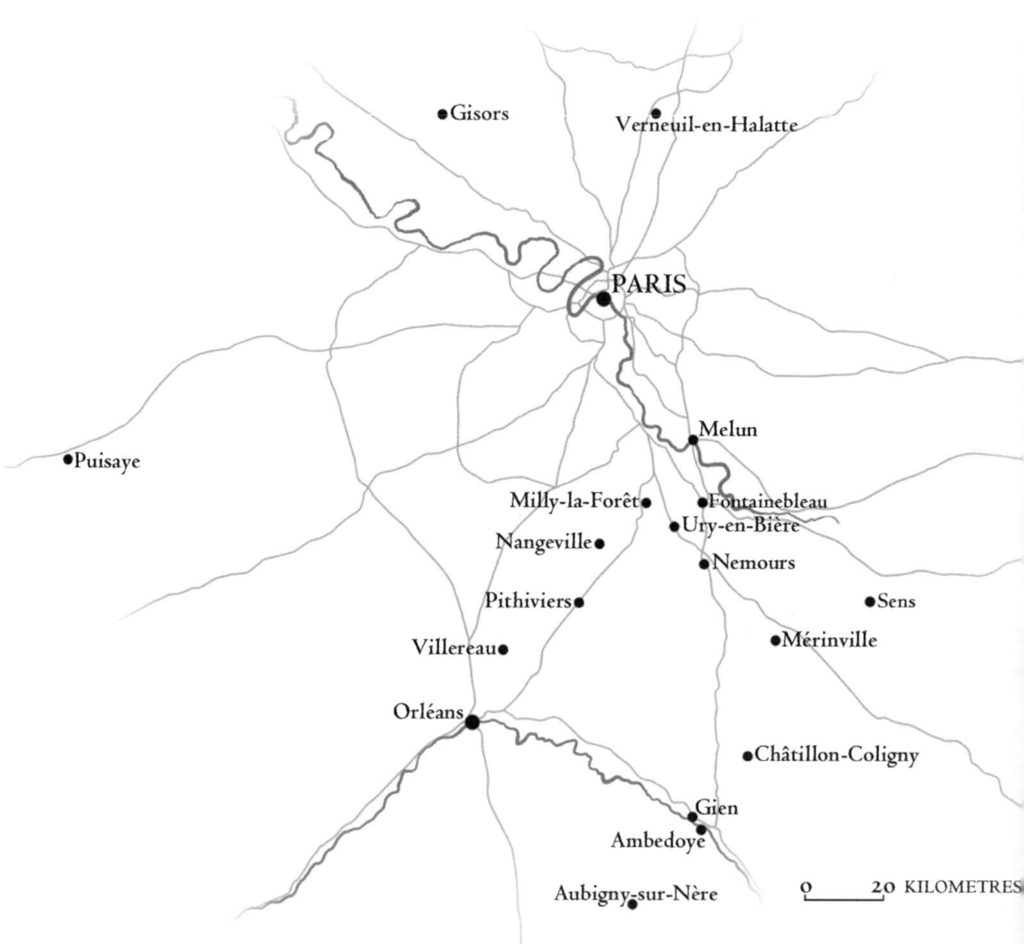

8) Local map showing towns and villages cited by François Rousset

Histories Reported by Trustworthy People

First, as far as the histories are concerned, since I have not trusted the histories of experiences furnished by others unless they were confirmed by my own, equally I have not wanted to ask that my own be believed without providing others with the grounds to trust them. I have carefully sought out similar ones from people who cannot be doubted. I shall report these other histories first in a concise manner, and then come to those which I call my own, some because I advised that the operations should take place, some because I witnessed them with my own eyes, seeing the exact way in which the incisions were made on the women, and this in their own homes, and confirmed by the testimony not only of the surgeons performing the operations, but also by the husbands, children, servants and witnesses who were present in large numbers.

First history[80]

Not long ago I was quite convinced of the truth of the history supplied by some worthy, older gentlemen near Milly in the area of Gâtinais,[81] which is not questioned locally. He said that the wife of a certain Godart living at Mesnil in the parish of Milly had some years previously given birth six times in this way, never in any other, and each time to living children. The surgeon was Nicolas Guillet, the barber in Milly, after whose death the woman also died because she

---

80. I am grateful to Gianna Pomata for bringing to my attention the significance of Rousset's repeated use of the term '*histoire*' (corresponding to '*historia*' in Latin), which I translate here as 'history'. It provides an important example in the French vernacular that corresponds to the rise of the publication of case histories (from the 1540s onward) in Latin by medical humanists. For a full discussion of the rise of the published '*historia medica*' or medical case history in the Renaissance, see Pomata's chapter 'Praxis historialis: the case of *Historia* in early modern medicine, in *Historia: Empiricism and erudition in early modern Europe*, eds. G. Pomata and N. Siraisi (Massachusetts: Massachusetts Institute of Technology, 2005), 105–146. Pomata has also demonstrated that case histories develop into a genre in their own right, frequently entitled *Observationes*, in which the case histories take center stage rather than, as previously, being confined to folds in the text of general accounts of diseases. See her discussion in: 'Observation rising: birth of an epistemic genre, 1500–1850' in *Histories of Scientific Observation*, eds. L. Daston and E. Lunbeck (Chicago and London: The University of Chicago Press, 2011), 45–80.

81. Milly-la-Forêt, a village at the western edge of Fontainebleau forest, in the former province of Gâtinais (between the Seine and the Loire).

no longer had his customary assistance when she was unable to give birth. It seems probable that this was a case of deep phimosis,[82] or a natural obstruction, the passage being sufficient to receive the seed,[83] but not to deliver the child.

Second history

In truth, I learned from Ambroise Le Noir, a most expert surgeon in our town of Pithviers,[84] and from Gilles Le Brun, that several times they had together extracted three living children from the side of a poor woman living near Mérinville[85] in Beauce. I wished to travel to her so that I could see the site of the incision, but I learned that a short time previously she had died of the plague, which was then very contagious and raging fiercely in that region.[86]

Third history

I have a learned epistle from Monsieur Aliboux,[87] a physician in Sens, who describes at length and in careful detail how Jean des Marais, a surgeon at La Chastre in the province of Berry, son of Loys des Marais, Ordinary Surgeon of the Archbishop of Sens, Salazar, extracted from the side of his wife a son named Symon des Marais, who also became a surgeon in his turn, and usher in the royal chamber of the Queen Mother. After this, she went on to give birth successfully again, this time naturally, to a daughter named Renée, who later married a grain merchant. This Symon (nicknamed 'the motherless') and Roze Gallardet had two daughters: Claude, married to François Artus d'Yssoudun; and Françoise, married to Olivier Gannier. Both of them

---

82. Rousset uses the term here to imply a constriction or adhesion affecting the vaginal labia.

83. For the male seed to enter the vagina so that conception could take place.

84. Pithiviers (as the town is now known) is in the Loiret department, some 30 km from Milly-la-Forêt, cited in the previous account.

85. A town some 70 km from both Pithiviers and Milly-la-Forêt.

86. For details of outbreaks of plague in this area, see Cyr and Baskett, 34, n. 53.

87. Jean d'Ailleboust (1532–1594), became First Physician to Henri IV; he wrote a Latin epistle, *The Monstrous Stone-Child, or the Putrified Embryo of the Town of Sens* [*Portentosum lithopaedion, sive embryon putrefactum urbis Senonensis*, Sens, Jean Savine, 1582], describing the discovery, during an autopsy after the death of the mother, of a calcified foetus which had remained in the womb for twenty-eight years.

attest to their father's birth, based on both local reports and on their father's regular accounts of it to the family.

Fourth history

Monsieur Pelion, a famous physician in Angers, having previously told Laurent Collot, a cystotomic surgeon[88] from Paris, of such an operation that had been performed in Anjou, testified again to the truth of it in a letter to Collot, which the latter sent to me. Monsieur Pelion declared that a certain surgeon, called Mathurin Debonnaire, had carried it out, but he gave no further details.

Histories Seen by Eyewitnesses

Dear Reader,
So that you will not accuse me of being unskilled or dull in devoting too much time to furnishing full histories with all the small details, I want you to know that the precise care I have taken to report these facts exactly has caused me equal trouble. But I have done this to reassure you, guaranteeing the truth so that if you wish you may check in the places that I have recorded for you, and also consult most of the eyewitnesses, if you have any doubts.

First history

At the hospital in Châtillon-sur-Loing,[89] a little before these first disturbances,[90] Monsieur Denys Armenault, a physician in Gien, and myself together saw a woman suffering from an unbroken fever, who had a large hernia on the left side of her lower abdomen, with a long scar and visible traces of the marks of a needle where the opening of this area had been sewn back together. She and her husband testified that some time previously a son — now aged approximately seven — had been pulled out from this incision since he could not be delivered in any other manner, and they showed him to us. This had been done by an elderly barber in their own village, in Burgundy,

88. A surgeon using a special instrument to make an incision in the perineum or bladder.
89. The town now called Châtillon-Coligny, in the Loiret department.
90. This refers to the Wars of Religion (a series of civil wars lasting from 1562 to 1598).

who, they said, was expert at such operations. I wrote down his name to enquire further about him through letters and friends, and to learn from him what practical experience of the operation he had acquired. But the difficulty of our age[91] caused me to lose the record of the place and of the person, and prevented my having the chance of learning what I had hoped to gain from it. In any event, she had not conceived or borne any other children subsequently, although she and her husband were both young. Those who worked with Armenault will have heard him tell this many times, since at first he found it unbelievable, as others did, but eventually he came to find it beyond doubt, and he determined that he would recommend the operation if necessity placed him in such a position.

Second history

Bernarde Arnoul, the wife of Estienne Massicauld, from Nangeville (which is between Estampes, Puiseaux and Pithviers), had been in full labor for four days to no avail. She got her husband to send for me in order to seek some urgent advice on how she could be saved, and was brave enough — in defiance of her husband's wishes — to allow herself to be opened. Indeed, once she had heard my counsel, she was in such a hurry to follow it that she would not wait for the said Ambroise Le Noir, whom I promised to send to her since he already had experience of the operation. (I happened to be unable to attend, being at the time confined to bed, seriously ill.) Instead, she used the first surgeon available, Jean Lucas, a young barber residing then, as he still does now, in Bunou, a neighboring small village, and he performed this operation, which he had never done before, with dexterity, watched by a group of people, some of whom, like himself, are witness to this fact. This took place on Easter Sunday 1556.

The incision (this should be noted as an example of how to proceed if necessary) started on the right-hand side of the abdomen, one fingerbreadth below the navel, and more than four fingerbreadths to the side of it. From there it went down directly almost to the pubis, without touching the rectus[92] muscles at all, remaining about

---

91. Ibid.

92. Cyr and Baskett (37, n. 62) identify the muscles thus, but they raise some questions about the consistency of Rousset's instructions.

three fingerbreadths away from them at the top, and slightly less at the bottom. After an incision had also been made, causing scarcely any bleeding, from top to bottom through the muscles and the peritoneum, the womb was clearly visible. He cut this separately, making quite a broad incision, so that the opening was large enough to be able to extract the living child easily, as well as its amniotic sack. Then he stitched the opening back up, not gastroraphically,[93] but like a common wound. He stitched not the womb, but the muscles and the peritoneum with five stitches, as I carefully noted, having gone, as soon as I was able to leave my sickbed, with the express purpose of examining the mother.[94] What I often had cause to note about her hereafter, since she came to me seeming to need treatment, was that she had something like a hernia that never went away, either because it had not been stitched up well, or because she had got up too soon after her operation, for she kept to her bed for no more than forty days in total after the operation. Approximately a year and a half later, her husband having died, she married Pierre Chanclou, who still lives there, and she became pregnant again and this time gave birth naturally, to a daughter. The daughter is now in her second marriage, living at Nangeville, where there are still some witnesses to this event.

Third history

At Ury-en-Bière, near Fontainebleau, two leagues[95] from Nemours, Collette Beranger, the wife of Symon de La Garde, was already beyond the tenth month of pregnancy and had for a long time been carrying a dead foetus in her womb without her lower parts opening to expel it. Finally she sent for Vincent Valleau, the surgeon in Nemours (who had previously been my assistant). He had no other obvious means of relieving her situation, and so, at the end of January 1542, he made an incision, not on the right-hand side as in the previous case, but on the left. It was made somewhat higher than in the case in Nangeville, as he cut through first the outer abdomen and then the womb. He then

---

93. With stitches used for sewing abdominal wounds such as hernias.

94. Cyr and Baskett point out (37, n. 63) that for a long time surgeons performing cesareans did not regularly suture the womb itself, as would now be the case.

95. The small town of Ury is some 12 km south-west of Fontainebleau.

pulled out the dead foetus, which was swollen and putrid,[96] together with the amniotic sack, which was already rotting. Then, without stitching the womb, he used five stitches (apparently having recourse to a desperate solution) to draw together the skin and a small part of the muscles, as is still quite apparent, with only the simple outer layer of skin having formed a scar over the intestines. I went there expressly, together with Pavie, the surgeon in Nemours, who was once the assistant of the said Valleau. I saw with my own eyes and touched with my own hand[97] the place of this terrible scar, which the woman bears without complaint, providing only that she has a light compress or bandage. It does not prevent her from working for her living as best she can, even though the injury is significant.

This case deserves to be known in order to demonstrate that in such circumstances it is not essential to imitate perfect surgical stitching, for there is a danger that one may spoil everything by trying to pretend to have a high level of competence in something about which one knows little, and where it is not really necessary.

The mother kept to her bed for a month and a half in total. Two years later, she gave birth, naturally, to a daughter and a further two years later to a son called Pierre de La Garde, who is now a blacksmith. She still lives in the village of Ury, and acts as a midwife, delivering children.[98]

Fourth history

Agnes Boyer, the wife of Jean Copain, who is still, as he was then, a farm laborer, living in Villereau, near Neufville-en-Beauce,[99] had had her body quite broken for four days by the incompetence of the midwives, all to no avail. She was then opened (as the other women were), on the right-hand side in her case, by Philippe Migneau, the barber in Neufville, in the year 1544. Her muscles and the covering

---

96. In many of the obstetric treatises of this period, physicians and surgeons warn of the dangers when a foetus has died in the womb but cannot be expelled. Ultimately, the decaying foetus would cause sepsis, endangering the life of the mother.

97. A formula reminiscent of the apostle Thomas touching the resurrected Christ (John 20: 24–29).

98. A useful indication of the way in which women who had themselves given birth could later become midwives, in rural settings often without receiving any formal training.

99. Now spelled Neuville (a town in the Loiret department).

skin were then sewn back by the barber as best he could. As far as her womb was concerned, she recovered quickly from the incision, but the damage the incompetent midwives had caused to her lower parts prevented the surgeons from curing her for more than seven months. She had given birth to a fine daughter who lived for more than seven months, in good health, but in the eighth month the child fell ill at the home of the wet-nurse, that was in the same village, and so died.

Soon after this, the mother became pregnant again, and almost all the time the child lay towards the hernia that she, like the other women, still had. It did not cause her any pain, but she could not deliver this child any more than the previous one, presumably for one or other of the reasons we have discussed above. And so, of her own accord, she asked to have an incision performed as before, but beg as she might she could not prevail upon the two new, young surgeons who had been sent to attend her from Neufville where they had taken over after Philippot had died of the plague. As a result, she and her unborn child both died pitifully because of their lack of resolve — unless it was cowardice or some other regrettable reason which prevented them from acting.

Fifth history

Again, in the year 1577, on the 22nd of July, at Ambedoye, near Saint-Brisson, in the region of Gien, Antoinette André, wife of the laborer Loys Garnier, was also opened. The operation was performed by Adam Aubry, a surgeon born in Pithiviers, and now living in Aubigny.[100] He reported it to me, giving precise details, and testified to its success, being grateful for my assistance in that, in the past, I had frequently discussed this operation with him. Knowing his skill and the success of the operations that he performed, I had advised him, following my own opinion, not to hesitate, if all else failed, to have recourse to this operation, despite the criticisms it occasions even from physicians themselves, provided only that he acted with caution, having made the decision after beseeching God's help. I had reminded him that, because of the haste which is occasioned by such urgent dangers, one cannot wait for the answer to requests for advice from afar, as one is

---

100. Probably the village of Aubigny-sur-Nère, some 17 km from Gien.

obliged to do in rural places or towns, where none wants, or dares, to support this opinion. Some respond negatively because they do not believe anything they hear about the operation, others for fear of being held responsible, as though they had caused the misfortune were things to turn out other than well.

Since then, the mother became pregnant again and gave birth naturally, but after a certain time she had to leave to follow her husband, both of them seeking the means of earning a living elsewhere in a time of famine.[101]

Sixth history

Even more recently, on the first day of February 1578, Jeanne Michel, from Argent, married to George Renauld, who lives on the outskirts of Aubigny, and who was well into the tenth month of her pregnancy, had been carrying her dead foetus for a long time, while still going about her daily business. Finally she was obliged to take to her bed, where she suffered in vain for a long time at the hands of the midwives. She sent for the said Adam Aubry,[102] and Guillaume Collas, a learned surgeon, who cut off one of the child's dead arms; it was livid and had been hanging out of the mother's private parts for a long time. But they were unable to obtain a hold on the rest of the body, so they made a slightly slanting incision in the mother's right side, quite a narrow opening in order to spare her. This caused the mother great pain when the child was extracted, since the womb could not release the child, because of the narrowness of the opening, and it followed the foetus as though they were trying to pull out the womb itself. However, this pain ceased as soon as the child and the afterbirth were extracted. Thus, after the ordinary discharges following childbirth, which flowed as well as if she had given birth naturally,[103] a little time later she left her bed. After five weeks she had her normal menses. Immediately afterwards, she became pregnant again, that is at the end of May, and she already became worried (remembering the recent

---

101. Rousset presumably includes this information to account for the fact that the woman can no longer be traced to act as a witness to the success of the operation.

102. See above, 43.

103. I.e. lochia, the post-partum vaginal discharge of uterine blood and some placental tissue, classically lasting between three and six weeks after birth.

past so clearly) about what would happen at the end of this pregnancy. When her time came, she gave birth naturally, and although the child presented initially with only one of its legs, which is a very bad start in these matters, nonetheless the midwife tucked the leg back in, and everything then turned out happily.[104] Since this time, she has become pregnant again, hoping that God would bring her as much help in the future as in the past, and at the present time she has been delivered naturally from this second pregnancy, and goes about her daily affairs as well as ever.

104. Rousset records, in a very mater-of-fact manner, the standard, early-modern technique for managing such malpresentations — in this case, a footling breech. The midwife would try to tuck the obtruding limb back into the womb to restore a more favorable position. Compare the recommendations given by Liebault (134-5) and Duval (277).

FOURTH SECTION

Citing, in Place of Authorities, Other Dangers to This Same Afflicted Part, Which Are Worse Than a Cesarean Section

Leaving aside the organ of the bladder — so as not to depart from the uterus — we shall compare this incision to some other operations that are more dangerous, yet are not inherently mortal. And we shall divide this discussion into the following five parts.

The first will treat pregnant women who did not think they were pregnant, but in whom the child had died and rotted, causing the womb to rot internally. Because they were not opened, they eventually died, whereas they would have lived had the problem been recognized and the operation performed in time.

The second will deal with women suffering from ulcerated wombs, both those who were giving birth, and those who were not. They were opened not by cesarean section but with actual cauteries[105] applied to the abdomen, without causing death or loss of fertility. This operation is worse than a cesarean.

The third will deal also with illnesses afflicting wombs which were rotten within, towards the top of the womb, and so thoroughly that the dead child, having left the cavity of the womb, moved towards the intestines, from which it was extracted through the epigaster, where it was thought there had simply been a huge ulcer. This happened without causing the mother's death, nor did it make her unable to bear children afterwards once the womb had healed of its own accord.[106]

In the fourth case, we have women whose wombs completely fell out[107] and rotted, and were entirely removed without causing death, either by section and cautery, or by means of ligature.[108]

---

105. White-hot irons applied to cauterize a site on the body. Cyr and Baskett (67, n. 114) find it impossible to establish from Rousset's account in this paragraph exactly what medical problem is being treated.

106. Cyr and Baskett (68, n. 115) speculate that this paragraph is describing cases of extra-uterine pregnancy.

107. A full uterine prolapse.

108. Either the womb was cut away and the remaining tissue cauterized, or the womb was tightly ligatured until it dropped off.

In the fifth case, we have women whose wombs had prolapsed and rotted, and then finally fell out on their own without causing death or any illness.

First Part, Containing Three Histories

First history

Loyse Pouppard, the wife of Nicolas Sevin, called Champgasté from Orleans, thinking that her menses were delayed just on account of a quartan fever,[109] for it usually happens in this case that the menses stop, had in fact conceived. However, she did not suspect she was pregnant, and so continued to use medicines and to have blood let and suffer other treatments that are common for quartan fever, as well as for hardness of the liver or spleen which accompany this malady. The child in the womb was taken to be these hard organs, not being recognized for what it was; it was judged to be some scirrhus or other lump caused by the apparent retention of the menstrual flow. Finally, once the child died and its softer parts began to rot, without there being any hint of delivery, the bones became detached in the womb over time and pierced it at the back near the large intestine. She gradually began to excrete them through her rectum when she passed motions, and among others she passed an entire bone from the leg. Having suffered in this manner for a long time, she died and was opened on the 6th of February 1565 by Florent Philippes and Michel Pichard, who found inside her only rotten bones, mainly those from the head. They were astonished that these should have survived for this length of time in this foul womb.[110] This woman could probably have been saved by having her abdomen opened had the problem been recognized in time, and had this remedy been approved and carried out promptly.

---

109. An intermittent fever, with a markedly raised temperature after about two days.

110. This description is similar to the better known case of the calcified foetus of Sens, which would be recorded in 1582 by Jean d'Ailleboust (in Latin) and by Simon de Provanchières (in French), in which a calcified foetus had been retained in the womb for some 28 years and was finally revealed only at the autopsy of the mother. It also anticipates the description in 1622, by Théophile Gelée, of a woman whose rotten foetus protruded from the navel and had to be cut out by surgeons.

Second history

Catherine des Fiefs, a gentlewoman from Oncy near Milly,[111] in her second marriage fell ill and at the same time became pregnant without realizing it. In Paris she was judged to be ill, as the other woman had been in Orleans,[112] undergoing a multitude of treatments including even the sweating regime. However, a midwife to the Queen[113] did consider her to be pregnant, noting all the signs of pregnancy, from the cessation of menstruation to milk in her breasts, from this time to the ninth month, at which point all the signs ceased, as did the child's free movement. The pains of labor commenced, but to no effect, and then immediately afterwards there followed all the signs of a dead foetus, but these were still ignored. Thus she returned from Paris[114] to her home, still carrying the dead child — for fifteen months in total, until the day of her death, in addition to the previous nine months in which it had been alive. The soft tissues rotted and were expelled from her lower parts, being judged, not without reason, by Monsieur Ponet, a learned physician from Melun, to be discharge from an ulcer on the womb. The remaining bones were thought to be scirrhus of the spleen. When she finally died, she was opened on the 3rd of October 1570 by Luc Champenois and Jacques Dazier, barbers in Milly, in the presence of Messieurs de Vertau and La Gainiere, and some others,[115] and much more putrid matter was found inside her. There was no womb, but all the bones of a child, some of them rotten, others whole, and among them was one of the clavicles which had already pierced the peritoneum and the muscles of the abdomen, leaving only the outer skin. It could not be seen on the left-hand side since it was already completely livid, something which had for a long time been taken for a scirrhus of the spleen. Had the suffering been thoroughly investigated

111. See 37, n. 81.

112. Louise Pouppard, in the previous account.

113. Presumably the midwife to Catherine of Medici (whose last children, stillborn twins, had been delivered in 1556), since Charles IX (reigned 1560–1574) did not marry until 1570, and his only legitimate child, a daughter, was born in 1572, well after the death of Catherine des Fiefs.

114. Cyr and Baskett mistakenly translate 'to her home in Paris' (69).

115. An example of the growing frequency with which autopsies were performed when the cause of death was uncertain, probably at the request of the family. Compare the discussion of this practice in Renaissance Italy in K. Park, *The Secrets of Women. Gender, generation and the origins of human dissection* (New York: Zone Books, 2006), 121–131.

(without holding to the first opinion which had been given too lightly), together with the succession of signs up to the death of the child during the pregnancy, and had the other occurrences which had been carefully noted in their order been recognized for what they were, I ask whether there would not have been a possibility, when she was unable to give birth, of saving her and her child by this section? Or at least after the death of the child, which occurred much later, of saving the mother by means of this same section, which by then offered the only and essential remedy?

Third history

A similar, sad outcome occurred in the case of a woman married to a surgeon, no less, from Montpellier itself, called Ausme. He had the advantage, as we can well believe, of care from the most famous physicians of this Faculty.[116] The woman, as Monsieur Rondelet records in chapter LXV of his *Method of Curing All Diseases*,[117] had a rotting foetus in her womb, parts of which were expelled, but the large bones remained unexpelled, so that a long time later she died from it. The cause of such a death should have been beyond doubt because of the earlier clear expulsion of some parts of the foetus, and because the rest had been retained, not having followed but rather remaining there in a state of putrefaction. Nonetheless, her husband acted well in wanting to be sure of this by the autopsy which took place.[118] But, since the situation was known earlier, it would have been more useful to extract the bones from the mouth of the womb if that had been possible, or, if it were not, to do so by means of cesarean section, If necessary, this new treatment would thus have been applied, as it should in all such cases of necessity, all objections being laid aside when all other options have failed.

---

116. In the second half of the sixteenth century, the status of the Faculty of Medicine of Montpellier rivalled that of Paris, with Chancellors of the caliber of Guillaume Rondelet (1507–1566) and Laurent Joubert (1529–1582).

117. *The Method of Curing all Diseases of the Human Body* [*Methodus curandorum omnium morborum corporis humani*, Paris: apud Jacobum Maceum, 1570].

118. As in the previous case, the autopsy results from the family's wish to establish the cause of death.

Second Part

Lest anyone doubt that these uteruses, which had suffered such trauma, could have been incised with a safe outcome for the mother and the delivery of the dead child — which was the related cause of such ulcers — in this second section I shall recount several true stories of such dangers being successfully overcome by the incision of the abdomen. I have drawn these from two esteemed physicians, although the women in question were not pregnant but rather had suffered heavily ulcerated wombs, which was worse for them. The status of both of these men, who are still alive, provides testimony and authority.[119] The first is Monsieur Aliboux from Sens, whose good and widespread reputation means that I need say no more about him; the other is Monsieur de Villeneuve senior,[120] residing at Valreas in Provence, who first taught me the practice of medicine after I had completed my studies and degree.

The letters in which Monsieur Aliboux, of Sens, and Monsieur de Villeneuve senior, from Valreas in Provence, extracted these details from their registers of their most important cures — something all good physicians should keep — were sent to me by themselves, and I shall include them here, having abridged the fine, rich Latin in which they were written in my translation into French.

Aliboux to Rousset, greetings

Close to my very house there occurred a case as strange as your cesarean section. A pregnant woman, either because she was already advanced in years, or having been unable for some other reason to deliver her child except in parts, had a very swollen lower abdomen on both sides because of the violence with which the surgeon's instruments had been applied.[121] She had all the signs of an ulcer from which discharges ran out into the lower passages. From this part of the abdomen, which was wide open after being cauterized, there came a copious amount of discharge, and more of the same substance and

---

119. Cyr and Baskett (70) wrongly take this sentence to refer to the women still being alive.

120. Also cited by Duval, 279.

121. Cyr and Baskett mistranslate '*ferrements*' (the surgeon's irons) as the woman's 'contractions' (71).

colour from the lower passages. She did not want to let me use my speculum[122] to see for myself what was hidden away within, but even so it was quite clear — from the various signs reported over the period of time and from the nature of the discharges — that the ulcer itself, and the opening of it, went right into the womb. The healing of both happened in the same way and at the same time. Since — as I have seen — this is so, what you are able to treat by your gastrotomy[123] is not so surprising; for it is more difficult for such an ulcer to heal than for a simple wound in such a place to do so. Farewell.

Second history on a similar subject from the same Aliboux

A certain Collette Symon, a baker's wife in this town of Sens, having suffered the violent application of the surgeon's irons to extract a dead foetus — but without then experiencing the discharges which should follow,[124] or expelling the afterbirth — within five days developed a very large swelling on both sides of the lower abdomen, with clear signs of an abscess. A cautery was applied, making a deep opening on one of the sides. The surgeon used his hand to pull out a mass of congealed, rotting and stinking blood, but the other side did not subside, nor could the surgeon extract any of the afterbirth in question.[125] For this reason, he made a new incision on the other side, from which he extracted the afterbirth. All this was not done without the greatest pain, in danger and despair,[126] for she remained half-dead and spent three years in bed. For the following two years she could move only on crutches, then with a stick, after which she gradually regained her strength such that she went on to have several children, one of whom, named Sebastien, still lives in this town. Farewell.

---

122. Instrument inserted in the vagina to allow the physician to examine the womb. This case is typical of many women's reluctance, on the grounds of modesty, to submit to internal vaginal examination by a male practitioner.

123. Surgical incision of the abdominal wall.

124. The lochia.

125. The retained placenta and foetal tissues putrefied, causing infection and swelling in the uterus.

126. Cyr and Baskett (71, n. 120) surmise that the description indicates the uterus was probably perforated during the original delivery or removal of the placenta.

Two other histories on a similar subject from Nicolas de Villeneufve

Nicolas de Villeneufve to Rousset, greetings. I am infinitely, etc.[127] But to come to the point, I confess that during my long life I have never seen this procedure, which you describe to me, of a woman delivered from the side and who has survived. I do remember clearly that all the lower part of Madame de Piles's abdomen was most tumerous, and I had Maurace, the surgeon in this town of Valreas, open it using an actual cautery, penetrating right into the cavity of the womb. More than seven pounds of the same putrid discharge came out both from the opening and from below.[128] So that we could see the site more clearly for ourselves, we dilated the lower regions using a speculum, and saw the size of the uterine ulcer, which we cured after six months. Since this time, she has given birth to a daughter who is still alive. This was in the year 1532.

Another history from Aliboux

I can also confirm to you the truth of a similar illness and cure, in the case of the wife of Brisset, the apothecary from Montelimar. I undertook this, with the consent of her husband, using a similar cauterization of the hypogastrium, against the advice of two physicians who were treating her. We cut right through to the inside of the womb, and putrid discharge from it poured out, landing beyond the foot of the bed, and at the same time, a marvelous quantity of similar putrid waste came out from below. She recovered within three months, and shortly afterwards conceived. Since then, she has given birth to three sons and a daughter. This was in the year 1558. I give thanks to God that, being beyond the 85th year of my life, I am, through His grace, in such health that I continue the exercise you used to see me undertake here, so that I am daily either out on my horse or on foot in the town, in as good a physical condition as you have kindly wished me to be. And for my part, I likewise desire you to be granted by Him an equally good and even greater span of years. Godspeed.

---

127. Abbreviated standard formula of salutation.
128. From the wound and the vagina.

Third Part

None of the previous histories in fact mention a woman who suffered both conditions at the same time, that is to say pregnancy and a section. The pregnant women were not incised, their children — being quite dead — having found a way out other than through an incision of the abdomen. Those who were incised were not pregnant, although they were in a worse condition, namely having abscesses in their wombs. It will therefore be more helpful to cite other cases in which the women suffered both pregnancy and the incision of the abdomen at the same time, even if the operation was not, as we are advocating, a cesarean to extract the child, but rather carried out with the aim of draining the abscess. In these other cases, there was, however, something else alongside the abscess, that is to say a complete foetus, or the collection of bones from a foetus long since dead. Therefore, just as in the other cases, because of the ulcer on the womb and other reasons, there was more danger than in our cesareans. And yet none of these women died. Furthermore, the majority of them went on to conceive afterwards, and carried a child to term. Now because three of the various stories which follow have been printed in a work by Mathias Cornax,[129] physician to the Emperor in Vienna in Austria, and another in the second book of surgery by Albucasis,[130] for the sake of brevity I shall leave out many circumstances which they cite, such as the place, year, day, persons concerned and witnesses.

[I omit the next six case histories (all drawn from other sixteenth-century or earlier sources, rather than from Rousset's own experience or contacts) and the cases of surgical removal or treatment of uterine prolapses. My translation resumes with the Epilogue in conclusion to the fourth section.]

129. He oversaw a 'cesarean' operation in 1549 in Vienna to remove a dead foetus from the living mother, who survived. This is recorded in the first of his *Historiae duae memorabiles* [*Two Memorable Histories*, Augsburg: per Johannem Zimmerman, 1555].

130. c. 936–1013, personal physician to Calif of Cordoba. His work on surgery (*Al-Tasrif*) was highly respected in medieval surgery.

Epilogue to the Preceding Histories

In conclusion, then,[131] the womb can develop such a severe abscess in its cavity that sometimes it has to be opened through the lower abdomen, which is more dangerous than if the incision were made higher up, as we do in the case of a cesarean, even with a red-hot iron. There can be such an extensive ulcer that the whole body, or all that remains of a dead child, can pass through it and end up in the intestines, whence it may come out either as a result of putrefaction or through an incision made in the abdomen; and yet the woman can recover without losing the ability to conceive. The womb can be removed, either cut away, cauterized or ligatured, without the woman dying; and after a longstanding prolapse, decay or gangrene it may come away and be destroyed without the woman either dying or falling ill. Therefore why can she not, if we take similar and even greater care as we artificially incise the womb, recover with the help we can give, and thereafter even conceive and bear a child to full term and deliver it through natural childbirth? This is unless some obstruction resulting from one of the causes discussed above prevents it, and makes it necessary to reopen the womb by means of a cesarean, but the second operation will be easier than the first.[132]

It would indeed seem that Nature has much cause to reproach her servant Surgery and those great masters who are responsible for the administration of it, seeing that we have demonstrated before their eyes, and they have touched with their hands, so many examples of this procedure that has helped humankind — whose care is their profession. We have pushed them forcibly, as though propelling them by the shoulder, to carry this out confidently and successfully. Yet, they are still unwilling, or do not dare, to approach it; rather those to whom experience, the mother of arts, has given this resource by virtue of their witnessing its obvious results are prevented or forbidden (as far as others can) from carrying out such an operation.

---

131. In the French, Rousset constructs a single sentence at the start of the chapter, culminating in the question '… natural childbirth?' The first three sentences in my English version correspond to four subordinate clauses in French, each of which is introduced by 'since' ('*puisque*').

132. Rousset is thus defending the principle of repeated cesareans for women who need them. (Cf. the account of the woman who survived a first cesarean but died when refused one while giving birth to her next child, 37-38.)

SIXTH SECTION

[My translation resumes with the final part of this sixth section, following Rousset's discussion of women's fertility after cesareans. In this conclusion to his treatise, he treats women's use of uterine pessaries, demonstrating the breadth of his interest in gynecological conditions.]

Of the Invention of the Pessary, and of Its Various Forms

It is not surprising if the Ancients never wrote anything complete on this subject, for women have used a multitude of small, effective ways to help themselves, being eager to look after themselves on their own in such illnesses and needs, and naturally ashamed to expose themselves before men.[133] Thus, they keep these ways secret, so that the majority of physicians do not know about them. I believe the pessary has been such a thing for a long time; however, today some surgeons write and teach about it, in various forms.[134] As far as pessaries used in the womb are concerned, they discuss what they are made from, their shape and their use.

Some make them just from wax, others from bored and hollowed silver and gold, still others from light cork. Some make them round, others oval, others triangular or like an uneven quadrilateral with obtuse angles. Some are shaped like a flattened heart, some round, truncated and oblong, yet others round and flat, with or without a hole in the middle. In addition, some insert a small string hanging from it so that they can more easily extract it when they need; others do not do this, and it comes out almost as easily, when anyone wishes, as if it had the string attached. Others never take the pessary out, as in the case I am describing. Even if it is within the womb, the women are not prevented from having normal relations with their husbands, who know nothing of it if their wives do not wish to tell them. This is because of both the generous, spacious place in which it is positioned and also its smooth, polished surface and the way it is shaped. It does

133. For a discussion of this commonplace in later medieval and early modern medical writings, see M. Green, *Making Woman's Medicine Masculine*, 31–36, 111–117.

134. Compare Bourgeois's discussion of pessaries for uterine prolapases in her *Diverse Observations*, Klairmont Lingo and O'Hara, I. 34, 'Remedies for a Prolapsed Womb'. Bourgeois, writing over a quarter of a century after Rousset, speaks as though the midwife would fashion and insert the pessary.

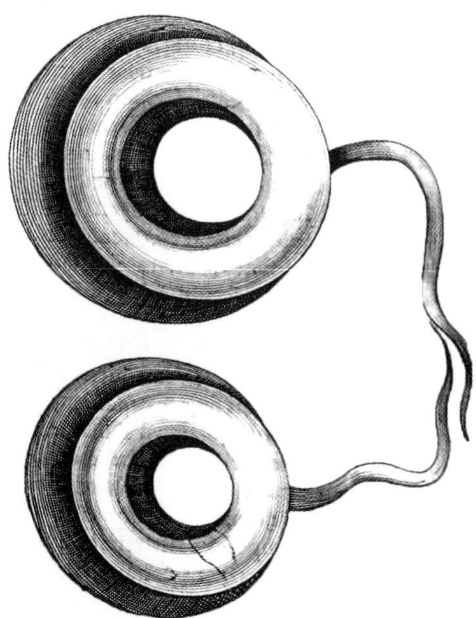

9) Uterine pessaries

Jacques Guillemeau, *De la grossesse et accouchement des femmes*, Paris, 1620
(Library of Royal College of Obstetricians and Gynaecologists, London)

not prevent them from conceiving and safely bearing a child, and giving birth; and is a marvelous and safe invention to help women deal with the troublesome condition of a fallen womb. Often, they are completely cured after having worn it for some time, without needing to continue using it.

It is also most useful in favoring conception if the women were previously subject to such prolapses. For if the epiploon[135] falls on the womb, as Hippocrates says in aphorism 46 of Book V,[136] and thereby prevents conception, what must be the effect of the womb falling and totally collapsing as though it intended to flatten itself under its own burden unless relief were provided? This is cured in other women by

135. Also known as the greater omentum: a fold of the peritoneum, from the stomach to the abdominal organs.

136. 'When unnaturally fat women cannot conceive, it is because the fat presses the mouth of the womb, and conception is impossible until they grow thinner.' (*Hippocrates*, trans. W. H. S. Jones, vol. IV (Loeb Classical Library, 1931). Rousset gives the locus as V. 56; I have amended this to reflect the numbering used in the Loeb and other modern editions. The same aphorism is also cited by de Serres, 338, n. 150.

making them lose weight, something we often achieve through an appropriate diet.

Histories about This Subject

Paradox concerning conception, and full-term pregnancy while wearing the pessary in the womb

I once heard the history of a woman from Puisaye[137] who had borne several children while wearing a pessary, and then I was again assailed with such histories by a midwife called Preignon, from Picardy, who is much sought after by the great households because of her long experience and her skill at her craft. Yet, I was unwilling to believe them, any more than others. However, I took pains to conduct such careful research in a number of places that I had occasion to be satisfied. Experience has once again shown the effects of this aid, which previously I myself found as incredible as once all the most learned men found the idea of the land below the torrid zone,[138] which however has been discovered and proved recently by the experience of simple sailors, disproving the writings of the most famous mathematicians and most outstanding cosmographers ever, which were generally held to be irrefutable.

In order to do this, in 1579, at Verneuil near Senlis[139] and the surrounding area, I ensured that I could meet, speak and talk privately with some women who have used it and still do so. The majority do not wish me to cite their names; those whose names follow do not hide the fact, since all their neighbors[140] already know it. In some other cases, even the husbands know nothing of it, and for this reason the names of the women must be concealed. There is Clemence Heraudié, the wife of the laborer Gervais Du Mont, who came to Verneuil from

137. Village in Normandy, in the Orne department.

138. Below the Tropic of Capricorn. A reference to the discovery of the spice route, from Europe to the Indian Ocean, in the earlier-sixteenth century.

139. Now Verneuil-en-Halatte, a village in Picardy, close to Senlis, some 50 km north-east of Paris.

140. In French the word is feminine, suggesting an informal social community between the women.

Gisors[141] a long time ago, daughter of Joannet Herauldié,[142] called Finet, previously a barber in Gisors. She had married very young and had a child before she was thirteen.[143] This may be the reason why her womb fell, given that, according to Galen in his *Book on the Natural Faculties*, it often falls during the strong pushing of childbirth.[144] Since it would not stay in place when it was put back, her father, being a surgeon, made her a pessary of the same kind as she now makes and furnishes for those who need one. She is often sought after to do this from near and far. She conceived, carried the child and gave birth three times while still wearing it. She used to put it back as soon as she had delivered, just wiping it, and recoating it with butter, without changing anything else. She has worn this same pessary in this way for more than 40 years, without any damage to herself, or any rotting of the cork, which has been recoated and refitted.

And the midwives in Verneuil, near Senlis, and the surrounding area — notably one known as 'la Mineuse'[145] — have repeatedly assured me they have in the past delivered several other women to whom she had given one of these pessaries, and especially one called 'la Nurette' who gave birth to a son, who was shown to me and is aged about nine at present. This pessary came out before the child and was put back on the fourth day after the birth since the womb had dropped again, and she wore it ever since, without any problem, until she died.

She also provided a pessary for another woman from Verneuil, called Geneviefve Salantin, who had suffered a fallen womb in her first marriage on account of a difficult delivery. She wore it for four years, and became pregnant while so doing, and kept wearing it

141. A village some 60 km west of Senlis.

142. I reproduce the two variant spellings (Heraudié/Herauldié) used in this paragraph in the original French.

143. Cf. De Serres' comments on the inadvisability of very early marriages, 338. The subject is also treated by Liebault in *Three Books dealing with the Infirmities and Illnesses of Women* [*Trois livres appartenant aux infirmitez et maladies des femmes*], I. 23.

144. 'In the case of the opposite (the eliminative) faculty, the os [bone] opens, whilst the whole fundus approaches as near as possible to the os, expelling the embryo as it does so; and along with the fundus the contiguous parts — which form, as it were, a girdle round the whole organ — cooperate in the work; they squeeze the embryo and propel it out forcibly. And, in many women who exercise such a faculty immoderately, violent pains cause forcible prolapse of the whole womb.' (Galen, *On the Natural Faculties*, section 3; cited from the Directory of Classic Literature, www.greektexts.com).

145. Literally 'the lesser'.

throughout the pregnancy. It came out on its own three weeks before her delivery — this is another remarkable thing for the discussion which follows, concerning the issue of the opening of the mouth of the womb in pregnancy[146] — and it did not cause her to give birth before her time. The child is presently three years old, and since then the mother has not had cause to have the pessary put back since the prolapse is cured, even though she has subsequently given birth to two large male twins, both living. This is a most remarkable thing for several reasons, which I shall leave the reader to deduce so that I remain brief.

[I omit the next 20 pages, in which Rousset produces further theoretical arguments in favor of pessaries, and then pursues the debate over whether the cervix can open during pregnancy. The translation resumes with the concluding pages of the sixth section.]

Answer to Several Other Objections, and That the Use of the Pessary is Not New, Although the Assertion of Conceiving while Wearing It is a New Practice[147]

This, dear Reader, is what I in truth discovered and wished to include in this treatise, as fitting the nature of my subject and the strange, paradoxical claims about it. And yet, this is the most essential truth, where the sentiments not of a single person but of all are erroneous, which nonetheless form the basis for the starting-point of an examination of what is true and what is false.[148] In addition, there is the benefit, even the necessity of using it appropriately, both for the comfort and support of the mother, and so that hope should not be lost of her still bearing a child while wearing it, which would not otherwise happen.[149]

146. Rousset devotes a section of his treatise to the question of whether the cervix could open during pregnancy.

147. I am grateful to Gianna Pomata for the suggestion that '*observation*' in French here corresponds to 'practice', one of the conventional medieval and early modern uses of the Latin term '*observatio*'. See Pomata's chapter, 'Observation rising: birth of an epistemic genre, 1500–1850', 47–48.

148. The French here is elliptical. Rousset appears to be defending uterine pessaries, even though their use or existence is not commonly acknowledged.

149. If she did not wear the pessary to correct the uterine prolapse, she would be unable to bear another child.

I have told you the truth, without prejudice, giving details of the places and people so that here and there you may make discrete enquiries, as I did, and satisfy yourself, while awaiting fuller proof in the future. I know that you will tell me that the Ancients or Moderns, who on all other subjects are most scrupulous, have never written it down as a precept. Nor has it been adopted or observed by a great number of very far-sighted surgeons. I freely admit this, in order to avoid a quarrel with those who would seek one, just as I do over our cesarean section, but you nonetheless see its importance.

Everything that was done in the past has not been written down; and everything that was written about unusual or secret things has not come down to us. There have always been some practices, especially as far as women's secrets are concerned, that served their private use and were handed down, as it were. The same was formerly true for the secrets of physicians themselves, even Asclepiades.[150] They would reveal some of their secrets only to their followers, as though bestowing an inheritance, and with a solemn injunction not to reveal them, as we can conjecture from the Hippocratic oath.[151] This is the more likely in the case of women, especially as regards those organs Nature gave them in order to bear us, given that even men, who feel less shame and modesty, are ashamed of these organs, only uncovering themselves at the last possible moment before their closest acquaintances.

Plutarch wrote about this in his book *On Curiosity*[152] saying that if Herophilus or Erasistratus or even Aesculapus, men who lived in a former age, holding the cures for illnesses and the instruments of health in their hands, came to a house and asked if they were needed by some man who was suffering in his rear parts, or some woman who had cancer in her lower regions, they would be sent away, like people enquiring into someone else's secret.

Now, these small yet important remedies, which are the only ones and are safe, are preserved and remembered by the common people.

150. Probably Asclepiades of Bithynia (c. 124–40 BC), who settled in Rome and established a new theory of atomic or corpuscular medicine — opposing Hippocratic humoral theory.

151. The oath contains the clause: 'All that may come to my knowledge in the exercise of my profession or in daily commerce with men, which ought not to be spread abroad, I will keep secret and will never reveal.'

152. Plutarch, *On Curiosity*, 7.

They are better content with such experience as they have than are those in famous places. Often we see the proud disdain of some learned but relatively inexperienced physician — who thinks that, like a lawgiver, he should give orders to Nature rather than serving her, as he should, with his dexterity and eyesight. Such a physician often manages only, because of his jealousy or contempt, to prevent one of a lesser standing from doing better than himself. This is the error which blinds us and often, to the cost of the greatest, removes the chance of our receiving good, effective help. Some people hope this help will be achieved from our treatments and bleedings — the latter often as barbarous as they are bloody if they are not overseen with careful deliberation rather than arrogant tyranny, as those who are learned, good, modest and experienced in the way they dispense health know how to do.

If we were to assume that up until now nothing of this has occurred, that no clever mind has invented what is required for the ordinary or extraordinary needs of women, as also happened with this cesarean section, even though people tell me that it may be possible by some chance,[153] nonetheless it would be a dereliction of our duty to allow any good thing to be wasted when God reveals it by such means and ministers as please Him, whenever this may chance to occur.

I would be willing to believe — as far as the support of the womb is concerned, but not in respect of the possibility of conception — that this is what Hippocrates referred to in Aphorism 47 of Book V, starting, 'If the womb ('*Si uterus*'), etc.',[154] if he had only mentioned it in some other place when treating particularly the cure of this prolapse of the womb, or if some other of the Ancients had ever written anything about it. Or if Galen's interpretation of this passage had not tended in another direction, pausing over the word 'suppurates'[155] which might

---

153. The construction of this sentence is obscure in the French. Essentially Rousset is advancing the argument that even if pessaries did not happen to have been invented by earlier physicians, he now has a duty to speak of them because of their usefulness.

154. 'If the part of the womb near the hip-joint suppurates, tents must be employed', *Hippocrates*, trans. W. H. S. Jones, vol. IV (Loeb), 1931; Rousset gives the reference as V. 48. Rousset's detailed argument here is based on a close reading of the Greek and Latin texts of Hippocrates and Galen, in order to postulate that it is just possible that Hippocrates was alluding to uterine pessaries in the aphorism cited.

155. Rousset gives the terms 'suppurates', 'jumps' and 'falls' in Greek, indicating to the reader his familiarity with the original commentary of Galen. We should note that he had

possibly have been replaced by 'jumps' or 'falls' so that the sense would be this: If the womb, which is situated between the hips, falls or jumps, a compress or stop must be placed in it. ('*Si uterus intra loxas situs deciderit*' or '*desilierit, necessarium est emmotum fieri*'.) The debate over the Latin words 'compress' or 'stop' ('*emmotum*' or '*linamentum*') would not invalidate this, since the same aid may be made from different materials.

But whether this is true or not, I refrain from contesting the authority of such excellent commentators as Hippocrates had, for I revere and wish to imitate them. Often, indeed, they did not fear to add their inventions, with modesty, to those of their forebears, for the service of those who would follow after them. Silently they taught us, as I here wish to do, to do the same for those who will come after us, especially when the truth is at stake. Being the daughter of time, truth has learned from her father not to produce everything at once, but whenever it may come, we must accept it like every other good thing, receiving it with a grateful hand when it offers itself to us in the fullness of time, in such ways, and by such means, as it pleases God, the ancient of days and Father of ages, to send it to us. To Whom be glory, honor and thanksgiving for ever. Amen.

---

used several Greek terms (printed in Greek characters) at earlier points in the text. Together with this detailed discussion of the Greek of Galen, the evidence suggests that he was one of the fairly limited number of early modern physicians with at least a working knowledge of Greek, as well as excellent Latin (the latter demonstrated by his works composed in Latin — see 6-7).

JEAN LIEBAULT

*Three Books Dealing with the
Infirmities and Illnesses of Women
(1582)*

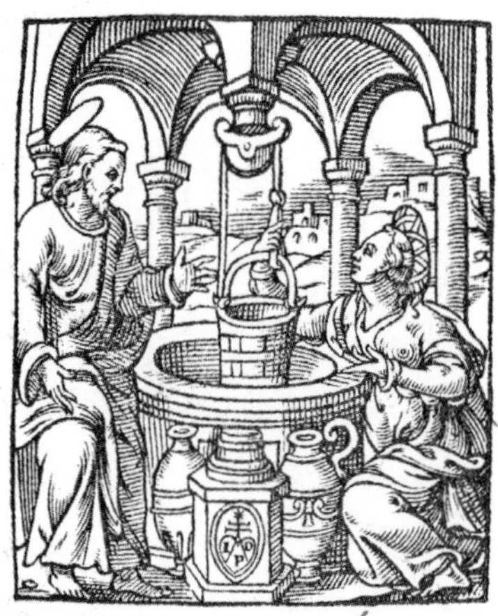

10) Title page: Jean Liebault, *Trois Livres*, Paris, 1582

(Library of Royal College of Obstetricians and Gynaecologists, London)

INTRODUCTION

TRANSLATION OF EXCERPTS FROM
THREE BOOKS DEALING WITH THE INFIRMITIES AND ILLNESSES OF WOMEN (1582)

INTRODUCTION

The compendium on women's health by Jean Liebault (or Liebaut, or Liebaud) — which would fall under the modern classification of gynecology and obstetrics — was one of the most enduringly popular works on this subject in the French language. To date, I have traced ten separate French editions, appearing at regular intervals between 1582 and 1674.[1] Its success was due in no small measure to Liebault's astute understanding of the evolving tastes of readers of vernacular medical treatises.

Life and Works of Jean Liebault

Born in 1535 in Dijon, Jean Liebault went to Paris to study medicine, and remained in the capital for the rest of his professional life. He married Nicole Estienne,[2] daughter of Charles Estienne, a physician, anatomist and member of the Estienne printing dynasty. Through the association with his father-in-law, Liebault's first publication was a French translation and continuation, in 1564, of Charles's Latin treatise on agriculture and domestic economy, *The Country Estate* [*Praedium rusticum*], which had appeared in 1554.[3] This French work achieved a very wide circulation, continuing to be published into the eighteenth century. It also set the style for Liebault's contributions to printed medical works in the vernacular: his method was to take an existing text which had already achieved popularity, and then translate, revise and extend it. In so doing, as his career progressed,

---

1. See *Les Traités d'obstétrique au seuil de la modernité*, 264–289.

2. A woman of letters, author of the poem 'The Sufferings of the Married Woman' ['Les *Misères de la femme mariée*', c. 1587], in which the poetess complains, among many other tribulations, of those of pregnancy and childbirth: 'I now leave aside the unbelievable sadness / Which this poor woman suffers in pregnancy; / The danger she faces in childbirth, / The burden of children, so heavy and wearying.' ['Je laisse maintenant l'incroyable tristesse / Que ceste pauvre femme endure en sa grossesse; / Le danger où elle est durant l'enfantement, / La charge des enfans, si penible et fascheuse.'] Whether Nicole's complaints were intended seriously or tongue-in-cheek is a matter of unresolved debate. For an analysis of her writing and of her marriage with Jean Liebault, see R. Reynolds-Cornell, '*Les Misères de la femme mariée*: another look at Nicole Liebault and a few questions about the woes of the married woman', *Bibliothèque d'Humanisme et Renaissance*, LXIV–1 (2002), 37–54.

3. The French version appeared under the title *Agriculture et maison rustique de M. Charles Estienne*.

he would increasingly obscure his debt to the original authors and promote the perception of himself as the works' creator.

This is already evident in 1573, when he produced a successful French version of another work originally published in Latin. The *Four Books on the Secrets of Medicine and on the Philosophy of Chemistry* [*Quatre livres des secrets de medecine et de la philosophie chimique*][4] were a reworking and elaboration of the second part of Conrad Gesner's *On Secret Remedies* [*De remediis secretis*], published posthumously in 1569. In choosing to concentrate almost entirely on the sections dealing with distillation, Liebault provided both physicians and apothecaries with a valuable resource, but Gesner's authorship is concealed in the work's French title, and the prefatory letter emphasizes Liebault's role in correcting and expanding on the original text. After editing a compendium of Latin medical writings,[5] and a Latin edition of recent commentaries on Hippocrates's *Aphorisms*,[6] Liebault next, in 1582, produced two French compilations: the *Three Books Dealing with the Infirmities and Illnesses of Women* [*Trois Livres appartenant aux infirmitez et maladies des femmes*] and *Three Books on the Embellishment and Adornment of the Human Body* [*Trois Livres de l'embellissement et ornement du corps humain*]. It was at this point that he took a final step towards claiming the credit for authorship, making it appear that the works had been translated by an unnamed person from his own Latin.[7] However, when in 1609 one of Liebault's successors, Lazare Pena, produced a revised and enlarged edition of the *Three Books Dealing with the Infirmities and Illnesses of Women*, he revealed that Liebault had drawn large sections of both his 1582 volumes from the writings of the Italian humanist and physician Giovanni Marinelli.[8] The exact relationship between Marinelli's text

---

4. Paris: Jean Sevestre for Jacques du Puys [Dupuis], 1573.

5. *Thesaurus of Health. Compiled from various authors.* [*Thesaurus sanitatis. Selectus ex variis authoribus*, Paris: Jean Dupuis, 1577]. The volume included works by Hippocrates, Jacques Dubois and Eucharius Rösslin.

6. *Jacob Houllier's Seven Books of Commentaries on Hippocrates's Aphorisms, edited by Jean Liebault* [*Jacobi Hollerii in Aphorismos Hippocratis commentarii septem par J. Liebantium in lucem editi*, Paris: Jacques Dupuis, 1582]. Houllier had been Regent of the Faculty of Medicine in Paris, 1546–1548.

7. See 79.

8. Father of the poetess and writer Lucrezia Marinella, and author of two books in Italian on women's health and beauty: *The Ornaments of Women* [*Gli ornamenti delle donne,*

and Liebault's reworking of it is discussed below, but what is most significant, in terms both of book history and of the circulation of knowledge, is Liebault's development over some 20 years of the technique of taking a medical or scientific text composed in another language and recasting it in French for a wider readership.

We have no details of the last decade of Liebault's career beyond the evidence of the continued success of his publications and his appointment as physician to Catherine de Bourbon, the sister of Henry of Navarre. The report by the historian Pierre de L'Estoile of Liebault's death in 1596, having collapsed on a stone in a road in Paris,[9] led to an assumption that he died impoverished. However, Reynolds-Cornell has challenged this with the plausible argument that the reference may simply indicate that Liebault was one of many victims of a virulent outbreak of the plague in this season.[10]

Circulation and Afterlife of the 'Three Books Dealing with the Infirmities and Illnesses of Women'

The French version of the *Three Books Dealing with the Infirmities and Illnesses of Women* remained in print in France for nearly a century after it first appeared, conferring on it a remarkable longevity in comparison with other vernacular treatises on women's health. The fact that it was sometimes republished under an alternative title is possibly a further indication of its commercial success. In 1585, it reappeared from the press of the original printer, Jacques Dupuis, with the new title *Treasure of Secret Cures for the Illnesses of Women* (*Thresor des remedes secrets pour les maladies des femmes*), inviting the reader to assume an association with the ever-popular medieval health book, the *Treasure of the Poor* (*Tresor des pauvres*).

In the early seventeenth century, we have seen that the work was given a second lease of life after the physician, Lazare Pena, edited

---

Venice: Francesco de Franceschi, 1562; 2nd extended edition Venice: Giovanni Valgrisio, 1574]; *Medicine pertaining to Women's Diseases* [*Le Medicine partenenti alle infermità delle donne*, Venice: G. Bonadio for Francesco de Franceschi, 1563; 2nd extended edition Venice: Giovanni Valgrisio, 1574].

9. See Pierre de l'Estoile, *Memoirs-Papers* [*Mémoires-Journaux*, ed. P. Bonnefon, Paris: A. Lemerre, 1888–96, vol. VII, 63–65].

10. R. Reynolds-Cottrell, '*Les Misères de la femme mariée*', 39–40.

and expanded it. He provided a new, explicitly neoplatonic preface[11] addressed 'to chaste young women', underlining the work's interest for a predominantly female, elite readership. Within the main text, his interpolations are clearly distinguished by the use of italic characters. They vary in length from short phrases to complete paragraphs. For the most part, they discuss further causes or signs of the illnesses Liebault had listed, while in places Pena also appends some of his own cures, making the work a fuller compendium of information. On several occasions, Pena introduces much longer additions, such as those in Book III chapters 45 and 46,[12] which allow him to develop his personal, neoplatonic understanding of the human condition in general and of the female body in particular.

Although there is no trace of any published English translation of Liebault, a manuscript version of a translation by W. H. Gent survives in Glasgow in the library of the eighteenth-century physician and bibliophile, William Hunter,[13] indicating that the work continued to attract some readers outside France nearly two centuries after it first appeared.

Structure of the 'Three Books Dealing with the Infirmities and Illnesses of Women' and Selection of Chapters for Translation

Liebault's *Three Books dealing with the Infirmities and Illnesses of Women* follow the essential divisions of Marinelli's work in that Book I deals with unmarried girls, or what would now be termed the pubescent female body; Book II with sterility and the female reproductive organs (notably the womb); and Book III with pregnancy and childbirth. In other words, the first two books survey the field of gynecology and the third provides an overview of obstetrics. However, whereas Marinelli's three books had 13, 32 and 16 chapters, Liebault's have 37, 66 and 51, and the additions reflect the areas that most interest the French

---

11. See 81-88.
12. See 122-6, 131-4.
13. Hunter was Physician Extraordinary to Queen Charlotte (1764–1783). The manuscript is held in the Special Collection of the University of Glasgow (GB 0247 MS Hunter 1–658).

physician.[14] Thus, the first 22 chapters of Book I are all Liebault's own composition, allowing him to develop his theories on the nature and illnesses of women in general and of pubescent girls in particular. Throughout Book II, he adds chapters on topical controversies, such as the nature of the cervix (II. 47–51 and II. 52–55), and shifts the emphasis from Marinelli's focus on sterility to his own interest in the anatomy of the reproductive parts.[15] At the start of Book III, he adds four new chapters on the nature of procreation, and a number of later chapters on irregularities of conception,[16] and on common ailments of pregnancy,[17] as well as expanding Marinelli's single chapter on the development of the foetus into six chapters.

In short, Liebault's compendium is a substantially larger and different work from the Italian volume that provided his starting-point. Whereas Marinelli addressed his volumes initially in 1563 to well-born women, and then in 1574 also to 'physicians, midwives and well-born ladies', Liebault is writing with a wider audience in mind, not least a male, lay audience, interested in questions of generation and sexuality, and likely to appreciate his regular addition of references to classical and contemporary humanist sources. As a result, Liebault's defence of, and sympathy towards, women may have been important in shaping the knowledge and attitudes of both sexes.

It is important to note that Marinelli is only one of Liebault's sources, and that as a humanist Marinelli had already summarized and drawn upon many of the classical sources to which Liebault also refers. The French writer readily cites additional classical, Arabic and recent European medical authorities, and in Book III he silently incorporates some sections from the popular birthing handbook by Rösslin, the *Rosegarden for Pregnant Women,* which was first published in Strasbourg and Hagenau in 1513, and then translated into Latin in 1532 and various vernaculars, including two translations into French

---

14. I indicate the additions of new chapters and major expansions in the notes accompanying the table of contents (90-97).

15. For example, the addition of chs. 36–40 on gonorrhea and on the cervix and womb, and of chs. 62–64 on the hymen, nymphae and clitoris, and the expansion of chs. 43–47 on diseases of the womb.

16. Superfetation and inherited defects, chs. 9 and 10; Monsters and hermaphrodites, chs. 12 and 13.

17. Ibid, chs. 24–39.

in 1536 and 1563.[18] The French translation, which continued to be published regularly throughout the sixteenth century,[19] was probably one of Marinelli's sources, and would have been familiar to many of Liebault's readers. In the translation of Liebault's chapters on preparing for birth (III. 45) and on difficult deliveries (III. 46), I indicate the obvious borrowings, which again confirm his facility as a compilator.

Liebault's and Pena's Arguments and Style

When examining how the *Three Books dealing with the Infirmities and Illnesses of Women* afford a place to the 'other voice', it is important to draw a distinction between Liebault's original work and Pena's later additions to it, for while Pena rarely abridges Liebault's text, he extends it in ways Liebault could not have anticipated.

Liebault's defence of women is rooted in his selective reading of classical medical authorities, with a predominant reliance on Hippocrates, accompanied by an equally discerning selection of Christian teachings favorable to women. Hence, while his prefatory 'Letter to the reader' shows all humanity to be wretched because of physical illnesses, and women to be more afflicted than men, this negative position is then cleverly reversed by the claim that women are superior by virtue of their ability to bear children (with the aid of physicians).[20] Liebault thus articulates the position that women's sexual distinctiveness confers on them potential greatness; refuting the Galenist and Aristotelian theories of women's innate inferiority, he argues that Nature purposely chose to make women different,[21] and praises the design of the female reproductive anatomy, notably the womb. Although, as a practicing physician, he is all too aware of the ills that may befall women, and devotes much of Book II to diseases of the womb, his ideological position consists of an uncompromising defence of the female body for the purposes of childbearing. Pena

18. For a recent account of the significance of Rösslin's work and a reassessment of his sources, see M. Green, 'The Sources of Eucharius Rösslin's *Rosegarden for Pregnant Women and Midwives*' (1513)', *Medical History*, 53–2 (April 2009), 167–192.

19. V. Worth-Stylianou, *Les Traités d'obstétrique*, 89–117.

20. See 78.

21. In this, Liebault implicitly dissociates himself from the view that the conception of a female is a mistake of nature.

grafts onto this a strongly neoplatonic strand, according to which Nature, which he loosely conflates with God, has designed the female body as an object of supreme beauty. Using language marked by many of the conceits and commonplaces of Renaissance love poetry, Pena eulogizes women's physical attractions and sexual powers. He is unusual among medical writers in placing the breasts alongside the womb as one of the key attributes of the female body, celebrating their eroticism in the context of a discussion of childbearing.[22] Yet, after praising the procreative forces Nature deploys in the female body (III. 45), in the following chapter Pena reverts to a less optimistic Christian perspective by reminding his readers that the pains of childbirth are a divine punishment for original sin.[23] The two arguments sit awkwardly together, but reveal a genuine tension in contemporary perceptions of women, who could be perceived at once as the finest objects in creation and the bearers of divine malediction.

Throughout the treatise, both Liebault and Pena move between abstract theoretical discussions and very practical advice on medical care. In this second sphere, the positions of the two physicians are close, and very similar to that of Marinelli — the ultimate goal is to relieve women's suffering as far as possible and to promote good health for the purposes of childbearing. All three writers imply that women must take a fair degree of responsibility for their own health. Following classical and medieval writers, they accord great importance to diet and regimen during pregnancy, each writer contributing to debates with his own favored recipes.[24] Yet Liebault, like many earlier writers and contemporaries, is particularly aware of the risk that pregnancy may unsettle a woman's tastes and produce strange cravings, beyond her control. Because he values the pregnant woman's mental serenity, which he believes to be essential to a successful pregnancy, he sanctions some dietary eccentricities, treating pregnant woman as potentially irrational but deserving of indulgence. While Liebault only cautions women against actions which may harm their pregnancy, such as

---

22. See 84-85.

23. See 132.

24. See, for example, Liebault's stipulation that quinces should be avoided and damask grapes consumed in their place, 109.

wearing over-tight clothing,[25] Pena, on the other hand, reserves some harsh satire for courtly ladies whose slavery to fashionable behavior risks unsettling the course of nature. His neoplatonic ideology in III. 46 rebounds unexpectedly to women's disadvantage, for while he claims that nature has endowed woman with ideal qualities, individual ladies ignore nature's ways at their peril. His sudden attack on women's gluttony, indolence and self-indulgence takes the reader by surprise. The arguments may be familiar from many contemporary moralists, and the physiological basis underpinning his observations is convincing, but the excursus provides a digression worthy of Montaigne. Like the latter, Pena reveals his nostalgia for the myth of the primitive races of women untainted by 'civilized' society, who apparently give birth without pain or difficulty.

However, such passages are not characteristic of Pena's contributions as a whole, and both he and Liebault are united in their wish to save French women from suffering in childbirth. If Liebault makes a standard reference to the insufficiencies of some midwives,[26] in general he anticipates that they will play a key role in deliveries.[27] He is notably flexible in his recommendations about positions for the birth: although advocating the use of the birthing chair, he acknowledges that other positions — lying, sitting and standing — may be adopted.[28] He and Pena also concur in their wish to see the midwife and physician try all other remedies before having recourse to the 'cruel instruments' of the surgeon.[29] What is Liebault's position in the crucial debate about saving the life of the mother versus that of the child, *in extremis*? In an earlier chapter on whether it is advisable to bleed women during pregnancy, he balances the physician's duty to both mother and child, advising that the physician must not think he can barter with God to save the mother at the expense of the child; instead he should have regard for both lives. Similarly, in chapter 49

25. See 105.

26. See 126.

27. There is some evidence of the developing role of male birthing attendants in deliveries by 1609: where Liebault instructed the midwife to ask a female attendant to press down on the mother's abdomen to hasten the delivery, Pena insists this should be done by a man (125).

28. See 119.

29. The phrase is used by Pena, 132.

of Book III,[30] on extracting a foetus by surgical means when normal labor has failed, he cites François Rousset as his authority, accepting that cesarean section on a living woman may be necessary:

> What I am here calling cesarean section or delivery by cesarean is a skillful extraction of the child through the mother's side when she cannot give birth other than through an adequate incision of both the outer abdomen and the body of the womb. This is done without harm to the life of one or other (unless they chance to receive any injury), and even without the mother being prevented from bearing a child thereafter. This is what is done when the child is still alive in the mother's womb.

Liebault has carefully chosen a procedure that, although controversial, allows the physician to avoid choosing between mother and child — the outcome of the operation he entrusts to God. The physician's role here, as throughout the treatise, is to assist the workings of nature for the benefit of women in childbearing. Pena chooses to develop this chapter on the extraction of the obstructed foetus substantially, making two separate, lengthy new chapters, which introduce much new material. He is even more emphatic than Liebault that, despite the risks, cesarean section should be attempted as a last resort on a living woman, to save mother and child, or at least one of the two — which one he does not specify. By the turn of the seventeenth century, the medicalization of difficult childbirth, in Paris at least, appears to be gathering pace, with an increasing confidence that surgery can, and should, offer some hope of escape.[31]

---

30. This chapter is not included in the translation for reasons of length.

31. See also the discussion in my introduction to Jacques Guillemeau (143), for evidence of increased surgical interventions in childbirth, at least among the elite, in early-seventeenth-century Paris.

TITLE PAGE [1582]

THREE BOOKS
DEALING WITH
THE INFIRMITIES AND
ILLNESSES OF WOMEN.[32]

Taken from the Latin[33] of Monsieur Jean Liebault,
physician in Paris, and translated into French.

IN PARIS,

From the press of Jacques Du Puys,[34]
at the sign of the Samaritan woman.[35]

M.D.LXXXII.

With the King's Privilege.

32. On the alternative titles used for some later editions of this work, see 68.

33. I have been unable to trace any original Latin version, and suspect this statement to be a cover for Liebault's unacknowledged reworking of Marinelli's Italian treatise: see 67.

34. The printer's device depicts Christ talking to the Samaritan woman by a well.

35. Jacques Dupuis worked as a printer in Paris from 1540 to 1589.

TITLE PAGE [1609]

THE ILLNESSES OF WOMEN
and remedies of these,
in three books,

By Jean Marinelli from Formia,
a learned Italian physician.

*Translated into French and extended by
Monsieur Jean Liebaud, physician in Paris.*

And in this latest Edition,
revised, corrected, and extended by one third.

By LAZARE PE.[36]
Dedicated to the ladies.

In Paris,
from the press of J. Berjon,[37]
at the Law Courts, by the prisoners' gallery.[38]

---

36. See 67.

37. Bookseller and printer in Paris from 1608 to 1621, son-in-law of the printer Denis Duval.

38. Although there is no date on the title page, the Privilege accorded to the printer, Jean Berjon, bears the date 23 March 1609.

[1582]

LETTER TO THE READER[39]

Although the human body is created with admirable art, and has all sorts of remarkable beauties and greatness, modeled on the most perfect divine pattern, and is endowed with a living heat stronger and fuller than any other, and is ruled and governed by a vigorous soul which surpasses all other, yet it is weaker, more delicate and fragile, less healthy and more subject to illness than any other animal's body. This is why Pliny berates Nature, calling it a wicked stepmother to men, but a mother to other animals.[40] For scarcely has man left his mother's womb than a host of illnesses start to surround him, seize him and threaten his health, and thereafter they follow him through life, until he draws his very last breath. Pliny counted up these illnesses and reckoned the total to be three hundred. However, if anyone wishes to examine all the particular forms of each kind of illness; all the calamities and damage to health which come from outside ourselves; all the symptoms which increase and come about daily without ever being seen, heard or noticed, and which cost us our lives; they will know that the number of illnesses that afflict the human body is far beyond not only three hundred, but several times ten thousand. The human body is so wretched that it is as though some predatory beast or bad spirit swore from the moment of its birth to undermine totally its health and life.[41]

Now this wretched state, which involves being subject to so many illnesses, is to be lamented more in the case of women's bodies than in that of men's. For, beyond the tens of thousands of illnesses which, in number and kind, torment women's bodies just like men's, but even more grievously, there are also an endless number of others, which

---

39. While the preface of the original 1582 edition appears to be written by the printer, it is not improbable that Liebault had a hand in its composition, given some of the detailed medical remarks. It is certainly quite distinct from Marinelli's preface of 1574, which was concerned mainly with defending the use of the vernacular for the circulation of medical knowledge.

40. See Pliny, *Natural History*, VII. 1. He remarks that to man alone Nature is at once a kind parent and merciless stepmother.

41. The French preface has no paragraph divisions. I have introduced some in the English translation to make the text more readable.

in addition cause women such fatigue that they might believe they would have been happier had they not been born or had they died immediately after birth.[42] Thus, it is certain that a woman's life would not really be a life, but rather a miserable existence, were it not for her fertility that makes her live on in the many bodies and minds of her descendants. This is why the Hebrews interpreted the name of the first woman, Eve, to mean life.[43] Not, I think, that she was destined to live, or indeed did live, more happily than those who followed her, but because her fertility made her live on, and made her name and that of her husband, Adam, immortal for posterity.

It is true that this happy fertility that makes a woman live on through her descendants would not be guaranteed unless she were defended against the attacks of so many tens of thousands of illnesses, which at all times wage mortal war against her. She is safeguarded and looked after in her sufferings by the art of medicine that was invented by God for this end, and by the particular remedies of learned and wise physicians. The divine Hippocrates, caring for the health and fertility of women and being charitably disposed to help them, wrote four books for their sake.[44] In one of these, he speaks of women's nature; in another of the diseases of virgins; in the third of the diseases affecting women who are of marriageable age or married; and in the fourth of the causes of sterility, the manner of ridding a woman of it and of restoring her fertility. Apart from these four books, in various sections of his *Aphorisms*, *Animadversions*, *Epidemics*, and almost endless other places he set down axioms, theories, experiences and histories of the nature, health, fertility, sterility, diseases, treatment and cure of ill women. Few later physicians, either classical or modern, have followed his example in this charitable endeavor, perhaps because the topic is so difficult and obscure, the subject as changing and unfixed as the object of it, so that it is very difficult to define a fixed, stable art, subject to firm precepts and laws. Rather, they have confined

---

42. Liebault is repeating the litany of complaints in the poem by his wife, Nicole Estienne, 'The Sufferings of the Married Woman' ['*Les Misères de la femme mariée*']. Given the uncertainty as to whether her original poem was serious or ironic, it is not clear whether his comments here are sympathetic or tongue-in-cheek.

43. Genesis 2:21–23.

44. In the Renaissance, Hippocrates was considered to be the author of *On the Nature of Woman*, *On the Diseases of Virgins*, *On the Diseases of Women* and *On Sterile Women*.

themselves to speaking of the nature, conditions and diseases of man, which they have found an easier and more predictable subject than womankind.

However, here is a new work that I have taken from the Latin of Monsieur Jean Liebault[45] and turned into French. I think that it omits nothing which could be encompassed within our knowledge of the nature of women of any age or condition — whether young, adolescent, old, virgins, marriageable, married or widows — nor concerning the various things that may befall her, occasioning sterility and preventing the bearing of children for which purpose she is ordained by the providence and will of God. It treats also the causes, signs and courses of all the illnesses which, apart from those common also to men, particularly threaten her good health. It also gives the best cures that may be of help to her, not only in the face of the countless illnesses and indispositions to which she is prone by virtue of her weaker nature and unavoidable misfortunes, but also in protecting her health, encouraging her fertility, and looking after herself wisely before and during pregnancy and childbirth. It is a most admirable work in all ways in its treatment of the health, fertility and cures of the illnesses of women, and so full of great learning and erudition, with so many remarkable observations and histories dealing with these subjects, that it will be judged admirable, enjoyable and profitable not only to women but to all people of good and sound judgment.

So, dear Reader, enjoy the labors, diligence and learning of Monsieur Jean Liebault,[46] and make no little use of this French work[47] which has been translated from Latin. But believe, please, that all the cures which you will find described in it (which, in truth, for the sake of the honor, excellence and standing of the art of medicine should not be divulged to the unlearned) will avail you little, even though they are most excellent, if you are not well versed in the mysteries and secrets of medicine, or if you are not guided in their use by a learned, wise and judicious physician. Otherwise, be content with the

---

45. From the 1585 edition onwards, the phrase 'of Monsieur Jean Liebault' is dropped. (On the putative original Latin text, see 67).

46. In 1585, changed to 'of the author'.

47. In 1585, changed to 'this French treasure'.

countless fine observations and memorable histories that you will find concerning the health, fertility and illnesses of women, in the hope that you may soon read three more books by the same author treating the adornment and embellishment of the human body.[48]

Godspeed.

48. This second volume was also published in 1582, by the same printer: see 67.

[1609]

LETTER TO CHASTE YOUNG WOMEN[49]

Preface

There is no knowledge that is more closely concerned with mankind than that offered by the physical sciences,[50] for, according to Avicenna, from whichever standpoint we look, they are at the center, the middle, the surface and the circumference of this microcosm.[51] It is impossible to turn our backs, to shut or open our eyes, without feeling and seeing them, both within and without. They dwell in this beautiful luminous palace through which the sun travels,[52] they reign over the moon, they control the elements; but, more nobly indeed than anywhere else and more gloriously, they hold sway over the human body. It is for this reason that, of all the parts of physical sciences, I judge the most useful to be that concerned with the physical form of man and woman; and that concerned with woman to be even more useful than that of man. It is as though Nature were displaying her power and majesty more fully among the lesser rather than the greater natures, as though (as one classical writer said) she takes more pride in the safekeeping of a single woman than in that of the whole sky. And in woman, who seems to be the last among all creatures possessed of reason,[53] there are more causes to wonder than in the whole realm of living creatures. For beyond what she shares in common with men, I would ask you also to consider the three parts by which she is particularly embellished, namely her face, her breasts and her womb. Here, Nature has attached such rich inventions and so many different qualities that the whole of Ancient philosophy is often hard put to account for them. Man is

49. The new preface by Lazare Pe [Pena], contained in his revised 1609 edition, and replacing the Letter written by Liebault for the 1582 volume, is essentially a neoplatonic manifesto.

50. Pena uses the term 'physical sciences' in the Aristotelian sense of knowledge about nature (τά φυσικά), or natural philosophy.

51. The microcosm refers to mankind, as opposed to the macrocosm, which is the rest of the universe.

52. The sky.

53. At the start of the seventeenth century, woman is still frequently considered to be inferior to man in her intelligence, a theory traced back at least to Plato (*Timaeus*, 90–91).

covered with distasteful hairs on his face and all over his body, his appearance is haughty and inhumane, his brow puckered, whereas a woman is as smooth as crystal, free of bodily or facial hair, her eyes are a reflection of celestial beauty that draws everything towards them. Unlike a man, she has a body which is most soft and pleasant to contemplate and touch: her flesh is supple; her complexion even and smooth, her skin fair; her bodily hair pale; her locks silky, shining and long; her face is completely bathed in beauty; her neck white as milk; her forehead broad and gracious; her eyes bright and shining with lively friendliness, and in all else she has such grace, refinement and elegance that there is nothing in Nature which can exercise a stronger attraction over a man's mind.

There are two things that make a woman attractive, her goodness and her beauty. Goodness indeed has strong and powerful chains, but it is the beauty that God has created in her face that, in the words of Leone Ebreo,[54] is a thousand times stronger. And who will describe them, asks Leone? Neither God, nor an angel, nor the sun, the moon nor an element. It is a magnet, a hidden force, a strength greater than that of the elements, a fifth heaven with magnetic and electric properties, capable of pulling a man towards it more strongly — yet without exerting any strength — than the trunk of an elephant. I would go further and say that it is not strength, knowledge or power, it is not like the water in a pearl,[55] the sparkle of a diamond, or the green of an emerald; what God and Nature have placed in a woman's face is an assembly of what is most potent and compelling in all the stars and heavens. It contains the sun. The stars and the moon have lent their brightness, fire its warmth, air its moisture, water its softness, the earth its grace. Just as, according to Alpharabius,[56] all the sun's rays and all the spheres united in one place light fire itself, so also all the strength of higher and lower Nature, brought together in this

54. Juda Abravanel, known as Leone Ebreo (or Hebreo), wrote the immensely successful *Dialogues of Love* [*Dialoghi d'amore*], which were published posthumously in Italian in 1535, and translated into French by Pontus de Tyard in 1551. These neoplatonic treatises on love develop Plato's theories (notably in the *Symposium*) on the ennobling qualities of love, and on the essential connection between beauty and goodness.

55. The series of images and antitheses, which Pena will develop, are commonplace in Petrarchan poetry.

56. Al-Farabi, a Muslim polymath, philosopher and scientist, c. 872–950.

single place, have made this attraction and charm. Thus, the Arabs, who were most skillful artists, painted woman with a look of amber, for having searched through all Nature's secret and public treasures, and having looked right inside the nature and origins of this one, they found that amber alone could express it, the ancient sages believing that all the enchantments, loveliness, beauty and everything most desirable in Nature were hidden in this wonderful crystal.

Now, what I am saying about female beauty is not vanity or affected praise, but the truth. Its attraction is even stronger than I can express in words, such that human wisdom, which seems to be the only shield against its spell, is weak and powerless against it. And even Plato, the most intelligent and moderate of all philosophers, loved women so much that he became their slave, composing whole works about their beauty. Xenophon, similarly, himself said that he loved his Clinia more than god, heaven or earth, while most Greek philosophers, being unable to enjoy the true, living Venus, often betook themselves to Cyprus to worship and kiss the buttocks of her image.[57] As for kings and princes, how often do they forsake their scepter to do homage to this new god lodged in the eyes of a woman? Even Alexander abandoned the most illustrious alliances of the East to marry a poor, yet beautiful barbarian,[58] far from all lands of his empire. But what I find most astonishing is that men are injured without being struck; neither sword, fire, nor a thunderbolt has touched them. The mere sight of this beauty has mortally wounded them, yet in a woman's face you see neither a dagger, acid, poison, nor fire. Whence comes this form of death? For death it certainly is; the man who has been struck dies hundreds of times each minute. It is a death even crueller than death itself because it does not let him die. This wound does not graze the surface, but enters deep within, striking the heart and the mind, causing the vital organs to wither, the flesh to shrivel, and the man will run through tombs and deserts seeking a cure, as though he were turned into a werewolf. But the only cure lies within the woman who had injured him. Thus we must recognize that Nature has granted something remarkable to women, which is denied to men, and that Nature has shown greater or better powers in women than in men.

57. Cyprus celebrated a particular cult of Venus, supposedly born from its seashore.
58. Roxane.

As for the breasts, how marvelous they are. For apart from contributing to the elegance and well-proportioned figure of a woman when they are sweetly shaped, round, firm, white as milk and set well apart,[59] how many purposes they serve. You see that Nature feeds the child in the womb on menstrual blood, but miraculously, as soon as the child is born, the blood rushes back up the mamillary veins, and fills the breasts, where it is changed into milk. If the blood is in the liver, it becomes red, but as soon as it is in the breasts it is whitened, the food becoming white chyle. Chyle becomes red blood, the blood becomes milk, the milk builds a new person. Nor is this all; one would think the blood ascends only via these two ordinary routes, but indeed all Nature, everything which is most noble and worthy in the whole body, pushes, drives and contributes to the food through these two channels, because the goal and purpose of Nature is to use everything, including every part of living beings, in order to protect the life of the new individual. Thus, not only the two ascending mamilliary veins, but also all the veins in the body, whether near to them or distant, deliver the food to the two vessels, whether openly, or at least through hidden connections and seepage. And just as in the procreation of the child, not only the brain, liver and testicles produce sperm, but all the parts of the body right down to the nails, according to the Rabbi Isaac Louris,[60] heating, digesting and contributing their essence and strength, so also in protecting the newborn child there is no part of the woman which does not provide it with food. And in this act, Nature is so powerful that, although usually women can scarcely digest strong food, they would be able to heat, digest and convert the most substantial of foods into milk. If foods are lacking, they could digest metals, and if these too were lacking, they would give the last drop of their blood to feed their baby.

These are the two celestial breasts of which the Ancients speak, which by their magnetic and permeable qualities attract all the strength of the planets and bring it to humans. They are the fountains of Nature, the receptacles into which Jupiter pours his nectar. Just as the

---

59. Pena is following stereotypical aesthetic preferences of the Renaissance, familiar from poets of the period, e.g. Clément Marot's poem 'On the beautiful breast' ['*Du beau tetin*'], 1535.

60. A Jewish physician (1534–1572).

soul derives nourishment by drinking ambrosia from two fountains, according to St Augustine, that is to say the Old and New Testaments, so also in order to nourish and take care of the infant, Nature has provided two breasts. While the child is bound to the dark prison of the womb, a symbol of the earth, he lives only on dirtied blood from the veins. But, as soon as he has escaped from the prison he runs to these two celestial fountains, which offer him the most perfect food. Just contemplate these miracles. The breasts provide food and they protect the heart, acting like a fortress, both warming it and being warmed by it, and keeping the child's victuals warm. They also serve, in the view of Aristotle, to incite the androgyne[61] to the act of love, for the male is captivated by the woman's eyes, and struck by this hidden fire he embraces and caresses her, kisses her and fondles her breasts. These urgent actions both warm the breasts and also stimulate the appetite of the womb because of the obvious relationship between the two, and so desire is kindled, together with the will to procreate.

Now if the nobility of the breasts is great, how much more so is that of the womb?[62] And if Nature displayed the richness of its creation in the first case, what shall we say of the second? The breasts are like the wet-nurse, the womb like the mother: the former raises and feeds what the latter has conceived and given form to. It is a miraculous thing that the womb can contain and lodge the child, so dilating in the course of pregnancy that its horns extend as far as the mother's sides. Yet if you pull and stretch it with your hands, applying force, it cannot be extended and it yields only to the demands of Nature. It will make room for up to four infants, however large and powerful their limbs may be. If another body were to be put within it, it could not be contained without damage to the woman, who would be torn apart.[63]

Look next at its form. An Arab will say that of all the parts of the body, it is that which seems most misshapen, base and least alive. Yet we should consider the artistry rather than its colour, its construction and not the appearance, its nature rather than its surface. Then we

61. Both man and woman.

62. Pena follows many French Renaissance medical writers in praising the womb above all other organs in the female body. Cf. Liebault's praise of woman for her fertility, 78.

63. Liebault assumes that a woman cannot bear more than four children, whereas many of his contemporaries delighted in apocryphal accounts of greater multiple pregnancies.

shall say that there is nothing more beautiful and more alive. Whence come the energy and powerful attraction it possesses, which allow it to draw from all directions, as though through thousands of mouths, the very food it desires and which travels through the veins, that are attached to it by the trunk of the seed-bearing vessels?[64] Is it a living being that attracts seed as though filling a sponge? Whence comes its obvious power to suck and voraciously devour the seed of a man, to enclose it, guard it so jealously that all men together could not match its zeal? What arouses such a fierce desire? Does it have a mind of its own, as Plato taught,[65] and another writer who compares it to a greedy tyrant who seizes everything he can from all around, and then hides his spoils in a cave? Not at all, for while it is indeed governed by 'the moon of the brain', as philosophers call the imagination, I think there is no direct connection between the head and this lower organ, for the former is in the higher sphere, and the latter in the lowest. Yet they are so bound together by shared feelings and hidden links that some people have believed the womb to rise up sharply towards the brain. It is true that it cannot act or accomplish its normal functions, attracting, drawing in, digesting, expelling, enclosing, unless it is helped by the imagination, which uses all the nerves of Nature, all the secret mechanisms of the body in order to make it react. And just as the moon causes the sea to rise and fall, and just as the lumerpa[66] only flies, sings and soars on high when the star of Mercury looks upon it, so too all these actions and movements of the womb derive not only from its own nature, but also from the force of the imagination which drives it where it pleases.

Where is the philosopher who will tell me the reason for this miracle, which allows the imagination to kindle love, set on fire all the desire of this organ when it was quite frozen? Does this happen through imagination, which is simply pure thought, which sees only the image of the thing, not the true thing itself, which has only a simple connection with the senses without really seeing? Yet, through

---

64. The fallopian tubes, commonly referred to as seed-bearing vessels, supposing an equation between the male and female reproductive organs.

65. *Timaeus*, 90–91.

66. A fantastic bird (described by Leonardo da Vinci, among others), supposed to shine so brightly that it absorbs its own shadow.

a strong impression, by a very strong force, it arouses reactions and movements, causing the counterweights that rule the noble organs to quiver, and warms and ignites the fire in the lower parts. Just as the sun produces heat by means of a sharp movement made by a strong reflection of light, so it is the imagination — the true fountain of love — which kindles cold things and cools warm ones. It is the imagination that makes us find ugly things pleasant, and pleasant things ugly. It is the imagination that governs this field in which the new infant is sown and conceived, and, finally, it is also the true image of the rational mind.

All these wonders together teach us that woman is one of the great miracles of Nature, and a subject in which philosophy finds more to study than in all the other things in creation. This is why I have concentrated particularly on woman, perusing all the authors who have dealt with her, both ancient and modern, and yet I could not find a single one who could satisfy my mind, for all lacked order and their words were marred by confusion, and I was left impatient until I chanced upon Giovanni Marinelli, an Italian from Formia, who sought not only to praise the excellence and perfection of this noble creature, but also indicated the way to preserve her beauty through putting right all the natural accidents which may befall her.[67] It was in Marinelli that I found what I was looking for; for he treated this subject so well that he carried off the crown in comparison with Ancients and Moderns alike. All the aspects of a woman, from greatest to least, are so clearly and specifically detailed, and with such learning. It is a worthy work, emanating from a worthy mind, as he has proved in everything. For he it is who has continued Arculani's commentaries on Rhazes,[68] writing four books on female beauty, and many other treatises, which both Italians and French have falsely tried to claim for themselves — as with this book on the illnesses of women, which Monsieur Jean Liebault appropriated. However, in comparing the two closely, I discovered that he had taken all his subject matter from

---

67. Pena is probably alluding here to Marinelli's other major work, *The Ornaments of Women* [*Gli ornamenti delle donne*, 1562], which discusses female beauty.

68. Marinelli had edited the *Handbook of John Arculan of Verona on the Particularities of all Diseases* [*Practica Ioannis Arculani Veronensis particularium morborum omnium*], published in Venice in 1560.

Marinelli, changing the order of chapters in places and adding some small things of his own the better to disguise it.[69]

But the honor must be restored to the original author, even though we may still accord some praise to Liebault for polishing and extending this book and translating it into French, together also with the volume on the adornment of women. It is one of the most useful tasks one can choose to undertake these days, and one of the best books there is on both theory and practice. This is why I readily selected it, corrected it in many places, developed it in others, where I judged the treatment of the subject matter to be too brief, and I have used Roderigo de Castro, the Portuguese physician famous throughout Europe, who fortunately assisted Marinelli in this task. The ladies will find herein things on which to feed their minds: the author tried hard to make clear to them everything regarding their health that is hidden in medicine. This is why he addressed the present work to them, and I continue in the same way, because of my great desire to serve them and to remain their,

Most affectionate,

Lazare Pe.

69. On Liebault's adaptation of Marinelli (for which Pena here gives him minimal credit), see 69-71.

[1582]

PRIVILEGE

Extract from the Privilege[70]

By letters patent from His Majesty the King, issued in Paris on 23 August 1581.

Monsieur de l'Estoille,[71] permission is given for Jacques du-Puys, the bookseller, sworn by the University of Paris, to have two books printed, that is to say: one containing *Of the Illnesses of Women*,[72] the other *Of the Adornment and Beauties of Women*.[73] And all other booksellers and printers are forbidden to print these same books or to have them printed for a period of nine years, as is also stated in these letters.

70. A Privilege is effectively an early form of copyright protection.

71. On Pierre de l'Estoile (or L'Estoille), see 68.

72. The title cited in the Privilege is less precise than that used by Dupuis when the book is printed in 1582.

73. Again, the title is modified when the volume is printed in 1582.

TABLE OF THE CHAPTERS OF THE THREE BOOKS ON THE HEALTH, FERTILITY AND ILLNESSES OF WOMEN

Where chapters are drawn from Marinelli, I indicate, in square brackets after the chapter title in Liebault, the corresponding chapter or chapters in the 1574 edition of *Medicine pertaining to Women's Diseases* [*Le Medicine partenenti alle donne*].

Of the First Book (p. 1)

Ch. 1   That woman is not a misformed or imperfect creature, but weak and prone to illness.[74]

Ch. 2   What are the illnesses of women, and the causes in general of these.

Ch. 3   The outline of the subjects to be treated in the three books concerning the health, fertility and illnesses of women.

Ch. 4   Retained menses in unmarried girls.[75]

Ch. 5   Pale, yellowish or dark colour in unmarried girls.

Ch. 6   Palpitations in unmarried girls.

Ch. 7   Bloating in unmarried girls.

Ch. 8   Unhealthy or abnormal appetite in unmarried girls.

Ch. 9   Loss of appetite in unmarried girls.

Ch. 10   Nausea and vomiting in unmarried girls.

Ch. 11   Shivering, stiffness and shock in unmarried girls.

Ch. 12   Unhappiness, sighs, moans, laughter in unmarried girls.

Ch. 13   Daydreaming in unmarried girls.

Ch. 14   Fainting in unmarried girls.

Ch. 15   Erratic fevers in unmarried girls.

Ch. 16   Thirst in unmarried girls.

Ch. 17   Hunger in unmarried girls.

Ch. 18   Sleeplessness in unmarried girls.

74. Chapters 1–22 are Liebault's own composition, not drawn from Marinelli's *Medicine pertaining to Women's Diseases*. See 69-71.

75. Liebault uses the term 'virgin' ('*vierge*') throughout these headings, denoting a girl not yet married. He is following the Hippocratic medical distinction between unmarried and married women, whereas Marinelli discussed only married (i.e. sexually active) women.

Of the Second Book (p. 160)

76. Not drawn from Marinelli.

77. Liebault uses the word '*fureur*', denoting both ardour and lack of control.

78. Not drawn from Marinelli.

Ch. 2   The types, differences and causes of sterility. *[Marinelli II.1]*

Ch. 3   The signs and indications of sterility. *[Marinelli II.2]*

Ch. 4   The same temperament in the man and the woman, a first cause of sterility. *[Marinelli II.3]*

Ch. 5   Flaws affecting some noble part, a second cause of sterility. *[Marinelli II.4]*

Ch. 6   Defects in the male seed, a third cause of male sterility. *[Marinelli II.5]*

Ch. 7   Flaws affecting the male member. *[Marinelli II.6]*

Ch. 8   Flaws and damage affecting the testicles. *[Marinelli II.7]*

Ch. 9   Excessive fatness or obesity of the body, a common cause of sterility in both men and women. *[Marinelli II.9]*

Ch. 10   Thinness of the whole body, a common cause of sterility in both men and women. *[Marinelli II.10]*

Ch. 11   Flaws and damage affecting the womb. First, its incorrect temperature.[79]

Ch. 12   Thickness of the womb.

Ch. 13   Pain in the womb.

Ch. 14   Inflammation of the womb.

Ch. 15   Erisypelas of the womb.

Ch. 16   Tumors of the womb.

Ch. 16[a] Tumors of the womb that have become absceses.[80]

Ch. 17   Scirrhus or hard tumor in the womb.

Ch. 18   Cancer in the womb.

Ch. 19   Ulcers in the womb.

Ch. 20   Fistulas in the womb.

Ch. 21   Rhagades in the womb.

Ch. 22   Condylomas in the womb.

Ch. 23   Hemorrhoids in the womb.

Ch. 25   Hardness of the womb.[81]

Ch. 26   Paralysis and slackness of the womb.

---

79. II. 11–29 in Liebault are loosely adapted from Marinelli II.8 and 11–13, but Liebault extends the discussion, demonstrating his greater interest in the physiology and pathology of the womb.

80. Erratum: the chapter I have designated 16[a] is wrongly numbered 19, after which the sequence resumes with 17, 18, 19, etc.

81. Erratum: there is no chapter 24.

Ch. 27   Inflammation of the womb.

Ch. 28   Hydropsy of the womb.

Ch. 29   Stones in the womb.

Ch. 30   Discussion of the occasion and reason for menstrual flow in women, its nature, kind and the usual duration of the flow. *[Marinelli II.14]*

Ch. 31   On the reasons for the corruption of menstrual blood. *[Marinelli II.15]*

Ch. 32   Suppression or reduction of menses. *[Marinelli II.16]*

Ch. 33   Excessive or immoderate menses. *[Marinelli II.17]*

Ch. 34   Menses that flow slowly. *[Ibid.]*[82]

Ch. 35   White flowers.[83] *[Marinelli II.18]*

Ch. 36   Gonorrhea or flow of seed.[84]

Ch. 37   An over-thick womb or neck of the lower regions.[85]

Ch. 38   An over-thin womb or neck of the lower regions.

Ch. 39   Whether the womb can be dislodged from its natural position. *[Marinelli II.19–20]*[86]

Ch. 40   Suffocation of the womb. *[Ibid.]*

Ch. 41   The wandering womb. *[Ibid.]*

Ch. 42   Ascent of the womb. *[Ibid.]*

Ch. 43   Convulsion of the womb. *[Ibid.]*

Ch. 44   The descent of the womb. *[Ibid.]*

Ch. 45   Prolapse of the womb. *[Ibid.]*

Ch. 46   Uterine frenzy. *[Ibid.]*

Ch. 47   Obstruction of the cotyledons.[87]

Ch. 48   What the true neck of the womb is.[88]

Ch. 49   The over-moist neck of the womb.

82. Liebault has expanded into two separate chapters subjects that Marinelli treated in one chapter.

83. The medical condition of leukorrhea.

84. Chapters 36–38 are not drawn from Marinelli. (In ancient usage, gonorrhea could refer to the sexually transmitted disease, but also to spermatorrhea or masturbation.)

85. I.e. vagina.

86. Chapters 39–46 in Liebault expand on II. 19–20 in Marinelli.

87. Chapters 47–51 are not drawn from Marinelli.

88. Liebault is distinguishing between the cervix, the 'true neck of the womb' ('*le vray col de la matrice*') and the vagina, which he treats in ch. 57.

Ch. 50   The thickened or hardened neck of the womb.

Ch. 51   The gaping or excessively open neck of the womb.

Ch. 52   The over-narrow neck of the womb. *[Marinelli II.21]*

Ch. 53   The obstructed neck of the womb.[89]

Ch. 54   The misshapen neck of the womb.

Ch. 55   The prolapsed neck of the womb.

Ch. 56   Pain, inflammation, erisypelas, abscesses, schirrus, cancer, ulcer, fistulas, rhagades, warts, condylomas, hemorrhoids in the neck of the womb.[90] *[Marinelli II.22–24]*

Ch. 57   What the neck of the lower regions is.[91] *[Ibid.]*

Ch. 58   The neck of the lower regions being over-moist, or fleshy, or thin. *[Ibid.]*

Ch. 59   The over-narrow neck of the lower regions. *[Ibid.]*

Ch. 60   The gaping and excessively open neck of the lower regions. *[Ibid.]*

Ch. 61   The closed neck of the lower regions. *[Ibid.]*

Ch. 62   The membrane called the hymen which blocks the neck of the lower regions. *[Ibid.]*

Ch. 63   Excessively large nymphae. *[Ibid.]*

Ch. 64   The penis.[92] *[Ibid.]*

Ch. 65   Pain, inflammation, erisypelas, abscesses, schirrus, cancer, ulcer, fistulas, rhagades, warts, condylomas, hemorrhoids in the neck of the lower regions. *[Ibid.]*

Ch. 66   Thyme warts. *[Ibid.]*

Ch. 67   Warts on the lower regions. *[Ibid.]*

Ch. 68   Gangrene of the neck of the lower regions. *[Ibid.]*

Ch. 69   Itching of the neck of the lower regions. *[Ibid.]*

Ch. 70   Intestinal hernia. *[Ibid.]*

89. Chapters 53–55 are not drawn from Marinelli.

90. Chapters 56–66 in Liebault expand on II.22–24 in Marinelli.

91. Liebault is pursuing the distinction between the cervix, which he discussed in ch.48, and the vagina. He refers to the latter as the 'neck of the lower regions', using the standard vernacular French term '*partie honteuse*' ('shameful part') to refer to it.

92. In reference to the clitoris, Liebault uses the word '*queue*' ('tail'), which normally refers to the penis, implying that the clitoris is analogous to the male member.

Of the Third Book (p. 524)

93. Chapters 1–4 are not drawn from Marinelli.

94. Erratum: there is no chapter numbered 6.

95. Liebault has expanded into two separate chapters subjects that Marinelli treated in one chapter.

96. Chapters 10–13 are not drawn from Marinelli.

97. In French '*mauvais germe*' (literally 'bad seed') is a common vernacular term to designate a hydatidiform mole.

98. Liebault has expanded into six separate chapters (14–19) the subject that Marinelli treated briefly in one chapter of Book III.

99. It was commonly believed that the foetus did not receive a soul until the third or fourth month after conception.

100. Not drawn from Marinelli.

101. The chapter number 20 is used twice. The title of chapter 20 [a] does not appear in the table of chapters. Chapters 20[a]–32 in Liebault expand on III. 5–7 in Marinelli.

102. Chapters 33–39 (treating breastfeeding) are not drawn from Marinelli.

103. Chapters 40–41 in Liebault expand on III. 8 in Marinelli.

104. Chapters 44–50 in Liebault expand on 11–14 in Marinelli.

105. Not drawn from Marinelli.

FIRST BOOK OF THE ILLNESSES OF WOMEN, AND CURES FOR THESE[106]

Chapter I: That Woman is Not a Misformed or Imperfect Creature, but Weak and Prone to Illness

In Book XIV of his work *On the Usefulness of the Parts*, Galen[107] speaks about the wonderful design of the human body, and compares the female body to the male's. He says that[108] a woman's body is misformed and imperfect, since Nature lacks sufficient and strong enough heat (the first and main cause of all actions and movements) to shape, bring to life and push out the parts of the female body, and so it has left most of these parts, especially those needed for conception, hidden within, in the same way that the eyes of a mole are hidden internally because Nature was too weak to push them out of the head. In this, Galen appears to follow the opinion of Aristotle who, in his book *On the Generation of Animals*,[109] calls man a supremely perfect creature and woman a flawed, misformed, weak creature, like a man who has been wounded, even a mistake and notable error of Nature. He explains that Nature is unaccustomed to create anything that is not large, excellent and perfect, and when intending to create a male from the available matter, she failed in her task either through weakness or some other obstacle, creating only a female.

---

106. My translation is based on the 1582 original text of Liebault. Where short corrections, or additions, were introduced in the 1609 edition by Pena, I indicate these in the footnotes. In the several places where Pena introduces lengthy additions, which could not be conveniently reproduced in footnotes, I include them in the text (signalled by a footnote), and use italic characters to distinguish Pena's contributions, as was the case in the 1609 text and in subsequent editions.

107. Liebault engages directly in this opening chapter (which does not derive from Marinelli) with classical and medieval theories of the physiological imperfection of woman, rejecting them in favor of his understanding of the physiological and anatomical distinctiveness of the two sexes. His views represent the advances in this field of mid-sixteenth century anatomists such as Falloppio, whose description of the female genitalia in his *Anatomical Observations* [*Observationes antomicae*] of 1561 was particularly influential. For a full account of these medical, anatomical and physiological arguments, see I. Maclean, *The Renaissance Notion of Woman. A study in the fortunes of scholasticism and medical science in European intellectual life* (Cambridge: CUP, 1980), ch. 3.

108. In the rest of the paragraph, Liebault summarizes Galen's argument in *Of the Usefulness of the Parts*, XIV. 6.

109. *On the Generation of Animals*, I. 20.

However, if we wish to examine things more closely, a woman's body is not misformed, nor imperfect, for the reasons that these two great writers advance. For we must believe that God, who creates and controls Nature, and who creates all living things, gave no less matter or power to Nature for the creation of the female body than for the male body. Should we say that there is something imperfect in the works of Nature and in what she creates just because they are not all of the same nature and kind, but rather of different and diverse natures, some more excellent than others? No, for the diversity and difference which may be present, and the excellence which distinguishes some above others, does not cause imperfection in some, and does not prevent each being perfect among its own kind in the eyes of the creator, and for the end for which He created them all. For far from thinking any creation or work of Nature is imperfect, on the contrary we should recognize that Nature shows herself more wondrous and displays her power and providence more greatly in this diverse range of creatures than had she produced only one sort, of a single excellence, even had it been the most excellent that could have existed. For a small ant is as perfect of its kind, which is the smallest of all animals, as an elephant of its kind, which is the largest. And so, Nature showed herself no less marvelous or admirable in the nature of this tiny creature than in that of the elephant. Thus we should not believe that Nature fell short of her goal in conceiving a female body, or that she wished to create a male but by some notable error created a woman. The aim of Nature in conception is to conceive a living being which can conceive and bear a living being of its own kind, and for this reason the body of a woman is no less whole or perfect than that of a man, since it possesses all the parts necessary for conception, shaped and situated in the right place in order to allow her to conceive and bear a child.

As for the hidden parts within the female body which Galen identifies as being so greatly misformed and imperfect,[110] we should rather consider this a greater perfection and more properly suited to their task, with the admirable foresight of Nature which neither wishes, nor can, nor should, push out the parts intended for reproduction, as is the case with the male body, for a man conceives within another,

110. See *On the Usefulness of the Parts*, II. 6, in which Galen argues that the female genitalia are imperfect because they are within rather than outside the body.

not within himself. But instead she hides them, and situates them in an appropriate place to receive the seed and thus conceive a living being; to carry it for a certain time and to expand as the child within does, without occasioning pain or injury to other neighboring parts, and in due course to release and expel the child.[111] *Moreover, the same providence of Nature has endowed women with an incredible appetite for sexual union, which brings extreme pleasure, so that as the two come together, the generation of their line ensues. Which shows that woman is not a mistake of Nature.*

Woman, like man, is endowed with reason. He is the principal instigator and first source of generation; she supplies the nature and the organs necessary for conception. This is the order of Nature, whose will is thus in all the things created. Thus, as the philosophers say, Nature gave two elements masculine characteristics, and to the other two passive, female ones;[112] in astrology, some signs occupy the masculine place, others the female;[113] and even in materials, those who study Nature recognize the two sexes, active and passive; the same is true of human nature. Aristotle,[114] Book I, chapter 2 and Book II, chapter 1.

For these reasons, the body of a woman is neither misformed nor imperfect. I willingly concede that it is imperfect when it is sterile, or bears no child, since Nature created it primarily to conceive and bear children of its own kind, not to remain sterile. This is why in the Old Testament married women who remained childless were looked down upon and considered unworthy to converse with the others.[115] I will also admit that a woman's body is weak and prone to illness. It is weak because of the lack of natural heat in comparison with that of men:[116] heat is responsible for physical strength, being what supports, sustains

111. The following sections in italic type (*'Moreover the same providence … book II, chapter 1'*) were added by Pena in 1609.

112. Fire and air are associated with the masculine; water and earth with the feminine.

113. The masculine signs are Aries, Gemini, Leo, Libra, Sagittarius and Aquarius; the feminine signs are Taurus, Cancer, Virgo, Scorpio, Capricorn and Pisces.

114. Aristotle, *On the Generation of Animals.*

115. Cf. Louis de Serres (see 307, n. 39), who, however, shows far more compassion for the plight of childless women.

116. Although Liebault has vigorously defended the specificity of each sex, he still follows the traditional classical assumption that women's humoral balance is naturally less hot than men's, thereby rendering women weaker. On evolving debates about relative heat and coldness in men and women, see I. Maclean, *The Renaissance Notion of Woman*, 33–35.

and drives all the actions of nature. A woman's body is prone to illness for the reasons we shall expound in the next chapter.

Chapter II: What Are the Illnesses of Women, and the Causes in General of These

It is not without reason that in a number of passages about the nature of women, Hippocrates writes that women are certainly more prone to ill health, and subject to greater and more serious illnesses than men.[117] For apart from their natural temperament, which is cold and damp; apart from their natural physical constitution, which is soft, flaccid, and rarely lends itself to exertion; apart from the superfluous excretions which abound in them; apart from the idle, sedentary and inactive life they are forced to lead because of the limitations of their bodies, they have in addition one organ which is so sensitive and so easily upset (that is to say, the womb) that the least indisposition of this organ results in endless, unrelated illnesses which are almost unbearable. For this reason, Hippocrates said that the most troublesome illnesses of women come from the womb,[118] or are within the womb itself, for it is from this part that there comes both life and the destruction of health.[119]

For if Nature created and shaped the womb to be the main organ in women, like a fertile garden, for the procreation of children in order to ensure the constant perpetuation of the human race (the individual members of it being inevitably subject to decay and death), we should not deny that for this reason the womb is one of the main, most noble

117. The first three chapters draw broadly on Hippocrates's treatise *On the Nature of Women*. For a detailed overview of Hippocratic gynecology and how it was understood in later periods, see H. King, *Hippocrates' Woman. Reading the female body in Ancient Greece* (London and New York: Routledge, 1998), ch 1. King argues that the texture of the flesh (loose-textured, spongy, wetter in women) is fundamental in defining the Hippocratic anatomy of female difference, 29–30.

118. In this chapter, Liebault relates most of the illnesses of women to the womb, a position characteristic of his adherence to the theoretical principle of the specificity of each sex. Although the womb is admired as the distinctive organ of the female body, its pre-eminence means that any illness of the womb affects the whole female body.

119. See Hippocrates, *Places in Man*, 47. Liebault opts for a simple, uterocentric reading of Hippocrates. However, King observes that other Hippocratic texts treat the womb as 'secondary to female difference', with the texture of the flesh determining the nature and function of the womb (*Hippocrates' Woman*, 33).

and necessary parts of a woman. Any injury to it, however slight, leads to wearisome consequences, affecting not only the womb but the whole body on account of its intimate connections with all other parts, such as the nerves, the spine, the membranes of the brain, and through the veins with the liver, and through the arteries with the heart. Hence the great philosopher Plato admired the nobility, movements, functions and marvelous effects of this part, and thought it was not only subject to the force and influence of the mind, which rules over the body, but also had its own individual mind, and he called it a living thing.[120]

Now the principal things — among many others — which cause the womb to be prone to illness and make it likely to be seriously afflicted are the two secretions it receives and which are sent to it from the whole body, that is to say spermatic fluid[121] and menstrual blood. If these are retained unduly, or flow excessively, they cause strange sufferings to women, even though, at the right time, the retention of them may enable the conception and fulfilment of the womb's purpose — the procreation and birth of mankind — and keep the body in better health. However, if they are retained at the wrong time, they cause the following undesirable sufferings: strangulations, palpitations, fainting, convulsions, disordered appetites, vagueness, suffocation of the womb, excessive sleep, starts, irregular movements, paleness, white discharge,[122] sterility, moles, colics, pains in the lower back, nausea, vomiting, inflammation, abscesses, ulceration, schirrus, swelling, hydropsy, rhagades, warts, erysipelas, cancers, hemorrhoids, and many other ailments. The excessive flow of spermatic fluid causes gonorrhea, nocturnal emissions, atrophy and sexual impotence. The excessive flow of menstrual blood causes sterility, hydropsy, cachexia, atrophy, loss of appetite, uterine prolapse, miscarriage, painful labor, difficult childbirth, and other dangerous symptoms, which we shall discuss individually.

These are the illnesses of women and the causes of them in general, which we have resolved to expound without intending to stray at all into other illnesses which are common to men as well as to women,

120. *Timaeus*, 90–91.

121. Liebault, like most of his contemporaries, assumes women secrete a seed-bearing fluid similar to male semen.

122. On leukorrhea, see 171, n. 65.

such as fevers, plague, apoplexy, paralysis, and others of which various great doctors have written at sufficient length.

Chapter III: The Outline of the Subjects to be Treated Here

The illnesses of women and the causes of these are in general such as we have described. So that they may be more easily known and recognized, I propose to treat them individually and to outline them as carefully as possible with regard to women according to their age, condition and position in life, in order that nothing which might help any kind of women, of any condition, should be omitted from our discussion. First, I shall describe the symptoms, and their cures, for unmarried girls from the age of 13 to 20, including nuns and others who have taken a vow of chastity. Secondly, I shall describe what may happen to newly married women, then the misfortune of those who, although married for a long time, remain infertile and cannot enjoy the fruits of marriage. Next, I shall describe how we should help women who are suffering when pregnant, in labor, or newly delivered, and then, finally, the decline that befalls widows or women who are nearing or have reached the age of 50. Thus, there will be little that has not been said about the illnesses and other misfortunes that can afflict women, whatever their age or condition.

THIRD BOOK OF THE ILLNESSES OF WOMEN

Chapter XX[a]: The Regimen That a Woman Should Follow during Her Pregnancy

Once there are definite signs that confirm that the woman is pregnant, here is the regimen that she should observe during the pregnancy in order that it may progress successfully and lead to an easy delivery, without much pain.[123]

Let her live where the air is temperate. She should avoid air and winds which are either too hot or too cold, for fear that if the air is unduly hot her body will be afflicted with excessive languor, sapping her strength, or that the cold will cause her to be afflicted with a cough, which will greatly disturb the child. If this disturbance is lengthy and incommodious, she will be in danger of giving birth before her time. Let her both sleep and be wakeful in moderation, but sleep more than she is awake.[124] She should avoid all sudden movements, exertions and strenuous exercise. She should not walk too fast, nor sit or stand up suddenly, nor run, and especially not jump, dance or on any account ride a horse.[125] She should not lift or carry any heavy load, nor stretch out or raise her arms or hands, or wave them around abruptly or frequently. She should not remain standing for any length of time, but take some gentle strolls, without tiring herself; she may take gentle and moderate exercise which in no way tires her or exhausts her physically, except when she is practically on the point of giving birth. For at this time walking to and fro, even if she is tired, will be of use.

---

123. This is the second of the two chapters of Book III to be numbered 20 (see 96). Liebault draws some sections of the chapter from Marinelli's treatment of the same subject in *Medicine pertaining to Women's Diseases* [*Le Medicine partenenti alle infermita delle donne*], III. 5, but changes the order of items and adds other material. It is a good example of his combination of translation, adaptation and expansion. I indicate all the sections drawn closely from Marinelli — the other sections are compiled by Liebault, the basic information being standard in classical authorities. Duval, in turn, derives some of his material on the same subject (ch. XVIII) from Liebault (see 260-275).

124. This sentence ('Let her both sleep… awake') is translated directly from Marinelli (*Le Medicine*, 1574, fol. 250^v).

125. The two sentences 'She should avoid…. horse' are very close to Marinelli's advice (*Le Medicine*, 1574, fol. 251^r). Most of the recommendations of this and the following two paragraphs are found in Aetius of Amida's *Tetrabiblus*, XVI. 12, which may have been one of Marinelli's and Liebault's sources.

The seats, chairs and stools on which she sits should be soft and comfortable rather than hard. Once seated she should not leave her feet unsupported, but place them a little higher, resting on some low support. She should avoid sitting or lying on the ground with her legs and thighs crossed or brought up against her womb, because sitting or lying on the ground in such a position often, as we have warned above, produces a deformity, or a child of monstrous appearance.[126]

She should avoid travelling in a cart, or even worse in a carriage, for numerous ladies have given birth before their time for this reason. If she really needs to travel, let her be carried in a litter.[127] She should dress lightly, her dresses should not be tightly laced nor constricting, so that the womb can adapt to the growth of the child; otherwise, if she dresses with more regard for her own pleasure than for the wellbeing of the child, she will give birth to dwarves, or to lame, hunchbacked, twisted, deformed children. I am referring to women who wear boned corsets and wish to have their bodies tightly laced.

She should abstain from lying with her husband, at least in the first months,[128] for this, more than all other forms of excess, provokes miscarriages. I know a number of women who gave birth prematurely for no other reason, and when I advised them to abstain totally or at least to have only very moderate relations, they started to carry their children to full term. Let her avoid all occasions which might give her cause to vomit or cough. She should avoid all unnecessary and sudden loss of bodily fluids, which are the main and best-known cause of miscarriage, especially nosebleeds or hemorrhage from hemorrhoids, or from any other place. For these, above all, are dangerous to pregnant women.

Let her especially be cheerful, not troubled by tears, weeping, worries, anger or sadness. Let her remain happy and of moderate and good spirits, for her joy and happiness of mind will make the child happy, arousing all its faculties and strengthening all the parts of its

126. On the Renaissance's preoccupation with what were identified as monstrous births, see A. Bates, *Emblematic Monsters. Unnatural conceptions and deformed births in early modern Europe* (Amsterdam-New York: Rodopi, 2005).

127. Standard advice in classical and Renaissance medical writers, also developed at some length by Soranus in his *Gynaecology* (trans. O. Temkin), I. xiv.

128. Marinelli gives more basic advice (*Le Medicine*, 1574, fol. 251ʳ), which Liebault develops substantially with reference to his own observations.

body.[129] Let her avoid all that might occasion shock or fear, and let her not be unsettled by any anger or other such disturbance of the mind. She should not contemplate nor fix her gaze upon any ugly, deformed or monstrous picture or portrait, but rather feast her eyes upon beautiful and excellent sights, by the careful contemplation of which her thoughts, understanding and imagination will be impelled to imprint the image of the beautiful things she has thought of or imagined upon the seed that she is forming, or upon the child she has recently conceived. When noble ladies are pregnant they are advised and enjoined not to look upon, or allow anything to be presented to them, or to think of or imagine anything that might harm them or cause damage as they conceive, or while their child is developing in the womb.

She should take care not to eat beyond moderation. She should certainly not bathe except when she is close to her time to give birth, for then bathing is good since it can relax the ligaments and open the mouth of the womb.[130] Let her take care to leave her womb fairly unconstrained, and if it is hard (as happens especially in the eighth and ninth months because of the tightening and compression which the fullness of the womb causes), she should favor foods which are able to soften the womb, such as thick soups, damsons, stocks made with bugloss, borage, herb mercury, violets, spinach, mallows with plentiful fresh butter; or such herbs as can be set in fresh butter.[131] She should also use for this purpose lettuces cooked in water, salt, wine and just a little vinegar. If despite all this her womb still does not relax, she should be given a suppository of honey and the yolk of an egg, or of venetian soap,[132] or a large pill, or better still, an enema made from veal or chicken broth (or broth made from sheep's intestines or head) in which you have marinated violets, mallows, marshmallows, but not

129. This sentence enlarges on Marinelli's advice (*Le Medicine*, 1574, fol. 251ʳ).

130. 'She should take care ... give birth' is taken from Marinelli (*Le Medicine*, 1574, fol. 251ʳ), but Liebault reverses the order of the two pieces of advice. Both authors give advice close to that of Aetius, *Tetrabiblus*, XVI. 12.

131. Marinelli also gives extensive advice on foods, both to eat and avoid (*Le Medicine*, 1574, fol. 250ʳ –252ʳ), but most of the details in Liebault's advice are independent of Marinelli's, partly reflecting the differences between French and Italian diets.

132. Also known as castile soap, and regularly used in the form of a suppository which acted as a laxative.

flowers of camomile since these are believed to stimulate the womb and cause a miscarriage, but rather flowers of sweet clover which are said to prevent miscarriage. In such broths you should blend some egg yolks and sugar. Or, instead of an enema, take a bowl with six drams[133] of cassia, and inhale it half an hour after a veal or chicken soup, not to prevent the cassia being digested and nature making use of it as some people think, but rather to dissolve and diffuse it in the stomach so that it can take effect more quickly.

In place of cassia, which sometimes relaxes, she may take two ounces of very good manna, in a capon broth. She should be fed on good foodstuffs, which are easily digestible and nutritious, such as bread made from white flour without the bran, because bran cleans out the body and provides little nutrition, or thick soups, or veal, mutton, partridge, pheasant, capon and chicken. It is true that thick soups and all delicate foods are unlikely to suit her in the early days of pregnancy, especially if she is nauseous and cannot stomach any foods. Fruit syrups, stewed fruits, panades, soft eggs, jellies, pearl barley will be very suitable for her, provided her stomach is not full of phlegm, and that she is not being constantly sick and is not of an over-wet temperament. For in that case, dry, hard foods would be much more suitable than moist, liquid ones. She should not eat too often because her natural heat, which is entirely directed towards feeding the child she carries and keeping it warm, will not suffice to digest too much food.[134] Her food may be flavored with cloves or nutmeg, which have the power to compress, and not with cinnamon or ginger, which may pierce and open.

Let her drink only very little, choosing fine claret wine that should not be watered down, but of moderate strength, not white or strong, and not flavored with cinnamon or spices, or diluted with water from the cistern or a goblet, just provided the tightness of her womb does not prevent this.[135] She should drink not at the start but rather at the end of meals, avoiding strong foods if her stomach is full of phlegm, which might require an incision. Thus, let her avoid garlic, onion,

---

133. A dram is an eighth of an ounce.

134. This idea is found in Marinelli (*Le Medicine*, 1574, fol. 251ʳ).

135. Marinelli is less cautious in recommending that pregnant women should drink good wine (*Le Medicine*, 1574, fol. 250ᵛ).

capers, horseradish, beans, mint, catmint and other such things. She should also avoid saffron, especially since it normally stimulates the menses, and windy foods or those that produce urine, and others that are too hot. She should eat very ripe and slightly astringent fruits to invigorate the stomach and stimulate the appetite, such as caramelized hazelnuts, court-pendu apples,[136] apples with a strong perfume, pomegranates, quinces, which are apparently able to give the child a good mind, a good memory and good perception, since this fruit has a drying effect, and dryness is most useful in helping us retain what we learn. When women consume this fruit, it often makes the child increasingly drier, even if it is flaccid while in the mother's womb. The drier the brain is, the more easily it retains information, so that it is said that to eat plenty of quinces during pregnancy gives the child a good mind, that is to say one that is retentive.[137]

However, I would advise that it may not be profitable to the mother or the child, for quinces will constipate the mother, and women are generally more prone to constipation in pregnancy; and they do nothing particularly valuable for the child, or which another food with drying properties would not do equally well. In addition, it is not good for the child to become dry, since natural pliability aids the growth of its body, which will remain short if the flesh is very dry. And a child who is born over dry is older,[138] and at the end of its time, which everyone wants to avoid as far as possible. Thus one sees that children born with such developed minds do not live a long time, for the main activities of a lively and very active mind dry out the body, which is almost continually overwhelmed by it; and while the dried body sharpens the mind, it will not last a long time. Thus we should not press nature too hard in anything, and since it is natural for a child to be pliable and moist, and this makes it grow and live longer, we should not worry about it developing a good mind, for the mind will be quite satisfactory if the temperament of the body is balanced. For the main quality of a balanced man is prudence, and a child is

136. A French variety of this period — possible an ancestor of Cox's Orange Pippin.

137. In 1609, Pena replaces the last phrase ('that is to say one that is retentive') with the following sentence: 'because of their scent and pleasant smell, which strengthens the brain and cannot cause the foetus to become dry because of the moistness which runs from all sides into the receptacle of the womb'.

138. What would now be called 'post-term'.

well balanced if it is born safely and is well nourished. So I cannot recommend that pregnant women should consume quinces. I prefer to advise them to eat damask grapes (known as '*passerilles*' or '*passes*' in the Languedoc). If the mother consumes them regularly, they are said to ensure the child has better eyesight, not that they really have the property to sharpen sight, but they are nutritious and thus make the blood pure, clean and good. The child nourished on this should have alert, fine and responsive senses, and a sharp and lively mind, more than if it had been nourished on thick, dirty blood.

If the mother's tastes are disturbed and she desires to eat foods which would be bad or of little use to her, she should not be prevented, but given them with great restraint, in small quantities.[139] If such foods are displeasing or not customary, they should be disguised, fried or roasted, or seasoned with some pleasing sauce. If you refuse pregnant women such foods, even though they are an abomination, you will cause the women to miscarry, for they run the risk of miscarriage if they crave something they cannot have, especially women who are prone to miscarry. For miscarriage can occur on account of troubles which assail the mind of the pregnant woman, or on account of her displeasure and anger when she cannot obtain something she strongly desires, just as it can occur from extreme anger, joy or sadness or other passions.[140] For passions or troubles which assail the mind are like winds and storms which whip up the waters of the sea and toss them hither and thither with great force. In the same way, our passions can so affect and disturb our humors that they toss them in all directions. So anger or displeasure can cause the menstrual blood, which was retained on account of the child, to be driven out, seizing the child and bearing it away with it, like a torrent sweeping away a large rock.

Thus it is very dangerous to refuse a pregnant woman something, especially when she is very given to strange desires, or has bad fits of anger and difficult pregnancies. Or on the contrary, it is dangerous

---

139. Renaissance physicians feared that denying a pregnant woman what she craved might be dangerous, either causing miscarriage (as Liebault goes on to explain) or leaving the physical imprint of the forbidden food on the foetus — a belief attested to in many Ancient writers, e.g. Hippocrates, *On Superfetation*, ch. 8; Galen, *To Piso*; Soranus, *Gynaecology* (trans. O. Temkin), I. x. Marinelli devotes a large part of a chapter (*Le Medicine*, 1574, III.6) to the subject of pica, or unnatural cravings.

140. Marinelli also cautions against excessive passions (*Le Medicine*, 1574, fol. 251ʳ).

for those women who are too patient and contain themselves, hiding their cravings, for their wishes and strong desires grow by virtue of being hidden. The Roman Emperor Marcus Aurelius[141] tells how Macrina, wife of the Roman consul Torquatus, died suddenly during pregnancy because of the strong desire she had to look at an Egyptian man who had a single eye in the middle of his forehead and who was walking down the street in front of her house. She dared not look at him because she did not wish to break her custom of not allowing herself to be seen at the window and even less to go out of the house while her husband was away (he being at war against the Volsci). The Senate greatly lamented the death of this virtuous lady, and some time later they remembered this tragedy, and among the privileges they granted to the Roman women who had shown great generosity towards the Republic at times of need, they included this one: namely, that a pregnant woman should not be refused anything which she asked for, provided it conformed with propriety and the law.

Ever since, the practice has been observed of complying with the wishes of pregnant women, and hence the common saying arose that refusing a pregnant woman something causes a stye in your eye, that is to say some punishment which, however small, will still be visible (like a blemish on the face). Not only would a man who refused to give a pregnant woman something she desired be punished, but the pregnant woman also, on account of the anger and displeasure she feels at her desire for some particular food not being met either during her pregnancy or while she was conceiving her child, would leave on some part of the child's body a mark of the thing she desired. Some have a mark like a cherry, others like a strawberry on one of their lips, or their nose or another part of their person. Some bear the mark of a fig, a melon, a cucumber or some other fruit on their thigh, leg, foot or other part of the body, all because the mother felt a strong desire for these fruits which could not be satisfied when they were out of

---

141. The anecdote appears in II. 89 of the immensely popular compilation by Antonio de Guevara, loosely based on the *Meditations* of Marcus Aurelius, which was translated into French in 1555 by Nicolas de Herberay des Essarts as *L'Horloge des princes*, and then from French into English in 1557 by Thomas North as *The Diall of Princes*. It is also cited by Duval: see 267-8.

season. Another may have a harelip or mouth, the head of a shad[142] or lamprey, because the woman desired them and could not have any.

One of my neighbors in the rue Calende was walking past a pie shop in the early days of her pregnancy and saw a piece of wild boar with the bristles on it hanging in the shop, and she wanted to eat some of the meat. Because her desire was not satisfied she gave birth to a child with a patch of black hair as large as the palm of your hand in the middle of its forehead. There is also a history of a woman who had a great craving to eat the flesh of a butcher when she saw his fleshy, bare, white arms.[143] Being overcome by this desire, she told the butcher of it, and he took pity on her, forthwith cutting a chunk of flesh from his thigh and giving it to her. The woman was delighted and immediately ate the raw flesh, and was fully satisfied. She gave birth to two boys, one of whom had a piece of flesh hanging from his lips, the other had his mouth permanently wide open. I have heard tell of another child, who had a deep red mark in one place on its hand, and this mark reddens and the colour becomes more apparent at the time of the grape harvest. It is said that when the mother was pregnant, she had a strong desire and an irresistible craving for new wine in mid-June[144] when it was impossible to obtain any.

Such marks on the child's body come, as we discussed in the previous chapter, from the strong imaginings or fears of the mother when she has experienced an extreme longing or desire, especially at the time of conception or throughout the time the child is taking shape within her womb — which can be about a month, according to Hippocrates, who says that thirty suns (or days) form the foetus, sixty give it movement, two hundred and ten perfect it.[145] And so it is, then, that the pregnant woman experiences her strongest cravings,

---

142. A river herring.

143. Liebault borrows this account from Levinus Lemnius, whose Latin work on *The Secret Miracles of Nature* (1559) had been translated into French. See *Les Secrets Miracles de nature* (Lyons: Jean Frellon, 1566), 66. Duval also uses this account: see 268.

144. Literally: on the feast of St John (24 June).

145. It was generally considered that the male child took shape over the first 30 days of pregnancy, the female over the first 42, the remainder of the pregnancy in both sexes being a period of growth of the foetus. See Hippocrates, *On the Nature of the Child*, 18. King offers an illuminating account of the Hippocratic understanding of conception as a gradual process (*Hippocrates' Woman*, p. 134).

having the greatest mass of retained excretory products.[146] In this first month, which is taken up with the conception and formation of the child, the strength of the imagination is such that it can imprint the shape of things on the seed which is conceived and starting to be formed, for it is malleable and easily takes on such imprints. When the child is fully formed, and when it is strong enough to move, it is no longer so subject to taking on these imprints if it is a question only of the mother's imagination, powerful though it may be. However, if this imagination causes suffering in the mother's body, it can cause such marks to appear on the child in the same place as on the mother. Now this imagining and desire for the thing the mother has wished for but been unable to have is so influential that, according to popular opinion, if while she suffers the desire the mother touches her own face, nose, eye, mouth, neck, throat or any other part of her body, a mark of what the mother desired will appear on the child in the same place. Thus some women advise a pregnant woman to put her hand on her behind if she cannot immediately satisfy her craving, so that the mark may be hidden, for it is better for the mark to be imprinted on the buttocks or some other area covered by clothing than to appear in a place where it would be seen. So a pregnant woman should not be refused anything at any stage of her pregnancy if she experiences desires and strange cravings, and especially not when she is conceiving or when the child is taking shape. This is what I had to say in respect of what she eats.

Immediately after her meals, she should rest on a comfortable bed, or in a low chair which leans backwards. For such rest allows the child to take its share of the food more easily. When it is not pressed by the mother's full stomach, it is strengthened by the energy the mother has derived from her food. Towards the eighth month, which is the most troublesome of all, she should restrain herself from eating and drinking as she is normally accustomed to do, because her stomach is growing, and she should start to take more vigorous exercise.[147] In the ninth month, it is good that she should bathe in order to relax the ligaments of the womb, and prepare herself to withstand with fortitude and forbearance all the pains and labors of the forthcoming

146. That is the retained menstrual blood and seed, which were believed to form the foetus.
147. Marinelli also recommends exercise at this stage (*Le Medicine*, 1574, fol. 252ʳ).

childbirth. She should also take care to keep her stomach and heart healthy, for these are the two organs of pregnant women's bodies that are most affected. To this end, it is good to prepare a powder or pill or opiate drinks of two corals, pearls, fragments of precious stones, preserves of roses, bugloss, borage and lemon peel, which should be consumed two hours before each meal. Or every morning she should take a slice of candied nutmeg or myrobolans. Externally, she should wear a stomach shield and rub her stomach with oil of musk, spikenard, wormwood, mastic, mint or nutmeg.

Chapter XXXII: Whether a Pregnant Woman Can be Bled and Purged without Danger

[I omit the earlier part of the chapter in which Liebault reviews classical advice on how much pregnant women should be bled, if at all, and at what stages of pregnancy it presents the least risk. The conclusion to the chapter is of most interest, since Liebault moves beyond other sources to express his own opinion on the relative sanctity of the mother's and the child's lives.]

We may therefore with confidence bleed pregnant women in case of urgent need when they are ill.[148] However, the quantity of bleeding needs to be decided with great care and prudence, with regard not so much to the extent of the illness and strength of the pregnant woman (according to which it might sometimes be necessary to let significant quantities of blood) as to the age and strength of the foetus. Since the foetus's wellbeing and health depend on a sufficient quantity of maternal blood to feed it, and allow it to grow and take shape, it cannot be protected if the letting of blood deprives it of its normal sustenance. For this reason, in the first months the bleeding should draw a small quantity, in the second trimester a still smaller quantity, and in the third trimester very little indeed, for the more the child grows, the more it needs to be fed.

Yet in judging the quantity of blood and bleeding, we should not be so concerned with the age and strength of the foetus that we neglect the health and life of the mother. Otherwise, even if you draw only a

148. Cf. the discussion of the same topic some 40 years later by Bourgeois at the start of the third and final volume of her *Obervations* (1626). She considers bloodletting in pregnancy as a relatively modern innovation, justified in cases of real need: *Diverse Observations*, Book III.

small quantity of blood, it will cause not only the miscarriage of the foetus, but will also thereby put the mother's life in danger. For there are some months during pregnancy when a woman who miscarries through illness necessarily dies, these being the eighth and fourth months,[149] as we have said previously, and in these months a mother miscarries for the least reason. This may result either from the nature of these months or from the great folly of the womb during these two months. Thus, during these two months, where possible, it is good to avoid bleeding her, as also (though less so) in the fifth and sixth months and those leading up to the ninth month. One may be bolder in bleeding the woman in the first three months for this same reason, for as miscarriage does not (generally) occur in these months,[150] when it does it is neither troublesome nor dangerous.

Yet experience shows that all miscarriages occurring during acute illnesses are dangerous to the mother. And we should not follow the misguided opinion of those who say that when the severity of the illness and other such circumstances require a great letting of blood, it is reasonable to draw a great quantity, and that it is better to run the risk of miscarriage by bleeding the mother than to expose the mother to death, and it is better to save the mother than to lose both the child and the mother. It is as though you were sure of the outcome of the bleeding, and as though you had made an agreement with God that if the child were lost the mother would be saved. For in addition to the fact that experience shows us that very few pregnant women who have miscarried during acute illnesses ever return to health, a pregnant woman who is seriously afflicted by a life-threatening illness which has affected her for a long time is often so weakened by this copious bleeding that she completely succumbs to the illness, and then cannot expel the child she has miscarried even when she is given the very best remedies.

149. Liebault is repeating general assumptions, drawn largely from Hippocrates. In particular, the danger of the eighth month of pregnancy (as opposed to the seventh or ninth month) is asserted in *On an Eight-Month Birth*, 2–3.

150. This statement blatantly contradicts current data on the rate of early miscarriage: up to three-quarters of miscarriages are now believed to occur in the first trimester. This difference in understanding may result from many early miscarriages having passed undetected in the sixteenth century.

Thus the greatest care must be taken in bleeding the pregnant woman right through her pregnancy, not only because of the risk of her miscarrying, but also to avoid undermining the health or causing the death of the mother. If the nature of the illness allows, and if the woman is strong enough to withstand the treatment, instead of bleeding her, it would be better to apply leeches or cupping to the armpits, groins or other such areas which allow the humors causing the illness to be cleared and drained. However, the thighs, legs and other lower parts should be avoided, for it would not be safe to rub these or to make an incision into the veins or scarify them, because such treatments could provoke the menses and cause the miscarriage of the foetus.

In place of bleeding, fasting may also be prescribed, by which I do not mean total abstinence and avoidance of food, but very great restraint, and very limited foods, such as just pearl barley, which can sustain the woman and the foetus for several days. It is better that such a fast should produce a baby which is weak, thin and sickly, but the mother alive, than that they should both perish, or at least risk an uncertain and perilous outcome. As for the regimen of a pregnant woman who is ill, it should be prescribed with regard to the strength of the woman and the kind of fever she has. If the fever is acute but she is possessed of good strength, restricted diet and activity are appropriate, especially since there are some pregnant women who were stout, plump and well fed before they became pregnant who can sustain such a diet for some time. If the woman is weakened, and if her strength is failing, she needs to be more generously fed, with frequent rather than large meals. In this way, the health of the mother and of the child will be protected.

Chapter XLV: The Way to Assist Pregnant Women When They Are Giving Birth

In order to assist women who are close to giving birth,[151] especially those who have very difficult deliveries, or who are fragile and

---

151. Marinelli has a chapter on the general regimen to be followed by women in the eight to ten days preceding the birth (*Medicine pertaining to Women's Diseases* [*Le Medicine partenenti alle infermita delle donne*], III. 9) and two chapters on the midwife's duties during

delicate, or who are expecting their first child, or who fear the pains and suffering of childbirth, the following methods should be used. They need to follow two kinds of regimen: the first over the period leading up to the birth, the other during it.

This is the regimen to be followed before the woman gives birth. She should eat nutritious and simple foods taking small portions but frequently. They should be foods which moisten without putting on weight, flavored with saffron and cinnamon, because cinnamon eases the problems of pregnancy and it is often mixed with the things a woman is given in case of a difficult labor, especially since the flavor of such drugs is fairly unpleasant. She should drink white wine or very good claret, mixed with a little water. She should avoid everything that can prevent labor as far as possible. If her abdomen is somewhat hard, whether it is naturally so, or as a result of the weight of the womb, or because of the hard matter which has accumulated in the bowels, she[152] should eat foods which have the power to soften and relax, like fresh figs, apples cooked in sugar and eaten on an empty stomach, especially if after eating them one drinks three or four mouthfuls of undiluted wine,[153] or if at least the cooked apples are soaked in the juice of sweet apples. If this does not cause her bowels to move, an enema of chicken or veal[154] stock will take care of the problem. Or a suppository of soap or animal fat, or egg yolk can be used, or a gentle medicine. Foods and sauces should be avoided if they have been roasted, fried or grilled, for some constrict, dry and constipate, or others produce a fluid which is rough and sticky, and they are difficult to digest.[155] Such foods include hard-boiled eggs, millet, panax, medlars, quinces[156] and other such

---

the birth (III. 10–11). Liebault's advice is not a direct translation of Marinelli, but covers some of the same areas, as indicated in the footnotes to this and the following chapter. Furthermore, like Marinelli, Liebault draws very closely in places on Rösslin's *Rosegarden for Pregnant Women and Midwives*. I indicate in the footnotes the sections where Liebault uses a verbatim translation of Rösslin; these can be conveniently compared with the modern English translation of Rösslin by W. Arons, *Eucharius Rösslin: when midwifery became the male physician's province*, 1994.

152. From this point, the text follows Rösslin closely (W. Arons, Eucharius Rösslin, 51), with some additions by Liebault, as indicated in subsequent footnotes.

153. Liebault adds to Rösslin's text the detail 'three or four mouthfuls of undiluted [wine]'.

154. Liebault adds 'or veal'.

155. The end of the sentence ('fried… digest') is an addition by Liebault to Rösslin's text.

156. Liebault adds 'medlars, quinces'. Compare his detailed recommendations on avoiding quinces in earlier pregnancy, 108.

things. She should rub her private parts, thighs, groin, lower back, and sacrum[157] with animal fat from capons, ducks or geese, or with a paste made from the seeds of quinces, fenugreek and mallow;[158] and she should apply to these parts anything which softens and relaxes, so that the birth passage becomes better lubricated, especially in women of an older age, since their private parts are already somewhat harder and drier.

A short while before the birth, when there are only two or three days left and when the pains are beginning to become sharper, the private parts, lower back and area around the perineum, in particular, can usefully be moistened. Or even better, the woman may once or twice get into a bath of lukewarm water in which leaves of mallows, pellitory, violet, artemisia, herb mercury, camomile, sweet clover, seeds of flax,[159] fenugreek and other such things have been boiled. And she should not bathe her whole body, only up to her navel. She should not remain in the bath for too long, but instead take baths more often. If she should not have the strength for taking baths, sponges soaked in an extract of this water should be applied to her loins, thighs, lower abdomen, private parts and all the body up to the navel. Steam baths should not be used on this occasion because they will weaken her too much. As she enters the bath she should inhale a chicken stock blended with egg yolk, a little saffron and cinnamon. When she gets out of the bath she should take one of the following crushed tablets.[160] Prescription:[161] of excellent cinnamon, one and a half drams; of fruit of cassia, bark of cassia, myrtleberry, half an ounce each, dissolved in water of artemisia; make an electuary. For tablets weighing two and a half drams, one to be taken on leaving the bath, followed by a very small draught of hippocras. Let her rub the parts of the body listed above with the fats listed above, or with this liniment. Prescription:[162] of oil of sweet almonds, two ounces; oil of lilies, fresh unsalted butter,

---

157. Liebault adds 'thighs, groin, lower back, and sacrum'.

158. Liebault adds 'and mallow'.

159. Liebault adds pellitory, violet, artemisia, mercurial, sweet clover, and seeds of flax to Rösslin's list.

160. The first part of this sentence ('As she enters …tablets') is added by Liebault.

161. In the French text, this prescription is given in Latin, with the abbreviations common to apothecaries' formulae. In all such cases, I have resolved the abbreviations in the translation.

162. In the French text, this prescription is given in Latin.

of each, half an ounce; of extract of nutmeg, linseed and fenugreek in water of camomile, one and a half ounces; with a very little wax, make a liniment. It would also be good for her to have this decoction injected into her lower parts, especially if she is thin or if her womb is dry and parched. She should also use perfumes made of musk, amber, nutmeg, musk wood, aloes,[163] and other things with a pleasing scent that have the power to open. On the days on which she does not bath, she should take a tablet of the electuary described above.[164] In addition, she should moderately exercise the body by walking, moving around, going up and down more than usual, shouting, becoming angry, handling things, stretching her arms, or travelling by carriage or on a gentle horse.[165] For such forms of exercise move the child around and greatly help it to be delivered.[166]

As for the regimen that is necessary at the time when she is giving birth,[167] that is to say once her labor pains have started and her waters broken, it is twofold. First, it should allow the child to be born easily, and secondly it should relieve the pains and travail of labor. So the woman giving birth should alternate between lying down to rest and walking to and fro, climbing up and down, jumping this way and that. She should hold her breath and hold in her lower bowels and abdomen, and take one of the tablets described above. And when she feels that her waters will run out with great force, then she should sit in a birthing chair intended for this purpose, which is open at the front, in which her body should be half reclining, as though half lying back so that she is neither completely prostrate nor completely upright.[168] Or she may be delivered in a bed to be more at ease, but her back should be slightly raised, so that she can breathe better and have the strength to push the child out. In addition,[169] she must keep her legs

163. Liebault adds 'aloes'.

164. Liebault adds 'she should take… above'.

165. Liebault adds 'becoming angry… horse'.

166. Many of these recommendations for stimulating labor are the direct opposite of the advice (104-13) for the regimen to avoid miscarriage in earlier pregnancy.

167. This section is also very close to Rösslin (Arons, *Eucharius Rösslin*, 53ff).

168. On debates about the use of birthing chairs, see xxvi-xxvii. Amongst ancient writers, Soranus described them particularly fully, recommending their use in straightforward labors (*Gynaecology*, trans. O. Temkin, II. ii). Marinelli also favors them (*Le Medicine*, 1674, III. 10, fol. 272).

169. The remainder of this paragraph ('In addition… pressing on them') is added by Liebault.

bent, her heels turned towards her buttocks, and her thighs apart, and she should press against a log of wood placed across her bed, having her buttocks slightly raised. Some women give birth standing up, being supported by several people, or resting their arms on the edge of the bed or on a bench. The best thing is for her to use a birthing chair designed for this purpose, *which should not be more than two feet above the ground*,[170] rather than on a bed or in another position, because the bones of the pelvis that must dilate at the time of birth will do so more easily if the woman is not lying or pressing on them.[171]

The midwife must be robust, careful, neither young nor old, accommodating, kind and strong.[172] She will stand in front of the mother, observing carefully her movements, the pains and laments of the woman, and she will comfort her, encourage her, assure her that she will be delivered safely and promptly; that her child will come out as it should; she will keep up her strength, giving her something to drink and eat from time to time. To encourage the mother, the midwife will tell her that she will have the child she wants, be it a boy or a girl.[173] She will touch her private parts and rub them with lily oil, linseed oil,[174] sweet almonds, or the liniment mentioned above.[175] When the mother has contractions, she will tell her to hold her breath, and to restrain herself as far as possible, and instead of shouting to block her nose and close her mouth.[176] A midwife may press down the upper part of the mother's abdomen, pushing the child down, for this greatly assists the delivery since she will not be so troubled by the contractions. If she is plump and rather fleshy, she should bend over

170. The specification 'which should... ground' is added in 1609 by Lazare Pena.

171. On the debate as to whether the pelvic bones actually parted during childbirth, see 32, n. 74.

172. This sentence ('The midwife ...strong') is added by Liebault. His advice conforms to the standard recommendations in other medical works, and builds upon common ancient recommendations. See for example Soranus, who opened his treatise with two chapters on the choice of midwife (*Gynaecology*, I. i-ii).

173. Marinelli says only that the midwife should promise a boy (*Le Medicine*, 1674, III. 10, fol. 273). This sentence ('The midwife ...strong') is added by Liebault. His advice conforms to the standard recommendations in other medical works of the period.

174. Liebault adds linseed oil to Rösslin's list.

175. Liebault adds the next two sentences ('When the mother... contractions').

176. This advice ('When the mother... nose and mouth') is also given by Marinelli (*Le Medicine*, III. 10, fol. 272).

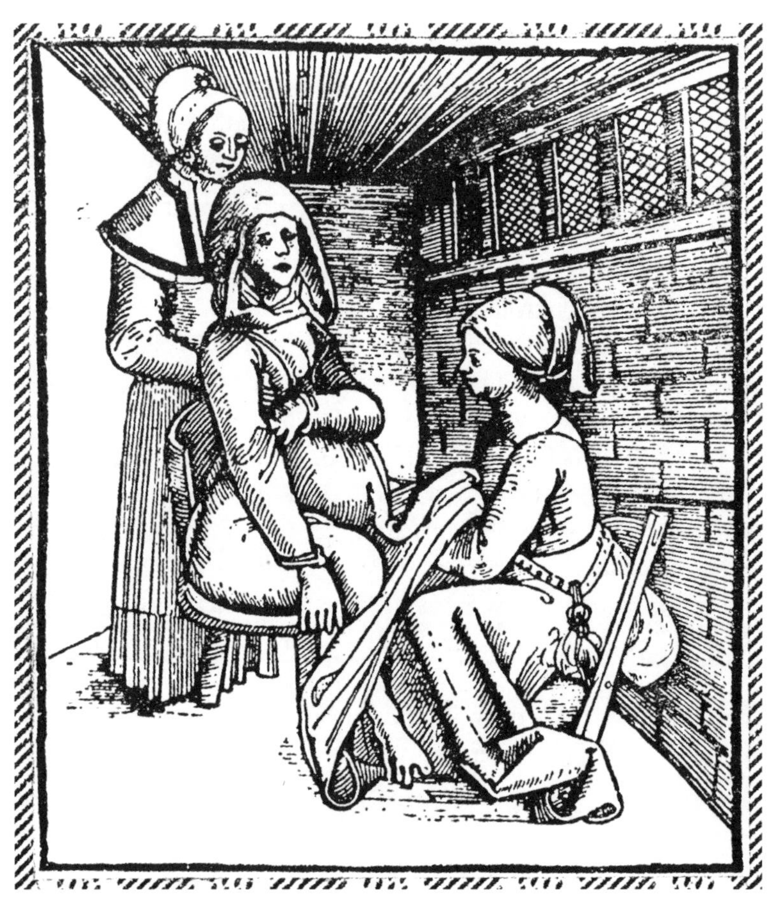

11) Woman giving birth in a chair

Eucharius Rösslin, *Der Rosengarten*, Strasburg, 1513
(Wellcome Library, London)

so that the womb is pushed and compressed further. If necessary the midwife should use her finger to open the birthing passage and relax it. If the waters have not yet broken, the midwife may tear the sack with the end of her finger or her nails so that the waters pour out and presently allow the child to be born.[177] If the waters have already broken, but the child has remained undelivered, the midwife should grease the woman's private parts even more so that they remain moist and become more open, for which she may use lily oil, linseed oil, etc.,[178] and she may also encourage the mother to sneeze. If the child's body or head is too big, she should do the same. The rest you may learn from midwives.[179]

If[180] you see that she is in labor for rather longer than either her strength or her delicate constitution can withstand, give her half a dram of the confection of alchermes,[181] blended in a drink with wine or water flavored with artemesia; or give her shavings of ivory, or heart of deer, or coral, or some of the inner partitions of the nutshells of unripe walnuts. Or the powdered droppings of a sparrowhawk finely ground with good red wine.[182] Or aetite,[183] or white magnetite,[184] fastened to the inside of the thigh, very close to the groin. Or the sloughed skin of a snake tied around the abdomen. Or a belt made of the skin of the animal the Poles call an elk, wound around the thigh.

177. Similar advice is given by most classical authorities, e.g. Paul of Aegina (*The Medical Works of Paulus Aegineta, the Greek Physician*, ed. and trans. Francis Adams, London: J. Welsh, 1834, 647).

178. Liebault adds linseed oil, etc.

179. Liebault is drawing a distinction between what physicians should know (the general procedures) and the specific expertise of midwives. Rösslin, apparently writing for midwives, gives some more details of helpful procedures. There are some similarities with Marinelli's advice (*Le Medicine*, III. 10, fol. 269), but Liebault is not providing a direct translation.

180. Compare Rösslin (Arons, *Eucharius Rösslin*, 64ff). Liebault and Rösslin offer many common recommendations, but Rösslin's advice is more detailed, and he lists the remedies in a different order. Duval draws some of his advice (Ch. XIX) from this section of Liebault (see 273-4).

181. A widely prescribed tonic, which could include raw silk, apple juice, ground pearls, musk, ambergris, leaf gold, rosewater, cinnamon, sugar and honey.

182. This remedy, and several of the following (the aetites and snake's skin), would be familiar from Pliny the Elder's *Natural History* (XXX. 44).

183. A stone traditionally used in Antiquity to prevent miscarriage and to shorten labor. In his pharmacopeia (*De materia medica*), Dioscorides, the Greek physician and botanist of the first century, recommends that the parturient mother should wear it attached to her thigh.

184. Again, traditionally employed to ease childbirth.

But as soon as the woman has given birth, remove the aetite, the white magnetite, the snake's skin, or the belt of the elk's skin, since it is said that such remedies have a secret power to draw the womb down.

See several more remedies in the next chapter. See also our work *The Country Farm* [*De la maison rustique*],[185] Book I, ch. 10, where we talk about a clear water that is marvelous for easy deliveries.[186]

There are even stronger and more powerful remedies, which learned and well-versed physicians do not know. The first kind lies within Nature itself, others within the skill and judgment of the physician. The third kind is known to few.[187] Nature is often her own remedy, she contains within herself the seeds of her own strength; she draws balm and elixir from her own treasure store. Within Nature, God has hidden everything that is necessary for such extreme action. Even if all the art a physician can imagine proved without strength, Nature would have the resources to ensure her own survival; provided she is not disturbed, she has her appointed time, her fixed season, to which she keeps before revealing her actions. This is her time of maturity, and for this reason she has her fire and her celestial flame[188] that are hidden; these are a source of heat and run through all the essential parts, the microcosm without and within, in the center and on the surface. Furthermore, this fashioning spirit, this divine source of creation which runs through all the limbs of this embryo and this shapeless mass, which fashions the noble parts of the foetus, is within Nature and comes only from Nature's providence. And since Nature has used only her own strength to shape the child, so too she applies no strength but her own to expel it, so that everything moves and shifts when Nature speaks.

185. Charles Estienne's original Latin text (*Praedium rusticum*) was published in 1554; a French translation, largely produced by Liebault, followed, under the title *L'Agriculture et maison rustique*, in 1564; it was then translated into English as *The Country Farme* by Richard Surflet in 1600.

186. In 1609, Pena omits this paragraph ('See several… deliveries') and instead adds a substantial new section to conclude the chapter ('There are even stronger… consult him on this', italicized in my translation). He expounds a neoplatonist view of the supremacy of Nature, with which the mother and physician must co-operate. Many of his ideas in this chapter develop the neoplatonist arguments expounded in his prefatory 'Letter to Chaste Young Women', 81-88.

187. This is the Wood of Life or Eloctis described on 125-6.

188. Throughout this section, Pena's language and imagery reflect neoplatonic concepts, such as the divine fire (the heat of which is present in the unborn child).

The womb, which had embraced the child like a captive or prisoner, and had seemed to hold it forcibly, powerfully rises up, relaxes, and pushes it as though by the shoulders; the pubic bone, the sacrum, the hipbones, which had compressed the foetus on all sides to prevent its exit, miraculously widen and open at the front. The whole body shudders marvelously; the face reddens, pain runs through all parts, above, below, in the groin, the womb, the loins; it is all gripped by the horror; Nature summons all her instruments, and deploys all her strength to give birth to what she has conceived. Thus, within Nature lies the strength to form, shape and expel. In addition, this same Nature, which caused the violent, agitated movement, calms it again with little help. Just as Nature opened it, so she closes it back up, reuniting the bones and the cartilage. Just as she fanned, so also she gives heat back to the tired limbs and restores them through a gentle rest. She had used her own strength, the human spirit; the heat of the heart; the air of the lungs; the spirit of the whole body, which is a strength concealed and hidden in all things created and which one Arab writer has called 'the spirit which preserves, retains and expels' the menstrual blood; the waters; the womb, and the strength of the child which itself instinctively pushes once it has reached maturity. The same Nature uses these same instruments to comfort, restore and cure.

Thus a woman's prudence lies in her respecting Nature in its entirety, without disturbing its workings, as far as she possibly can. Everything depends on this harmony and order, as a philosopher has said. If she learns from a physician to harness and control her disordered appetites, to live without dissipation or excess of sweetmeats; if she restrains her desires, her mouth and her harshness, she would experience almost no pain. If[189] a woman eats in a single day a hundred types of food, all differently disguised,[190] if she overburdens her liver with a cock's testicles and crests, sparrows, larks, testicles of small fish, mushrooms, lizard's or crocodile's liver, wines, cinnamons, sugars, various sauces, fish disguised in three hundred ways, as in the kitchens of Pius V,[191] are not these

189. In this sentence, Pena effects the transposition from his exposition of general neoplatonist philosophy to a satirical attack on women who live at odds with the rules of Nature.

190. I.e. presented with rich sauces.

191. Pena probably cited Pius V (Pope 1566–1574) because the Pope's personal chef, Bartolomeo Scappi, had written a very popular five-volume *Works* [*Opera*, 1570], treating

enemies of Nature? Moreover, a woman will stay in bed for 15 hours without expending any energy, whereas Nature requires movement, exercise, and a change of air. She then spends the rest of her time combing her hair, looking in her mirror, colouring her skin, and does not leave her chair as she imagines castles of love on the Cape of Hope.[192] If she does bestir herself, it will be to undertake some delicate movement underneath her bedcovers, shamelessly douching her womb with various distillations of different kinds that corrupt it and make it smell as foul as a carcass.[193] In short, all her excesses lead only to the ruin of Nature and undermine all her strength. Which means that in childbirth, women are subject to cruel symptoms and strange attacks, for in this extraordinary action, Nature finds herself so weak, exhausted, devoid of all power that she cannot push out the child, and often causes these women to suffer a cruel death; whereas, if you go to Arabia, Macedonia or Egypt, which are warm, burning countries, and where women have very narrow wombs (whereas here in northern countries, and especially in Paris, the girls are rarely ever virgins), nonetheless, because these women are full of energy, work, do not spend 15 hours lazing in bed, and do not fill their stomach with so many sweetmeats and various sauces, they give birth almost without pain. You will even see some Arab women deliver their child on the sand, without crying out or moaning, and then they themselves wash the child in the river.[194] Even here in villages of France, you will see peasant women give birth without great trouble, whereas these precious ladies, whose wombs are amply able to stretch and are as large as the wombs of three Egyptian women together, moan like the Greek Furies.

This is because they do not respect the order and harmony of Nature; if care is taken of her, Nature is her own cure. You will have no need of drugs or of a physician; Nature needs little, she lives on natural things, she detests all false sophistication, she loves movement, exercise and air, she seeks out what is natural not artificial; she wants the truth not a mask. Thus the woman must learn from her physician the regimen to follow,

---

Italian cuisine, including recipes for elaborate feasts, and with a predilection for marinades and sweet spices.

192. An ironic allusion to women's taste for reading romances.

193. A reference to the practice of douching the vagina with medical or cosmetic treatments.

194. Pena, like many of his late Renaissance contemporaries, subscribes to a version of the myth of 'primitive', distant countries in which women are reported to give birth naturally and without pain.

consult him often; tell him all our[195] *physical and mental sufferings so that by mature, wise advice he may teach her the remedies of Nature. And if it happens that Nature is not strong enough to relieve the patient, as often occurs in extreme cases, the physician will immediately provide suitable remedies, such as the following. He will instruct the husband or another person (it must be a man)*[196] *to put his hand on the navel and to push down with moderate force; he will apply comforting epithemes*[197] *to the heart, and by mouth he will give her viper's water or theriac, and after this the strongest concentration of red cinnamon water, celestial water. He will use everything necessary to reinvigorate and restore warmth to the heart, for in the whole of Nature there is nothing which has such a strong expulsive force as the strength and might of the heart; if you let it become weak, you will see only misery result. In Egypt, two men, one each side, take the woman's arms, and apply pressure under her armpits, which has the power to push the foetus down. It has been proven that there is nothing which helps push so well as the following drink: one grain of ambergris, two grains of musk dissolved in aqua vitae, in which infuse equally small quantities of betony water and chicory water.*[198] *This draught achieves a marvelous effect without harming the patient's health. There is also a salve that has the same effect of relaxing the areas around the womb. Prescription:*[199] *one ounce of butter, one ounce of grease dissolved in aqua vitae and blended as well as possible. Then smear the whole region from the navel to the groin, and repeat frequently. You will see a miracle. There are a myriad of remedies to be found here, there and everywhere, but the majority of them are useless and the prudent physician will avoid them.*

And if ordinary medicine cannot cure this cruel state, yet there is some other hope before the surgeon's irons need to be applied: it is the Wood of Life, sometimes called Eloctis, which comes from the Indies. This wood is celestial green in appearance, although in fact it contains all colours and is no single colour. Fierce snakes and poisonous, dragon-like

195. The use of the first person plural form of the possessive adjective is surprising, but suggests that Pena is referring to the sufferings that are the lot of all humanity.

196. Here Pena blatantly contradicts Liebault's earlier instruction (119) that a midwife or female assistant should apply pressure to the top of the womb to hasten the birth.

197. I.e. poultices or lotions.

198. In the French text, this prescription is given in Latin.

199. In the French text, this prescription is given in Latin.

lizards guard it.[200] *Those who would obtain it cover themselves from head to foot and over one hand wear an iron gauntlet, while in the other they carry a phial of clear water with which to dampen the dragons' fury. When they have taken the branch from the tree, they prepare it in an extraordinary fashion, and then give some of it to their wives. After this, the women give birth without pain. If you come across it, keep it most carefully for your lady, for she will conceive without difficulty. Its strength is such that the merchants who bring it to Europe do not suffer from sadness or fall prey to despair. It so strengthens the heart and the noble organs that it powerfully drives out anything which is damaging to the health, and it is especially effective for women giving birth, for just the scent of it makes a woman deliver immediately and without pain. No one has described it and known it other than the Babylonian writer Avicenna, so we must consult him on this.*[201]

Chapter XLVI: Difficult Births

Difficulties in giving birth[202] come mainly either from the mother, or from the child. Often they come from the outside air being too cold or too hot.[203] Sometimes they come from the ignorance of the midwife.

200. This may be one of the earliest references in western European writings to the komodo dragon (a member of the monitor lizard family, found in various Indonesian islands).

201. I have not been able to trace a reference to the term *'Eloctis'* in Avicenna or any other obvious source, but suspect Pena is referring to agarwood (known in Latin as *'lignum aloes'*). Although it is not specifically mentioned in the section of Avicenna's *Canon* that deals with difficult births (Liber III, Fen 21, tract II, ch. 31), it is listed in the treatise on medical cordials [*Libellus Avicennae de medecinis cordialibus*] at the conclusion of sixteenth-century editions of the Canon, where it is specifically said that *'lignum aloes'* relaxes all limbs (Avicenna, *Liber canonis*, Venice: apud Iuntas, 1562, fol. 564ʳ). The resin from agarwood (the resinous heartwood produced on aquilaria trees as a reaction to mould) was increasingly exported from Southeast Asia from the 1580s onward, and valued for its medical powers when burned as incense or used as the basis of essential oil.

202. Compare Rösslin (Arons, *Eucharius Rösslin*, Ch. 3), which lists 18 reasons for difficult births. This chapter owes little directly to Marinelli (who listed more causes of difficult births in *Le Medicine*, 1574, III. 9, fol. 269); I indicate the few small borrowings where they occur. Instead, Liebault draws parts of his advice from classical sources which discuss difficult births, notably Hippocrates, *On the Diseases of Women*, I; Soranus, *Gynaecology* (trans. O. Temkin), IV. i-iv; Aetius of Amida, *Tetrabiblus*, XVI.

203. Rösslin cites these as the 13th reason for a difficult birth (Arons, *Eucharius Rösslin*, 48).

They come from the mother[204] if she is too fat, misshapen, too short, too thin, too young,[205] too old, naturally weak or weakened by illness like hemorrhage, delicate, sickly, fearful, prone to give birth prematurely, or very late such as in the eleventh month.[206] Or if she has consumed astringent foods during her pregnancy,[207] she has been sad; she suffered from hunger or thirst; she often inhaled musk, amber, civet or other such scents that, as we said before, draw the womb upwards.[208] Or if, during her labor, she suffers from contractions that do not compress the womb, but stop around the navel.[209] Or if her womb is misshapen, the birth canal too unyielding, hard, narrow and constricted; she has some tumor, pain, ulcer, wart, rhagades or hemorrhoid at the top of her lower parts or in one of the neighboring parts, such afflictions preventing these places from being able to open fully.[210]

They come from the child when the membranes around the child are so tough that they do not break in the course of labor; or when they are so weak that they break at the very onset of labor, which means that later these parts are not moist and well lubricated.[211] Sometimes also, the placenta comes first, and such deliveries are called '*filius ante patrem*' ('the son before the father'), and they are the most dangerous of all.[212] Sometimes when the placenta is broken it causes blood to pour out and fill the womb so that the mother cannot push the child

204. Marinelli also divides his causes into those coming from the mother and those from the child (*Le Medicine*, 1574, 269).

205. Cf. Rösslin (Arons, *Eucharius Rösslin*, 46), who cites as the first reason for difficult childbirth a small uterus when the woman has become pregnant before the age of 12.

206. This list is similar to what Rösslin (Arons, *Eucharius Rösslin*, 46) cites as the fifth reason for difficult childbirth; Rösslin also specifies premature or post-mature deliveries as the tenth reason (*Eucharius Rösslin*, 47).

207. Rösslin cites this as the 14th reason for a difficult birth (Arons, *Eucharius Rösslin*, 48).

208. Rösslin cites this as the 17th reason for a difficult birth (Arons, *Eucharius Rösslin*, 49).

209. Rösslin cites this as the 18th reason for a difficult birth (Arons, *Eucharius Rösslin*, 49).

210. Cf. Rösslin (Arons, *Eucharius Rösslin*, 46), who cites as the second reason for difficult childbirth afflictions which prevent the uterus and vagina from opening fully. The third and fourth reasons in Rösslin concern specific injuries to the bladder or anus (such as hemorrhoids).

211. Rösslin cites the excessively hard or weak chorion as the 12th reason for a difficult birth (Arons, *Eucharius Rösslin*, p. 48).

212. Liebault is describing the condition now termed *placenta praevia*, in which the placenta occupies the lower segment of the uterus, partially or completely obstructing the opening of the birth canal.

out, just as when the bladder is too full and one cannot urinate. If the child is too weak it is unable to help the mother.[213] The same is true if it is too large, or if its head is too big, or it is misshapen, or if it does not present with the head first with the hands by the side, but rather both feet first, or just one foot presenting first, which is more dangerous, or one or both of the hands presenting first, or if it presents badly, doubled over with the buttocks first, or in a transverse position with one side first, or the stomach first.[214] All of these positions for birth are contrary to Nature, for the natural position for a child to come out of the womb is head first, for, as Hippocrates says,[215] the upper parts are the heaviest. If the child is female,[216] if it is stillborn,[217] if it is a twin,[218] if it is accompanied by a mole, or if the womb is filled with stones, grit or sand, a difficult delivery can be anticipated. So too, when the waters in the allantoid membrane run out long before the child comes out, or if a hemorrhage happened a long time previously, or if the labor pains occur separated by long intervals, are weak because the cotyledons have scarcely broken and the membranes of the amniotic sack take a long time to break away from the wall of the uterus.

The signs of a difficult delivery can most often be recognized only from the account of the woman in labor and from several other indications. It is possible to tell if the child has died in the womb from the coldness of the womb, the dull eyes, white flecks in brown eyes, bad breath, decaying matter running out of the lower parts.[219] The height of the child can be determined from how tall the father is and how short the mother is, thus you will work out the rest.

213. Cf. Rösslin (Arons, *Eucharius Rösslin,* 47), who cites a baby that is too small or too large as the seventh reason for a difficult birth.

214. Liebault has listed here all the major irregular presentations, illustrations of which commonly circulated in treatises such as Rösslin's. These presentations are cited by Rösslin as the ninth reason for a difficult birth (Arons, *Eucharius Rösslin,* 47).

215. On cephalic presentation, see Hippocrates, *On an Eight-Month Birth,* X. 2.

216. Rösslin cites as the sixth reason for difficult childbirth (Arons, *Eucharius Rösslin,* 47) the delivery of a girl rather than a boy.

217. Rösslin cites as the eleventh reason for difficult birth (Arons, *Eucharius Rösslin,* 48) a very weak or dead foetus.

218. Rösslin cites as the eighth reason for difficult childbirth (Arons, *Eucharius Rösslin* 47) the delivery of twins or of babies with two heads.

219. Rösslin deals at length with detecting foetal death, listing these and other signs (Arons, *Eucharius Rösslin,* 87–88).

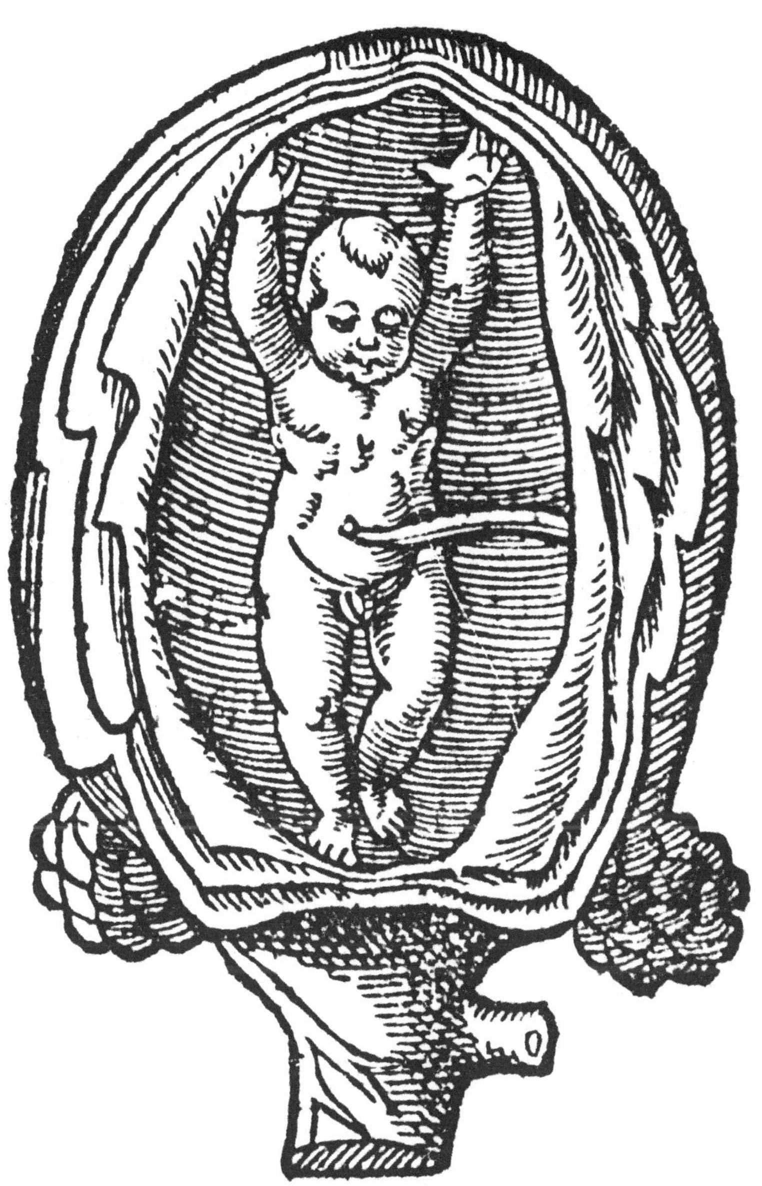

12) Foetal malpresentation: footling breech

Jacques Guillemeau, *De l'heureux accouchement*, Paris, 1609
(Bibliothèque nationale de France)

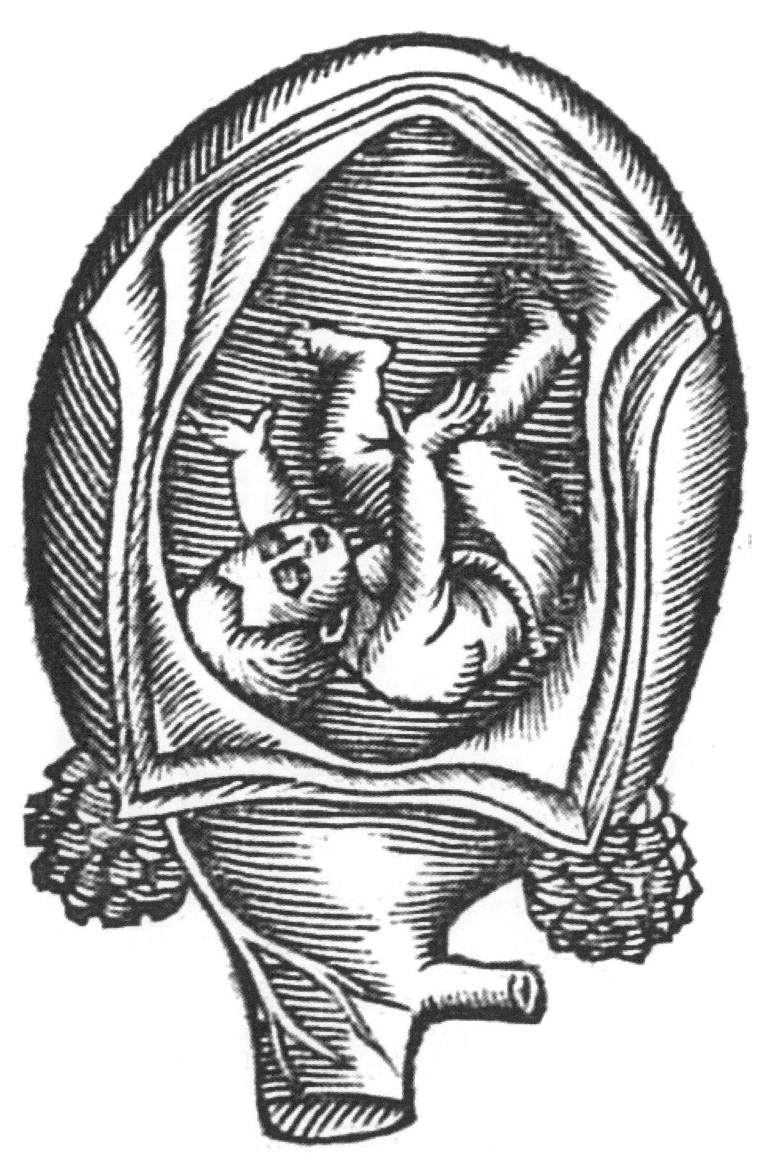

13) Foetal malpresentation: transverse lie

Jacques Guillemeau, *Les Œuvres*, Rouen, 1649
(Library of Royal College of Obstetricians and Gynaecologists, London)

If the pain[220] is situated in the chest and the internal parts near the womb, in a healthy woman this is a sign the delivery will be successful, especially if she is of good courage and has powerful breath. But the mother and child face great danger if the opposite signs are present, for all difficult deliveries cause all kinds of other problems, as well as the risk to life. Often there is a violent force which causes the peritoneum to rupture near the navel and groin, so that the intestines spill out, and a hernia develops, or the vein of the chest or the womb bursts, causing them to collapse, and phthisis results with spitting of blood and coughing, and sometimes the pupils dilate and the vision clouds over, as Avenzoar[221] noted. In his book on The Secrets of Women, *Albert the Great says that some births are so difficult that all the bones break, and a gash runs right from the rectum to the womb, as I have often observed, and yet it is not a rupture but rather a tear in the skin.[222] This is much worse, for with my own eyes I saw quite a strong woman suffer such a dreadful concussion because of Nature's powerful efforts that her eyes came half out and her bones were completely exposed, and the abdomen above the womb was torn apart from the neck of the womb to the very top of it — the damage was evident, and the child and the mother died two hours later.*

It must be acknowledged that there are natural causes cited above, and, over and above these, excessive passions which consume all the strength and power of material, living, natural spirits, and which deplete and drain the basic moisture,[223] which narrow the passages to the liver, or in the same way cause the womb to shrivel, and so totally destroy the foetus that all that is left is a lump of dry stone, so devoid of energy and health that it cannot ever leave the womb without violence and danger for mother and child. And moreover, if one taps on the outside of the abdomen of the mother about to give birth, the same rigidity results,

220. The following paragraphs from 'If the pain is situated …' to '… servant of Theology' (italicized in my translation) are added by Pena in 1609, and reflect both his medical training and his theological beliefs.

221. Avenzoar, or Ibn Zuhr, a famous Muslim physician of the twelfth century who practiced in Seville.

222. See H. Rodnite Lemay, *Women's Secrets. A Translation of pseudo-Albertus Magnus's 'De Secretis Mulierum' with Commentaries* (Albany: State University of New York Press, 1992), 107.

223. I.e. upsetting the balance of humors. In childbirth, desiccation is the imbalance most commonly cautioned against.

an example of which was seen in Chambery.[224] *For the violence of a blow so altered the child's position and posture, and so astonishingly undermined the strength of both the womb and the child that at the time and for two months afterwards the womb was quite unable to open, and the child (which was still alive) did not have the strength to move or be born. And so all the cruel instruments*[225] *had to be applied to seize the child, and after this Nature has allowed this woman to conceive again.*

Nature has her order and her rules, she relies on weights and counterweights. If you unbalance these, you will produce only confusion. Furthermore, Avicenna teaches that in the very matter of the womb there is an innate force, as though it possessed its own intelligence which would act to expel the foetus, and if it loses this strength, the child will die in its prison and will not be able to escape without the use of violence.[226] *Thus anything which takes away this strength makes the delivery painful and difficult, and anything which increases it makes it easy and unlabored.*

Now apart from these natural causes, there is a higher cause that must be acknowledged, which surpasses every cause and effect in nature, and that is God's anger at man's sin.[227] *For the lamentations, cries, distress and horrible pain that woman suffers in childbirth, and the misery and danger man endures in being born are precisely the scourges of God's just vengeance which chastises both in their flesh for man's rebellion. Mohammed said that at this moment*[228] *the Devil plunges his claws into the woman's entrails and tears her apart to the point of death, and that he rains blows on the child like a torturer sent by God to punish this crime. If this is not literally true, it is true as far as the pain is concerned for, as one of the Fathers of the Church says, it seems that all of Nature gathers together in this mortal body all the afflictions and cruel sufferings it could imagine. There are a million wild animals on earth, all of whom give birth without help or assistance, without groaning or writhing. They have no drugs or doctors, they are not covered by any blankets or*

224. Presumably an allusion to an unusual case of this kind witnessed by, or reported to Pena.

225. I.e. surgeons' irons and knives used to extract an impacted foetus.

226. See the section of Avicenna's *Canon* that deals with the anatomy of the womb (Liber III, Fen 21, tract I, ch. 1).

227. Pena refers to the condemnation of woman to pain in childbirth because of original sin (Genesis 3:16).

228. I.e. of giving birth.

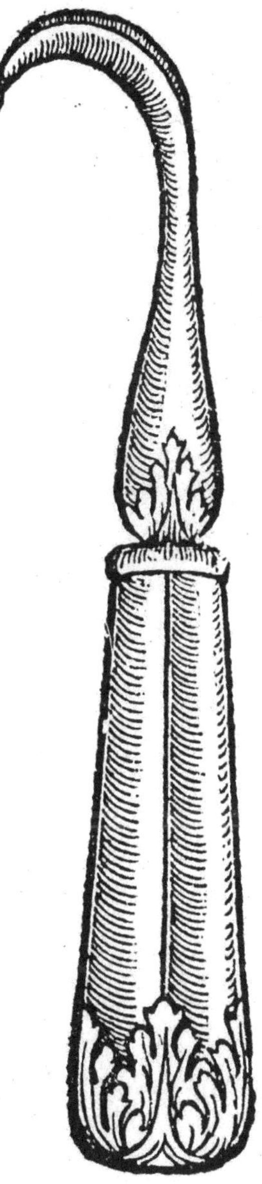

Illustration of a knife to cut into the swollen part. It should be of a size such that it can be easily held in the hand in order to incise and open the head, chest or abdomen.

14) Surgeon's knife

Jacques Guillemeau, *De la grossesse et accouchement des femmes*, Paris, 1620
(Library of Royal College of Obstetricians and Gynaecologists, London)

curtains in rooms kept at the temperature of eternal spring. Rather, they give birth in the middle of the countryside, in winter, surrounded by the snows, and they labor with no danger to their own life or that of their offspring. Yet woman, who is made in the image of God, who rules over these animals, is not granted this privilege by the heavens. Thus, in this act her status seems much lowlier, as though she were lower than the animals. This is why we must so admire the greatness of God's judgment, and accept that Medicine is only the servant of Theology.

In order to manage difficult deliveries in general, you will need to follow the method I described for births, in addition to which I would add that women in labor should often hold their breath, not constricting the throat, but pushing against their lower parts. Let them walk up and down, move about, go up and down and make vigorous movements. You should cause them to sneeze, as is recommended in aphorism 35 of Book V (*'Difficulter partenti superveniens sternutatio, bonum'*).[229] Let them be given pungent enemas in order to clear the mass of excrements, and during the contractions which they will experience, let them try to combine those of the bowel and of childbirth. Let them make regular use of the common remedies, which I shall now describe: let their private parts be rubbed frequently with the oils, greases and liniments mentioned above. As for specific remedies, they should be followed according to the cause of the problem.

If the problem lies with the mother, think about her and prescribe what is appropriate for her condition, which is the cause of this difficult labor. If she is weak, feed her little and often. If she is frightened, embolden her by giving her good hope, and do likewise for other conditions. If the amniotic membranes have broken and the waters all run out, you should frequently moisten the private parts with oil, grease, and a moistening decoction.

If the problem lies with the child, because it is feeble and weak, which you can tell because its movements will be feeble and delayed, the woman must make a strenuous effort to push the baby out with the contraction of her abdominal muscles. If the problem is caused by the baby's bad position, the midwife should try to correct it, partly by pushing, partly by pulling, partly by bending and partly by guiding

---

229. Hippocrates writes, 'Sneezing occurring in a woman affected with hysterics, and in difficult labor, is a good symptom.' (*Aphorisms* V, 35)

it in a straight line.[230] If the hand or the foot presents first, do not try to pull the child by this limb, for you will either wedge it lower in the womb, or you will dislocate or break the foot or the hand. Instead, put the foot or the hand gently back into place with your fingers.[231] If the child does not present straight in the birthing canal, push it back into the womb, then turn and position it so that it can come out straight. If the child's body, head, buttocks or chest are too large, try by every means you can to moisten the womb and the neighboring parts, both internally and externally. If the amniotic membranes are too tough and will not give way, you will have to puncture them with your fingers or cut them with scissors, but without damaging the child.

If, despite all these remedies, and others which you and the midwife may try according to what you judge necessary in each case, the child still does not come out, do not, I beseech you, resort to the hand of the surgeon unless you are sure that these methods have been often repeated yet are ineffectual, and that the hand of the midwife cannot do anything more. Remember that God works great miracles, and Nature achieves incredible things, and that very often Nature, as Galen says in the second book *On the Causes of the Pulse*, will use every means she possesses when she senses that the situation is extremely grave. Here are some remedies you may try before you have recourse to the surgeon.[232]

Give her this medicine. Prescription:[233] squeeze two and a half ounces of excellent theriac, infused in the juice of parsley, with one scruple of cinnamon and dissolve in it castoreum; and one scruple of powder of bark of cassia and one ounce of syrup of artemisia; make a potion.

Another prescription: bark of flower of cassia, date pit, cartilage, the center of a nutmeg, of all of these one scruple; make a very fine

230. Rösslin looks in detail (Arons, *Eucharius Rösslin*, 56–62) at handling each of the common foetal malpresentations, accompanying his recommendations with the illustrations borrowed from Soranus. Liebault gives very similar recommendations.

231. This is standard advice, found in most classical writers from Hippocrates onward (*On the Diseases of Women*, I. lxxv).

232. Liebault recommends that both physician and midwife try everything before allowing the surgeon to intervene, indicating that he views the actions of the surgeon as a threat to the life of either the mother or child. Unlike Marinelli (*Le Medicine*, 1574, III. 11, fol. 284–5), he does not recommend the reciting of prayers and psalms.

233. In the French text, his sequence of prescriptions is given in Latin.

powder with two and a half ounces of the juice of sweet parsley with white wine. Make a potion.

Another prescription: cinnamon, bark of cassia flower, dittany, of all of these one scruple; make a powder to be taken with a concoction of linseed.

Another prescription: bark of cassia flower, two ounces; chicory, blackberry, half a minim; boil with equal parts of white wine and water, adding at the end two drams of savin; prepare for one dose; dissolve cinnamon, half a dram, of saffron six grains; make a potion.

Another prescription: root of blackberry tincture and round birthwort, of each one ounce; dried leaf of calamint, pennyroyal, savory, thyme, lesser centaury, of each half a minim; make a decoction in watered honey.

The perfumes of laudanum, belladonna, alipta moschata, amber, artichoke applied to the womb. Perfumes made from foul-smelling things applied to the nose. It is said that the perfume of an ass's nail applied to the womb, although foul smelling, delivers the foetus from the womb.[234] Fomenations and liniments, moisturizing and relaxing baths of the private parts, loins, lower back, thighs and other areas near the womb. Bitter, moisturizing enemas introduced either into the rectum or the womb. Pessaries made of powdered juniper and aristolochia, powder of the electuary benedicta laxative, powder of white hellebore, powdered pigeons' droppings mixed with mercury honey,[235] adding myrrh, castoreum and asafoetida.[236] Apply cataplasms to the lower abdomen. Prescription:[237] of the decoction of pulp of bitter apple, one pound; juice of rue and of savin, of each three ounces; mix with lupin flour; make a plaster from the navel to the pubis and right to the groin.

It is said that one should attach coral, aetite, weeping storax,[238] or green coriander, or root of buckwheat to the right thigh; and let root of henbane be attached to the left thigh. Let a vulture's feathers be tied

---

234. This advice ('Perfumes… womb') is also found in Marinelli (*Le Medicine*, 1574, III. 10, fol. 278).

235. A compound of equal parts of honey and the plant mercurialis.

236. A spice also known as devil's dung.

237. In the French text, this prescription is given in Latin.

238. A scented resin.

under the soles of the foot in order to bring about easy childbirth.[239] If despite all these remedies the child does not come out, recourse must be had to the hand of the surgeon, which may be used in two ways. The first, by pulling it out. The other, by cesarean section, which we shall speak of hereafter.[240]

239. This recommendation derives from Pliny the Elder's *Natural History*, XXX. 44.

240. Chapter 49 of Book III is devoted to the methods of extracting the foetus from the womb, and is largely derived from Rösslin and Ancient sources. However, while talking mainly about techniques to deliver a foetus vaginally, Liebault acknowledges that in the last resort cesarean section may be attempted to save the life of the mother: 'The manner of these three incisions has been fully described by Charles Estienne in his *Anatomy*, and after him by the very learned François Rousset in his book on cesarean delivery, and we advise you to read this book in order to learn how you should conduct such a dangerous undertaking.'

JACQUES GUILLEMEAU

On the Safe Delivery of Women
(1609)

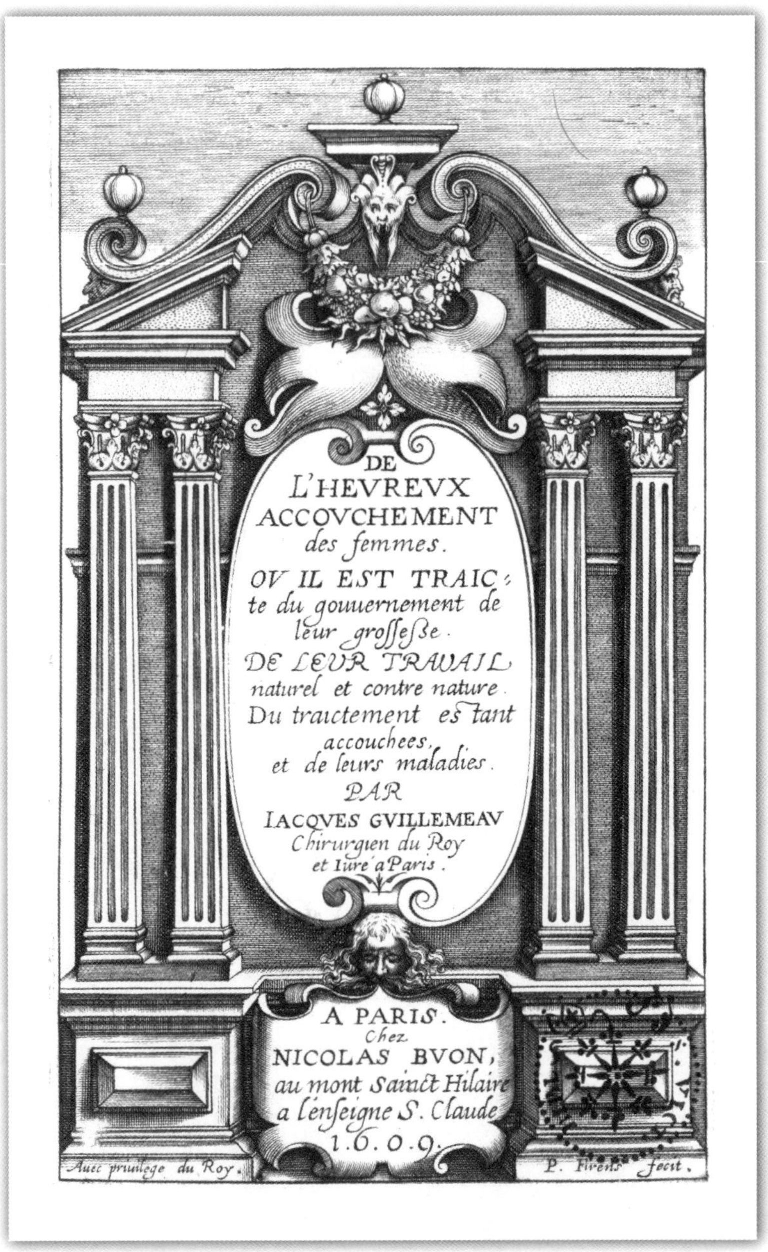

15) Title page: Jacques Guillemeau, *De l'heureux accouchement,*
Paris, 1609

(Bibliothèque nationale de France)

INTRODUCTION

TRANSLATION OF EXCERPTS FROM
ON THE SAFE DELIVERY OF WOMEN (1609)

Preliminary texts

Book I

Book II

Book III

INTRODUCTION

Guillemeau's treatise on obstetrics and neo-natal care appeared the same year as the first volume of the *Diverse Observations* by the royal midwife, Louise Bourgeois. It provides a particularly valuable insight into a respected and well-educated surgeon's perception of childbirth, at a time when specialist surgeons were adopting an increasing role in deliveries in Paris.

Life and Works of Jacques Guillemeau and of His Son, Charles Guillemeau

Jacques Guillemeau was born in Orleans in 1549, and grew up in an established family of surgeons.[1] He learned his skills from his father, who worked alongside Ambroise Paré as surgeon to three successive kings, Henri II, François II and Charles IX, until his death in 1569.[2] Paré then accepted the young man into his household in Paris, and although Guillemeau spent periods studying in Montpellier (the other foremost center of medicine and surgery in France), Paré's influence remained formative; Guillemeau cites his mentor with great respect in his own writings. As a skilled anatomist, Jacques Guillemeau was one of the surgeons who took part in the autopsy on the body of Charles IX in 1574, but it was not until 1577 — after some three years as a surgeon to the armies of Philip II of Spain in the Netherlands — that he was appointed as a royal surgeon, under Henri III. During the 1580s, Guillemeau took up permanent residence in Paris, working at the Hôtel-Dieu hospital when not at court. After the death of Henri III in 1589, his position as royal surgeon was — exceptionally — reconfirmed by Henri IV, whose autopsy Guillemeau also conducted in 1610, and then by Louis XIII. In the last 15 years of his life, as Paris emerged from the scars and chaos of civil wars, Guillemeau appears to have enjoyed a stable and rather successful professional life, which allowed

1. For a full account of the lives of Jacques and Charles Guillemeau, see the older biography by F. Poulain, *La Vie et l'œuvre de deux chirurgiens: Jacques Guillemeau (1550–1613) et Charles Guillemeau (1588–1656)*, (Montpellier, 1961), and the more recent one (which has corrected the date of Jacques Guillemeau's birth) by P. Dubard, *La vie et l'œuvre de Jacques Guillemeau* (2006).

2. See Dubard, *La vie et l'œuvre de Jacques Guillemeau*, 32.

him to buy an elegant residence for his family in the rue des Billettes (now the rue des Archives). Of his five children who survived infancy, Charles — born in 1588 — followed in his father's footsteps, becoming surgeon to Louis XIII in 1618, and then continued his social ascension by qualifying as a physician in 1627.

Both father and son took a particular interest in obstetric surgery and medicine, and Guillemeau was one of a small group of Parisian surgeons who appear to have been summoned by noble or elite families to attend difficult deliveries,[3] either alone or with Monsieur Honoré, the foremost 'accoucheur' of the early-seventeenth century. It is also undoubtedly proof of Jacques Guillemeau's high reputation that he was called to deliver Mlle Simon, daughter of the late Ambroise Paré, when she was in danger of dying from an acute hemorrhage during labor.[4] There are even indications that in some cases families would routinely have Guillemeau attend a birth, rather than simply relying on a midwife, even if no complications were anticipated.[5] Through Guillemeau and Honoré, we witness the first signs in early-seventeenth-century Paris of what would, over the next 50 years, become the fashion for delivery by experienced male surgeons.[6] It is notable that at the birth of the Dauphin in 1601, Guillemeau was present, as royal surgeon, although Louise Bourgeois actually carried out the delivery. When the Queen had a breech delivery in 1607, the king ordered Honoré to stand by also, even though in the event his intervention was not needed.[7] These surgeons were clearly specialists

3. See for instance his reports of the delivery of Mlle Danzé, in 1603, in *On the Safe Delivery of Women* [*De l'heureux accouchement*, 1609, 224]. This episode and others not included in the present volume are available (in English trans) on my research website: www.birthingtales.org.

4. *On the Safe Delivery of Women* [*De l'heureux accouchement*], 1609, 221.

5. He cites a case in which, after the midwife had overseen what appears to have been the routine delivery of a baby, he delivered the placenta, only to discover the mother was about to give birth to a second child: *On the Safe Delivery of Women*, 285.

6. On the much wider movement towards medicalized deliveries undertaken by surgeons in the following century, see J. Gélis, *La Sage-femme ou le médecin. Une nouvelle conception de la vie* (Paris: Fayard, 1988), 291–327.

7. See the reports of the royal births by Bourgeois, *A true account of the births of my lords and ladies the children of France with the noteworthy particularities thereof* in *Diverse Observations*, O'Hara and Klairmont Lingo, Bk II. See also my analysis of Bourgeois's report of the birth of the dauphin: 'La théâtralisation de la naissance du dauphin (1601) chez Louise Bourgeois, sage-femme de Marie de Médicis', in *Le «Théâtral» de la France d'Ancien Régime*, ed. S. Chaouche (Paris: Honoré Champion, 2010), 137–154.

in the field of obstetrics, even if their experience could hardly have matched Bourgeois's claim, in her *Observations*, that she had attended more than 2,000 births.[8]

We know of Jacques Guillemeau's practice primarily through his impressive series of books on surgery and medicine, which owe more than a little to his apprenticeship under Paré.[9] Despite his good knowledge of Latin, Guillemeau, like Paré, chose to publish only in French, a decision that ensured his writings were accessible to his fellow surgeons.[10] His works fall into two categories: comprehensive overviews of anatomy and surgery,[11] and specialized treatises on the two areas that particularly interested him, ophthalmology,[12] and obstetrics and neo-natal care. In the latter fields, his two volumes, *On the Safe Delivery of Women* [*De l'heureux accouchement des femmes*], a weighty tome of some 450 pages, and *On the Care and Upbringing of Children from the Very Time of their Birth* [*De la nourriture et gouvernement des enfans, des le commencement de leur naissance*], comprising just over 200 pages, both appeared for the first time in 1609.

Circulation and Afterlife of
'On the Safe Delivery of Women'

Jacques Guillemeau's two volumes achieved a relatively wide circulation in French in the half-century after their first appearance, initially being reprinted three years later (1612) as part of his *Works on Surgery* [*Œuvres de chirurgie*]. After his death, both works were taken

---

8. *Diverse Observations*, O'Hara and Klairmont Lingo, I. 14.

9. Dubard points out that we have very few documents relating to Guillemeau's earlier life in Orleans or his life in Paris before he acquired a house in 1597 (*La vie et l'œuvre de Jacques Guillemeau*, 2 and 107), hence the particular importance of his published writings.

10. Although it was assumed for a long while that Guillemeau was responsible for the translation into Latin in 1582 of Paré's *Œuvres*, it is now agreed that his role was limited to oversight of the work of the anonymous translator. For a comparison of the French and Latin versions, see I. Pantin, 'La traduction latine des *Œuvres* d'Ambroise Paré', in *Ambroise Paré (1510–1590). Pratique et écriture de la science à la Renaissance. Actes du Colloque de Pau (6–7 mai 1999)*, eds. E. Berriot-Salvadore and P. Mironneau (Paris : Honoré Champion, 2003).

11. *Anatomical Tables* [*Les Tableaux anatomiques*, 1586], a work heavily indebted to Vesalius, and *French Surgery* [*La Chirurgie française*, 1593], extended and republished as *Works on Surgery* [*Les Œuvres de chirurgie*, 1598].

12. *Treatise on the Diseases of the Eye* [*Traité des maladies de l'œil*, 1585].

over by his son, Charles, who significantly extended them for a new edition in 1620.[13] The first volume bears a slightly revised title, *On the Pregnancy and Delivery of Women* [*De la grossesse et accouchement des femmes*]. Charles added to it a short treatise of his own, in French, on impotence.[14] Further editions of the revised works appeared in 1642–3 and 1649, suggesting that it continued to find a ready public before the volumes of Mauriceau came to dominate the vernacular market in the later-seventeenth century.

Jacques Guillemeau had dedicated both volumes to two leading court physicians, whom he numbered among his close colleagues and friends,[15] but specified in his prefaces that his work was addressed above all to young surgeons, especially those living outside major towns (and thus away from the centers of medical instruction). However, he included a preliminary letter to women in *On the Care and Upbringing of Children,* exhorting them to breastfeed; this points towards both a professional male readership and a lay female one. Charles Guillemeau is even more explicit: while still aiming to instruct inexperienced young surgeons, in his preface he also addresses his work to those ladies who are too modest to uncover themselves in the presence of their physicians, and to midwives in need of some tuition.[16] Thus, professional medical women join the two previously designated groups of readers.

Charles Guillemeau extends his father's two treatises on an even more substantial scale than that of Pena's additions to Liebault's text.[17] The 1620 edition of *On the Safe Delivery of Women* is almost

13. Some reissues of the 1620 edition are dated 1621.

14. *Treatise on Errors which are committed in Legal Proceedings concerning Male and Female Impotence* [*Traicté des abus qui se commettent sur les procedures de l'impuissance des hommes et des femmes*].

15. *On the Safe Delivery of Women* was dedicated to André du Laurens (first physician to the Queen, Marie de Medici, and then also to Henri IV), and *On the Care and Upbringing of Children* to Jean Héroard, the physician to the royal children.

16. Charles Guillemeau's terms suggest that he considers some midwives to be inadequately trained, an attitude which is also reflected in his sharp criticisms of Bourgeois for apparent errors in delivering the placenta after Madame, the king's sister-in-law, had given birth in 1627, and which he believes caused her subsequent death. Yet, ironically, Bourgeois's *Diverse Observations* had precisely appealed to physicians and surgeons to provide anatomical training for midwives, as Klairmont Lingo shows in her section on the 'Organization, Style and Tone of the Three Volumes' in Bourgeois's *Diverse Observations*.

17. See 68-69.

double the length of the original version, and includes engravings (for example, of the surgeon's hook and knife[18] and of various foetal malpresentations).[19] As far as the additions are concerned, Charles Guillemeau has both interpolated his own comments into many of the chapters written by his father, and included many new chapters. Thus, where the three books of the 1609 edition by Jacques Guillemeau contained 18, 25 and 11 chapters respectively, in 1620 they stand at 22, 28, and 48, while *On the Care and Upbringing of Children* has grown from 28 to 39 chapters. It is clear that Charles Guillemeau's major contributions occur in the third book of *On the Safe Delivery of Women*, and they reflect his particular interest in post-partum and neo-natal care, with, for example, nine new chapters about the breasts and fifteen about diseases of the womb. As to the chapters authored by his father, it is only rarely that he excises anything; instead, he adds new material ranging from a half sentence to several pages, most often in order to develop a medical explanation of a condition.

An English translation of Guillemeau's original 1609 edition was published in London, printed by A. Hatfield, within three years, entitled *Child-birth or, The happy deliverie of women: Wherein is set downe the government of women. In the time of their breeding childe: of their travaile, both naturall, and contrary to nature: and of their lying in. Together with the diseases, which happen to women in those times, and the meanes to helpe them. To which is added, a treatise of the diseases of infants, and young children: with the cure of them. Written in French by James Guillimeau the French Kings chirurgion.* It provides a very close translation of the French text, the anonymous translator describing his work in the short Translator's Preface as 'the shadow' of the French original.[20] It is clear from the preface that the English translator is more uneasy about the need to use direct language to speak of the woman's reproductive organs than Guillemeau had been — even though Guillemeau's language is relatively chaste and restrained in comparison with the styles of, say, Paré, Joubert or

---

18. 238 and 245 respectively.

19. 249, 253, 258, 265, 266, 269,272, 276, 278, 280, 284, 287. These are modeled on the Muscio illustrations, which had been used in the French translations of Rösslin.

20. I quote from the online version of the 1612 edition available at Early English Books Online.

Duval.[21] However, vernacular books on reproductive health were still a rarity in early-seventeenth-century England as compared with France, hence the translator's apology for addressing not only 'the literary common-wealth of Physicke', and surgeons and midwives, but also those female readers who hesitated to consult a physician on matters of such delicacy. We may surmise that the book also found a receptive audience in England, since there was a reprint of the translation in 1635.

It is quite possible that but for Mauriceau's rise to pre-eminence with the publication of his *Diseases of Women with Child and in Childbed* [*Maladies des femmes grosses et accouchées*] in 1668 and the ensuing popularity of his works, Guillemeau's treatise might have continued to circulate for longer. In the event, Guillemeau is drawn upon by Mauriceau as a source, both openly acknowledged and also silently pillaged, and some of Guillemeau's case histories in particular[22] are thus given a further lease of life.

Structure of 'On the Safe Delivery of Women',
and Selection of Chapters for Translation

Whereas each of Liebault's three books dealt with a different state of womanhood (unmarried, married but not yet pregnant, and pregnant or giving birth) and combined the treatment of what would now be termed gynecology and obstetrics, Jacques Guillemeau selects his material mainly from the field of obstetrics, discussing pregnancy (Book I), delivery (Book II) and the health of the mother and child after birth (Book III). It is noteworthy that he hardly discusses conception, a subject that preoccupies most of the physicians writing on the subject of pregnancy and birth. Inevitably there are overlaps between Liebault and Guillemeau, but their approaches are primarily distinguished by their different professions — physician and surgeon. Even when Charles Guillemeau revises the work in 1620, he is still writing as a surgeon (albeit nurturing aspirations to become a physician), and his

---

21. The translator claims, 'I have endeavored to be as private and retired in expressing all the passages in this kind as possibly I could', 8.

22. E.g. Madame Du Pescher voiding a bucketful of waters.

style is not markedly different from his father's in the way Pena's was from Liebault's.[23]

Given the length of Guillemeau's treatise, I have needed to be selective in the choice of extracts for inclusion in this volume. In order to provide useful comparisons with the other writers, I have concentrated on chapters from the first and second books, rather than those dealing with post-partum and neo-natal care in the third. I have given priority to Guillemeau's general advice applying to all pregnancies and deliveries, since this displays most clearly his particularly caring attitude to his patients. However, I include several chapters focused on his surgical expertise, namely the delivery of a dead foetus, and the excision of a living foetus from a dead mother.

Guillemeau's Arguments and Style

It may seem paradoxical that a surgeon, who would normally be called to intervene only in difficult labors, should devote so much of his manual to normal pregnancies and deliveries as well as complicated ones. However, Guillemeau's title, *The Safe Delivery of Women*, expresses well his over-riding concern: that the mother and child should both survive the birth, whether this be, in his terms, 'natural' or 'against nature' ('*contre nature*'). Hence, his advice concerns both straightforward and complex cases. It is particularly important to note that at various stages in the treatise, in a manner reminiscent of his mentor Paré, he states that a safe birth depends ultimately on God's help:

> If they do this, women will be confident of being delivered
> safely and joyfully, and they will know that with the help of
> God they will bear their fruit to its full term, and it will be
> born into the world without great difficulty, assuring them
> of a prompt and safe delivery.[24]

23. In the analysis that follows, I draw primarily upon the parts of the work written by Jacques Guillemeau, since his approach and style still determine the character of the volume re-edited in 1620.

24. See 178. Cf. the remark in Book II, ch 5: 'For in this way the mother and child will regain their strength and the child will be ready to be born at the hour ordained by God'.

This conception of the surgeon as assistant to God or Nature accounts for the notably modest tone of Guillemeau's writing, which distinguishes him from most other contemporary authors of medical works.[25]

However, his diffidence — coupled with a wish to avoid unnecessary controversies — is counterbalanced by a quiet confidence in his own judgments, for he clearly believes himself well qualified to provide advice both for midwives and surgeons, as well as indirectly for pregnant women. His assertion that he has attended over five hundred deliveries over forty years[26] would suggest an average of some twelve a year, although I would conjecture that he undertook more deliveries in the last decade of his career.[27] Thus, while he has less first-hand experience than Bourgeois, he could nonetheless draw widely on personal observations as well as theoretical expertise.

His usual approach is to proceed from general physiological axioms, and then support or develop these with reference to classical authorities or case histories, while being prepared on occasion to nuance or even correct his sources.[28] At a minor level, for example, he gives general advice on how much sleep is needed by the pregnant woman, citing Hippocrates in support of his warning that she should not linger too long in bed in the morning, but finally making the personal concession that 'she may rest until nine o'clock'.[29] However, in the same chapter, he argues against Hippocrates's dictat that

25. See, for example, the self-effacing language at the start of chapter 6 of Book I, when he advises the woman on how to conduct herself during her pregnancy (the italics are mine): 'Now that I have prescribed the regimen a pregnant woman should follow throughout her pregnancy, she should also follow, *if she judges it good*, the recommendations I shall set out *which are not entirely necessary, but useful and helpful* to preserve her beauty and also her health.' De Serres's style is comparable to Guillemeau's in this respect (see 301-2).

26. See 187.

27. Most of the accounts of specific births in *On the Safe Delivery of Women* relate to the preceding decade or are described as 'of recent memory'. This fits with the fact that Guillemeau now spent more of his professional time in court circles, and also reflects the fact that the practice of summoning surgeons specialized in childbirth appears to have become increasingly common in Paris around the turn of the seventeenth century.

28. As will be seen in some of the footnotes accompanying my translation, Guillemeau's references to classical sources are sometimes inexact. It is probable that in such cases he was relying on memory (or an erroneous secondary source) rather than writing with the primary text before him. For a surgeon, the principles and practical recommendations seem to have been more important than the classical authorities.

29. See 175.

pregnant women should not be purged from the fourth to the seventh month, maintaining that 'today physicians ignore this when necessary' since they use weaker drugs for the purpose.[30] Even on the most controversial of subjects, such as cesarean sections on living women, when he puts forward strongly held views, it is still in very measured language, without any disparagement of his adversaries. He frames his opposition to the procedure with an objective and dispassionate choice of words: 'Some believe that... I cannot advise this... I know that it may be argued that...'[31]. On another divisive question, the choice to be made in extreme cases between the life of the mother and the child, Guillemeau takes care to state the arguments neutrally, while urging the surgeon to delay as long as possible before ever extracting a living child with the hook. Ultimately, he simply acknowledges the heavy responsibility such an operation imposes, deliberately leaving the theoretical debate to the theologians.[32] His careful wording suggests that in the last analysis he would save the mother over the child, but he is not prepared to take sides openly in this most contentious of issues.

How far does Guillemeau's advice on the conduct of pregnancy and delivery match the calm tone of his style? First, this is a surgeon who would rather wait as long as Nature requires for the delivery to be accomplished without intervention. He would rather act only when necessary, and even then always with due concern to minimize suffering on the part of the woman. Secondly, it is the safe delivery and the physical and mental wellbeing of the mother that lie at the heart of his work, so that the reader instinctively believes him when in his introductory epistle to the reader he claims that he wrote his work because:

> I have sought a means of helping [pregnant women] in their labor, whether natural or contrary to nature, and of supporting them in the accidents that may occur during their delivery.[33]

30. Ibid.
31. See 205, 214, ibid.
32. See 211.
33. See 159.

Like other surgeons and physicians, he certainly finds occasion to castigate midwives (and relatives) who delay too long in summoning a surgeon for a difficult delivery,[34] but he is even more insistent that 'the midwife's duty is not to rush or hurry anything'. The waters should not be broken, nor the membranes stripped, and the midwife needs to establish that the woman is in true labor before urging her to use her contractions.[35] Above all, the midwife, like the surgeon, must carry out her tasks with a combination of gentleness and dexterity. Hence, Guillemeau repeatedly advises the midwife to lubricate her hands with greases before performing internal examinations, and when the head crowns, he emphasizes the need for her to act 'gently' and 'neatly':

> [...] the midwife should cradle it gently between her hands, and when it is delivered and the mother's contractions increase, she should pull the shoulders out neatly, slipping her fingers under the armpits, choosing the opportunity and moment when the contractions are intensifying and she can gently grasp the child.[36]

Given the growing role of expert surgeons in deliveries in Paris around this time, it is important to emphasize that nowhere in the treatise is Guillemeau looking to medicalize normal deliveries, or to suggest that the tradition of a normal delivery supervised by a midwife assisted by several women is unsatisfactory. Rather, he urges the surgeon to verify whether any intervention is needed, and to ensure that all those present are convinced of the necessity of his actions. It may seem surprising that much of the introductory epistle to the reader is devoted to an extended comparison between surgical interventions in obstructed childbirth and other surgical operations. Yet Guillemeau is writing as a general surgeon, who seeks to demonstrate that, *when necessary*, surgical intervention in childbirth is as essential as other surgical operations — and requires even greater skill because of the difficult conditions of conducting operations (via the vagina) without clear vision of the affected part.

34. See Liminary Epistle to reader, 158.
35. See 201.
36. Ibid.

However, it should be noted that in the chapters on extraction of a dead foetus — a procedure undertaken in order to save the mother's life — Guillemeau writes in a vein radically different from Liebault the physician.[37] As a skilled operator, he has no fear of the hook or irons: while stressing that the foetus should be handled 'gently', to minimize trauma to the mother, he insists that 'if [the mother's] strength is visibly fading, the safest thing is to intervene manually'.[38] Despite furnishing very precise instructions to the surgeon-reader on the conduct of this gruesome operation, Guillemeau remains sensitive to the mother, advising that the surgeon should take his cue from her contractions, and urging that she should be given 'the chance to regain her strength' between the delivery of the head and the rest of the body. The patient is referred to sympathetically as 'the poor woman'; she is to be given some wine, to dull the pain, and above all, she is to be encouraged by the surgeon and those present. Emergency deliveries may sometimes require skilled technical intervention on the part of the surgeon, but the birth is not thereby depersonalized in Guillemeau's eyes.

Indeed, the large number of anecdotes of actual deliveries throughout the work — with both happy and sad outcomes — are testimony to Guillemeau's conviction that childbirth is an experience that profoundly affects individual women. He may be giving general guidelines, but he is well aware that they will be applied to specific cases. Equally, although he has his own preferences on subjects such as diet, exercise or position for delivery, he allows that different women may exercise a degree of personal choice. Thus, although he personally believes women are more comfortably and will be more safely delivered lying in a bed — a view that was to come to prevail over the next century — this is accompanied by the acknowledgment that 'it is quite certain women do not all give birth in the same fashion'.[39] The prescriptive tone and approach of many later 'accoucheurs' are certainly not present in Guillemeau's treatise.

How far can we surmise that Guillemeau's particular style of writing contributed to the success of the work over the first half of the seventeenth century? In answer, it is important to bear in mind his key

37. See 135.
38. See 208.
39. See 195.

readerships: less literate or less experienced surgeons, midwives and interested lay readers. On the one hand, the work can be understood without the level of professional or technical expertise that much of Rousset's treatise anticipates. Nor, on the whole, is the physiological discussion as specialized as in Liebault; rather, Guillemeau seeks to make his knowledge accessible to a wider readership. On the other hand, he does offer some very detailed instructions to both midwives and surgeons — how to tie the umbilical cord, how to perform podalic version — but this is achieved without the use of overly technical language. On occasion, he also draws analogies with common objects to allow the reader to grasp his description, such as advising the midwife that the bulging bag of waters prior to the onset of full labor will resemble 'a bottle, or rather a bladder that protrudes and is full of water.'[40] In addition, the various case histories make the work more readable and memorable, and give readers the strong impression — rather like Bourgeois's *Diverse Observations* — that they are being allowed a privileged professional insight into the world of childbirth in early-seventeenth-century Paris.

40. See 200.

TITLE PAGE [1609]

ON THE SAFE[41] DELIVERY

of women. In which is described
how to look after them in
pregnancy, and in labor both
natural and contrary to nature.
On the care of them when they are
delivered, and on their illnesses.

BY JACQUES GUILLEMEAU, surgeon
to the KING, and sworn in Paris.

IN PARIS,

From the press of NICOLAS BUON,
at the Mont Saint Hilaire,
at the sign of St Claude.

1609.

41. The English translation in 1612 used the cognate form 'On the *Happy* Deliverie…', and recent critical studies in English have usually continued to refer to the work in this way. However, in modern English, the phrase 'safe delivery' seems more accurate. I am grateful to Alison Klairmont Lingo for her comments on this point.

TITLE PAGE [1620]

ON THE PREGNANCY AND DELIVERY OF WOMEN.
On looking after them and the manner of treating the accidents which befall them.

BY the late Jacques Guillemeau,
surgeon to the KING.

Revised and expanded with illustrations from
engravings. And on several secret illnesses.

With a treatise on impotence
BY Charles Guillemeau,
ordinary surgeon of the King.

IN PARIS,

From the press of ABRAHAM PACARD,
at the rue St Jacques,
at the sign of the Sacrifice of Abraham.

M.DC.XX.[42]

---

42. Unusually, the title page of the 1620 edition (like the 1621 reissue of it) makes no reference to the Privilege that the volume contains.

PREFATORY EPISTLE [1609]

To Monsieur du Laurens,[43]
Sieur Deferriere, Counsellor to the King,
and First Physician to His Majesty

The greatest satisfaction that man can have is to live in good health. Those who are in ill health simply languish; not only are their humors altered, but also their behavior. For the person who is naturally good and even-tempered will be made irritable, cross and hateful by illness. This led Galen to believe and write that our manners often follow the temperament of the whole body. This is why if each of us is charitable, we should try (as far as lies within us) to ensure the health of our neighbor. This charitable design has led me to publish this book so that, just as previously (when young) with my hand, so now with my pen, I may help pregnant women, including through the offices of our young surgeons dwelling at a distance from the advice and help they can obtain from good towns. They will find in it what may usefully assist them not only to deliver the women safely, but also to relieve them from some accidents and events which may befall and trouble them after the true labors of their delivery.

Now as I often chanced to be under your authority in such matters, notably serving the greatest ladies of the realm,[44] and as I observed and learned, both from your learned and wise counsels and from your weighty writings, various lessons and good rules pertinent to this matter, I thought that I should be failing in my duty and guilty of the vice of ingratitude if I did not acknowledge in my turn that, as the main inspiration of this undertaking, you are owed the chief honor for all this work. I dedicate to you all I have written on the subject, as though to a god who, acting as protector through the splendor and magnificence of his guarantee, will be able (this

---

43. André Du Laurens (1558–1609) was a celebrated anatomist and professor of medicine at Montpellier before becoming physician to Henri IV and Marie de Medici.

44. An allusion to Guillemeau's presence at the deliveries of both the Queen, Marie de Medici, and of other noble women at court. For futher details see my article, 'La théâtralisation de la naissance du dauphin (1601) chez Louise Bourgeois, sage-femme de Marie de Médicis'.

I beg in all humility) to defend it against jealous attacks from all ill wishers.

Your most humble and most affectionate servant,

Guillemeau.

Paris, this 1st April 1609.

[1609]

LIMINARY EPISTLE, TO THE READER

Although man is the most perfect of animals, nonetheless by his nature he is so weak and so subject to various accidents that the great Hippocrates judged that from his birth man was illness itself. He cannot, he said, be useful in anything while he is still being suckled, since he relies on the help of another. Then, as he grows, he becomes bad and unruly, needing a master to instruct him; and when he reaches the flower of his youth, he becomes audacious and proud; then, in his decline, he is wretched, left with only the memory of his misspent labors.

Pliny[45] comments, and experience demonstrates to us, that just the noxious smell of a snuffed-out candle can cause the child to die in the mother's womb; or she may miscarry and deliver him before his time, and he will not have the strength to resist and defend himself. And even if he remains in the womb until the time appointed by nature, most frequently he would not be able to be born safely, even if he presents naturally, without the help I do not say of the mother, nor the help he can give himself, but also that of the midwife and of the several other people present with her, receiving and caring for him. And what is worse, if he is badly positioned, feeble or weak, and the midwife's knowledge is exhausted, in order to save the child and also the mother from death, the surgeon must be called to deliver the mother and bring the child into the world. This, let me say in passing and without reproaching anyone, is often done too late because of the stubbornness of relatives and midwives.

And even if the child is born by his own efforts, without the help of the surgeon or any midwife, he still brings his death with him, as it is said, which he clearly demonstrates by the cries and wailings he makes as soon as he sees the light of day, seeking help and succor. For if he remained in the state in which he comes forth from the mother's womb, accompanied by his afterbirth (or 'bed')[46] which he brings with him, doubtless this afterbirth would putrefy and infect the child, and

---

45. *Natural History*, VII. 7. 43.

46. In middle French, the afterbirth is popularly called the '*lit*' or bed.

in the end this decay would cause his death. In addition, often if a drainage passage were not made in his rear or his penis, or in a girl's private parts, which are sometimes obstructed, he would be unable to suckle or to dispose of his excrements, nor would a girl (when she reached the right age) be able to have her menses. This would cause them to choke and suffocate. Often, also, his head and other parts of the body, like the arms and legs, would be misshapen, or even broken and dislodged from their sockets, and it would never be possible for these limbs to return to their rightful and natural place. So it is most necessary that the surgeon apply his hand, acting with great dexterity, so that everyone can clearly see that the operation is essential and well-founded, for the first operation which was performed in the world was an omphalotomy, or cutting of the umbilical cord, which Adam and Eve performed on their firstborn.[47]

This is what prompted me to publish this book and in it to deal with various illnesses which befall pregnant women. I have sought a means of helping them in their labor, whether natural or contrary to nature, and of supporting them in the accidents that may occur during their delivery. I was further spurred on to this by reading the lament of Soranus,[48] who said:

'O male occupatum virorum genus, occidimur nos, non morimur: et ab illis qui inter vos peritissimi existimantur perperam curatae: vos de qualibet levissima vestrarum affectionum libros ex libris facientes, bibliothecas voluminibus oneratis, et nostris interea diris ac difficillimis cruciatibus nulla vel exigua mentione facta.'

['Oh race of men, you use your time ill; we are driven to the point of death, we do not die. And by those amongst you who are considered the most expert, we are wrongly treated. You write book upon book on the slightest of your afflictions, you fill libraries with heavy volumes,

47. Genesis 4:1 records the birth of Cain, but with no mention of the cutting of the umbilical cord, although the previous chapter contains the oft-quoted verse, 3:16, in which God condemns Eve and her descendants to suffer pain in childbirth as a consequence of her disobedience in the Garden of Eden.

48. Soranus of Ephesus (93–138), whose important treatise on gynecology was available in manuscript in Heidelberg in the early-sixteenth century (and thus possibly consulted by Rösslin), but remained unpublished until the nineteenth century. Various Latin translations and Greek epitomes preserved significant fragments of it, so that Renaissance physicians or surgeons such as Guillemeau knew it indirectly, largely through the abridged translation by Caelius Aurelianus.

and we, meanwhile, are tortured with the direst and most grievous pains of which you make not the slightest mention.']

I had intended, some 15 years ago, to write something on this subject in my work on surgery,[49] but after reflecting at length I thought it more expedient to make it into a separate treatise, since the subject merited it on account both of its inherent difficulty and of my great wish to discuss a number of things which can occur in these circumstances. And in truth this operation is greater, for its antiquity, and the importance and the skill required, than all the others that are carried out on the human body.

As to its antiquity, without doubt the first operation that was performed in the world was the omphalotomy or cutting of the umbilical cord, which Adam established, as we said above, when he performed it on his firstborn.

As far as its importance is concerned, some may perhaps advance the claim that delivering women is not as important as the following operations: stopping hemorrhages, whether from veins or arteries; trepanation; opening an oedema; cutting someone suffering from dropsy, or skillfully drawing blood from a vein. As far as hemorrhages are concerned, it must indeed be said that if they are not arrested, through the loss of blood one will eventually lose one's life. However, we need to consider that often they stop of their own accord, and nature (which is wise and provident) usually controls and stops them. I have found myself in various battles, though a long way from the actual hostilities, in which I treated injured men who had had the large vessels of their bodies cut and broken, having lost a large quantity of blood on the battlefield, but the bleeding had stopped by itself.

Someone will object that if a man is wounded such that the bones of his head are cleft, he is in danger of dying unless the blood, which has spilled out of the wound onto the membranes, is removed by means of trepanation, for this blood would completely putrefy, and thereby cause decay in the brain, the main site of life, the use of which is more than necessary. Yet, we see how in some cases the filth comes out of

---

49. Guillemeau's volume on *French Surgery drawn from Ancient Physicians and Surgeons* (*La Chirurgie françoise recueillie des antiens medecins et chirurgiens*) had first been published in 1594.

the nose, the ears or the mouth without any need for trepanation, or it may even pass right through the bones.

We can say the same about emphysema and hydropsy. A person suffering from the first has his chest full of rotting matter; in the second case the abdomen is full of water. Both would suffocate unless the surgeon makes an opening to perform paracentesis or to drain the pleural membranes. Yet, often the person suffering from emphysema gets rid of the rotting matter through his mouth or in his urine — the exits are obvious and nature uses them. The person suffering from hydropsy gets rid of the liquid in his urine or his stools, and even in his sweat or through some little vent furnished by nature, such as in the navel or the legs. Experience has shown us that this is true for many people. Thus you see that such operations are not always essential.

As for the letting of blood, you will say that a person runs a great risk of losing his life in a short time if, when suffering from severe pains in the head or the side, he is not bled promptly, since the blood which courses through his veins asks only to be let out. I would answer that often nature does so through the nose, the mouth, the eyes, the ears, the seat and other parts of the body, for the wellbeing of the patient.

But in the case of childbirth, this is not true, for if the entrance to the womb is closed, as I have seen in some women, whether because a thick, tough membrane naturally obstructs the passage, or because some scar in this area has thickened and obstructed the walls of the neck of this womb, it is impossible for nature to part and break through these obstacles. For, in the first case it is difficult for even a tiny stylus or a probe the width of the shaft of a small feather to pass through, and in the second case, you cannot introduce a small probe as wide as a needle through the little hole in the middle of the membrane. Experience demonstrated this to me in the case of two women both of whom were pregnant, as I shall discuss later. So in such cases it is necessary that the hand of the surgeon be used, otherwise the child and the mother will perish wretchedly. It might be objected that the mother herself could have opened the door, tearing the scar and breaking the membrane. But, what would you say to me in the case of a woman whose baby is badly positioned, doubled up inside the womb, or a woman who has convulsions or a hemorrhage, or both together? The mother would be unable to turn the baby or pull it out, least of all if the child's head is stuck between the pubic bones such that it is impossible to turn it safely. The surgeon is obliged to use his skill to pull it out.

As for the dexterity required, there is no comparison with other operations, for there are no surgical operations in which it is not necessary to see clearly, either by daylight or by the light of a candle, and in which the part one is treating and handling does not need to be exposed and visible to the eye. Yet in this operation, both because of those who are present and because of the fear the woman might feel, we are forced to hide the very entrance where we put a hand, and when this is done to find the child in whatever position it occupies without being able to see it.[50]

If there are two, three, four or even five children (and Albertus Magnus insisted that in Germany he had seen a woman who gave birth to 65 children, five every year),[51] I leave you to judge what skill the surgeon must display so that if they present badly he can bring them out one after another.

Furthermore, every time a woman is delivered well by the hand of a surgeon, two lives are saved, both the mother's and the child's. For this reason, as a great authority said, 'in childbirth, God's help is invoked, for the safety of the mother and the child is sought.' ['*In partu invocatur Dei auxilium, quaeritur enim et parturientis et nascentis salus.*']

Now in all other operations, even if they fulfil their aim, only one person can be saved at a time. Thus, we can judge that such an operation is the most desirable of all for its antiquity, importance and the skill required.

In order to make it easier and to instruct the young surgeon, I have brought together everything I have been able to, from my observations over more than 40 years, in which I have practiced and observed others in the greatest houses, both within and outside this kingdom,

---

50. On the prevailing consensus that the male surgeon or physician should not look at a woman's genitalia, even to perform an assisted delivery, see Klairmont Lingo's analysis, 'Authorizing the text', in her introduction to Louise Bourgeois's *Diverse Observations* (Klairmont Lingo and O'Hara). She provides evidence, however, that for certain procedures, such as the use of the speculum, the male practitioner might occasionally break the taboo.

51. Albertus Magnus, *De Animalibus*: cited by H. Rodnite Lemay, *Women's Secrets. A Translation of pseudo-Albertus Magnus's 'De Secretis Mulierum' with Commentaries*, 175, n. 78.

which, thanks be to God, I have served. In addition, I did not disdain to enter the humblest abodes, partly out of charity and partly to gain further experience. I compared what I was able to observe with what the ancient Greek and Latin writers and modern authors wrote about it. Having assembled it all, for the service of the young surgeon, I wrote this in French for the sake of those who are less learned and who do not have knowledge of the Greek or Latin languages.

Someone will say, diminishing the small honor I might have had for this labor, that the ancients had written about most of this. But let them heed the words of the great oracle, which says that it requires no less intelligence or powers of understanding to be able to judge well of things which were previously written than to be the first to produce them.

I know that my learning, and even more so my powers of expression, will be found wanting on various accounts, but I beg of the reader to accept the book in the same good faith in which I present it. And in the same way, I desire those who are more experienced than I am to improve it. I am satisfied that my mistakes should be pointed out in a friendly manner. I shall not refuse to retract them willingly, just as the divine Hippocrates did, freely confessing his faults, and saying in public that he had earned more shame than glory in practicing medicine.

[1609]

EXTRACT FROM THE KING'S PRIVILEGE

By grace and privilege of the King, it is granted to Nicolas Buon,[52] bookseller in Paris, to print, or to have printed, as many times as he wishes a book written by Mr. Jacques Guillemeau, surgeon to the King and sworn in Paris, *Treating the safe delivery of women and the manner to look after them in their labor both natural and contrary to nature. On the care of them when they are newly delivered and during their period of lying-in.* With prohibition to people of whatever rank or condition to print it or have it printed, to sell or distribute copies other than those printed by the said Buon, or with his consent; nor to extract individual treatises to print them separately or in other works, on pain of a fine of 100 ecus and the confiscation of the books which shall be found to have been thus printed at the expense of the said Buon, as is set out more fully in the original of these letters established in Paris this 25th day of March 1609, signed and sealed with the great seal in yellow wax.

De Brigard.

---

52. Traded between 1598 and 1628. See P. Renouard, *Imprimeurs parisiens* (1898), 54.

[1620]

EPISTLE TO MONSIEUR HEROARD

*To Monsieur Heroard, Seigneur de Vaugrigneuse,
Counselor of the King in his Councils of State and
Privy Council: and first physician to His Majesty.*

Monsieur,[53]

This small work by my late father was dedicated to you from its birth. Like an inheritance, it obliges me, as now it is reprinted and enlarged with much research on related topics, to offer it to you, its owner. For France honors you for the excellence of your knowledge, which brings mankind close to the gods, and, as it were, you bring back from the grave those whom daily infirmities would consign to death before their time. I know that your graciousness will measure the sincerity of this undertaking rather than the value of the gift, which could only be worthy of you if it came from you yourself. For my part, it suffices that this lowly attempt, passing from father to son, should build on our wish to honor such a person, whose good esteem is like a rich, precious treasure. So accept this gift, if you will, Monsieur, bestowing on it your protection, and allow me ever to remain,

Your most humble and very obedient servant,

Guillemeau.

53. Charles Guillemeau is following the example of his father, Jacques Guillemeau, who had dedicated his other treatise of 1609 (on the care of infants) to the same Héroard, physician to the royal children, notably the young dauphin — later Louis XIII — and an expert in what would now be termed pediatrics.

[1620]

EPISTLE TO THE READER

To the Reader

Greetings.

Dear Reader, this book which my late father intended for the public good has been well received, treating as it does a quite difficult subject, which ordinarily causes many problems for the most skilled. I am having it reprinted for you with the addition of copperplate illustrations and of a treatise on impotence, and with much detailed research and many secrets, which are necessary for the understanding of the most hidden illnesses of women. Not that I would be presumptuous enough to wish, as the proverb says, to illuminate the sun, that is to say to instruct the learned, but here the young surgeons who have little experience of such learning, or who are scattered here and there, far from the towns, will find both the cause of illnesses and the cures for them. It will be Ariadne's string to lead them from a labyrinth reputed to be mortal both to anyone who does not know its paths and to the health of women who suffer the consequences of dangerous ignorance.[54] Midwives may also benefit from such a gift, and instead of vainly flattering themselves that they can rely on their skills, recognize in truth certain flaws in their handling of births and of the care of newly-delivered mothers. Indeed, it may go so far as to serve some well-born women whose decorum does not allow them to uncover themselves before surgeons, and who will now be able to help themselves. Let all these groups be grateful for this work, and benefit from these fruits intended for the public good, the goal towards which the actions of all good people should be directed.

---

54. Bourgeois had used a similar reference to Ariadne in the dedicatory epistle to Marie de Medici which accompanied the first edition of her *Observations* in 1609: see *Diverse Observations,* O'Hara and Klairmont Lingo. Charles Guillemeau (probably the anonymous author of the pamphlet launching a vitriolic attack on Bourgeois following the death of Louis XIII's sister-in-law shortly after her delivery in 1627) may well be deliberately echoing her to reclaim the voice of authority for himself.

[1620]

EXTRACT FROM THE KING'S PRIVILEGE

By grace and privilege of the King, it is granted to Abraham Pacard,[55] bookseller in this city of Paris, to print or to have printed by such printer as he wishes a book entitled *On the pregnancy and delivery of women. On looking after them and the manner of treating the accidents which befall them. Together with the care of their infants. By the late Jacques Guillemeau, surgeon to the King. Revised and expanded with illustrations from engravings, and with various secret illnesses. With a treatise on impotence. By Charles Guillemeau, surgeon to the King.* With prohibition to any printers, booksellers or other people of whatever rank, status or condition, to print or have printed in any part of this kingdom the above-mentioned book, for a period of 10 years, on pain of all the expenses, damages and other greater pains stipulated by this privilege, notwithstanding any objections or appeals and other letters contradicting this one. For this is the pleasure of his Majesty. Issued in Paris this 8th day of September 1620. Signed by the Council.

De Verneson.

And sealed.

---

55. According to P. Renouard, Abraham Pacard worked in Paris as a printer from 1600 to 1619, and then went to Charenton. However, this preface suggests he was still in Paris in September 1620 (*Imprimeurs parisiens*, 286).

[1620]

TABLE OF THE CHAPTERS

Of the first book (p. 1)[56]

The care of the pregnant woman during the nine months of her pregnancy, and the manner to treat the illnesses which may befall her during, and outside, this time.

Ch. 1	The signs that a woman is expecting a child.
Ch. 2	The signs to tell whether a woman is expecting a son or a daughter.
Ch. 3	Signs that a woman is expecting twins.
Ch. 4	On false conception.
Ch. 5	On the regimen that a pregnant woman should follow.
Ch. 6	How the pregnant woman should conduct herself during the nine months of her pregnancy.
Ch. 7	On various accidents that may befall women during their pregnancies.
Ch. 8	On the abnormal appetite, called *pica*.
Ch. 9	On toothache.[57]
Ch. 10	On nausea and hiccups.
Ch. 11	On sickness which affects pregnant women.
Ch. 12	On pains in the stomach, sides and abdomen which befall pregnant women.
Ch. 13	On pains in the lower back, hips and loins and on difficulty in urinating which affects pregnant women.
Ch. 14	On palpitations and flutterings of the heart, and on faintness which affects pregnant women.
Ch. 15	On coughing.
Ch. 16	On a tight and constricted abdomen which affects pregnant women.
Ch. 17	On diarrhea which affects pregnant women.

---

56. I list here the contents of Books I-III, but not those of the separate volume on the care of infants.

57. Ch. 9 of Book I is added in 1620.

Second book (p. 135)

The way to care for the pregnant woman during her labor, whether it be natural or not.

58. Ch. 19 of Book I is added in 1620.

59. Chs. 21 and 22 of Book I are added in 1620.

60. Chs. 1 and 2 of Book II are added in 1620.

61. Ch. 14 of Book II is added in 1620.

62. In 1609 the chapter title was only 'The way to extract the child when it has become swollen and bloated in the womb'.

Third book (p. 309)

The treatment of the newly delivered mother, and the accidents that may befall her during her lying-in.

Ch. 1   On the regimen of the mother after delivery.

Ch. 2   What must be done to the stomach, breasts and private parts of the mother after delivery.

Ch. 3   On the accidents which may befall recently delivered women. And first on contractions.

Ch. 4   On the hemorrhage which occurs in some women immediately after they are delivered, and other accidents.[63]

Ch. 5   On the over-abundance of milk which occurs in newly delivered women.

Ch. 6   On tumors in the breasts, and first on inflammation of the breasts.

Ch. 7   On flatulent tumors in the breasts.

Ch. 8   On oedematous tumors in the breasts.

Ch. 9   On scrofulous swelling of the breasts.

Ch. 10   On schirrus of the breasts.

Ch. 11   On cancer of the breasts.

Ch. 12   On the size and droopiness of the breasts.

Ch. 13   On prolapse of the rectum and womb.

Ch. 14   On the bruises and grazes which birth causes to women's lower parts.

Ch. 15   On hemorrhoids.

Ch. 16   On hemorrhoids of the womb.

Ch. 17   On the excessive flow of lochia from recently delivered women.

Ch. 18   On the excessive flow of menstrual blood.[64]

Ch. 19   On red, bloody, orangish or yellowish flow.

Ch. 20   On the white flowers[65] in women.

Ch. 21   On gonorrhea.[66]

63. Chs. 4–12 of Book III are added in 1620; in 1609 Book III consisted of only nine chapters.

64. Chs. 18–22 of Book III are added in 1620.

65. The medical condition of leukorrhea, producing excessive or offensive white discharges from the vagina. (French uses the term *'fleurs blanches'* — 'white flowers' — distinguishing it from the menses or *'fleurs rouges'* — 'red flowers').

66. See 93, n. 84.

67. Chs. 24–26 of Book III are added in 1620.

68. This chapter and all the remaining ones (chs. 28–48 of Book III) added in 1620.

[1620]⁶⁹

BOOK I

Chapter 5: On the Regimen That a
Pregnant Woman Should Follow

So that the pregnant woman may enjoy perfect health, she must carefully follow the rules and recommendations concerning the six things which are not natural,[70] that is to say: air; eating and drinking; exercise and rest; sleeping and waking; fullness and emptiness; and troubles of the mind.

First, she should choose her dwelling in good air, a temperate climate, neither too hot nor too cold, nor watery, without being exposed to mists or winds, especially the southerly one, for, as Hippocrates says,[71] when such winds blow, pregnant women miscarry for the slightest reason. The north wind is equally bothersome to them, for such winds cause catarrh, sweats and much coughing in pregnant women, leading them to give birth before their appointed time. The same is true for winds that bring bad smells and mists, which are drawn into the lungs along with air when we breathe, and often cause unpleasant, troublesome diseases.[72]

In respect of food, pregnant women should eat nourishing dishes which produce a good digestive juice, and which are moderately drying. They should eat enough for themselves and the children they carry, and in this state will be dispensed from fasting at any period of the year, for too much abstinence sometimes makes the child frail and sickly, and often causes it to be born prematurely, since it seeks sustenance which it cannot obtain from the mother's body. Equally,

---

69. I use the 1620 French text as the basis for my translation, but indicate in the footnotes where this differs from the 1609 original text.

70. I.e. which are within the woman's, rather than nature's, control.

71. More precisely, Hippocrates claims that southerly winds in winter followed by dry northerly ones in the spring make women likely to miscarry (*On Airs, Waters and Places*, X).

72. The 1609 edition had the following additional sentence: 'Aristotle says that the smell of a snuffed-out candle may cause a pregnant woman to miscarry, so she should avoid all bad air, and live in houses which are well aired and pleasant, avoiding bad smells as far as she can.' In the Liminary Epistle to the Reader, 158, the same warning is attributed to Pliny.

if the mother consumes too much food, it can often cause the child to suffocate, or make it grow so large that it can no longer remain in its place. This causes it to be born, or it becomes ill, since such foods, which allow the child to feed and grow, decay. In his work *On Crises*,[73] Hippocrates writes that the sister of Caius Duellius ate so excessively when pregnant that she miscarried.

All foods which are too cold, hot or watery should be avoided, and especially at the start of a meal. Dishes which are over-salty or over-spicy are not to be permitted, nor are baked foods. Aristotle and Pliny write that if a pregnant woman eats over-salty food, the child will be born without nails, which is a sign that it will not have a long life.[74] Her bread should be made from good wheat and be well kneaded, light and well baked. As far as meats are concerned, she should choose chicken, pigeons, doves, pheasants, larks, partridges, veal and mutton. For vegetables and herbs, she should choose lettuces, endives, borage, bugloss and sorrel, and she should avoid uncooked salad. At the end of the meal, for dessert, she should eat pears, quinces, either cooked or preserved in jelly, or cherries and damsons. She should avoid all foods that are diuretics, causing the urine and the menses to flow, as well as those provoking flatulence, like peas and beans. Nonetheless, pregnant women often have such a perverted appetite, because of some bitter or salty humor contained in the membranes of the stomach, that they wish to eat coal, chalk, ashes, wax, salted fish which is raw and has not even had the salt washed from it, and they drink verjus[75] or vinegar, or even the dregs of wine, and it is impossible to prevent them from tasting and eating these things. But they must abstain as far as possible since such rubbish can seriously damage their health and that of the child. Yet if they cannot contain themselves so greatly, they may take just a little in order to satisfy their cravings, for fear lest worse befall them. For I have seen women who had been forbidden to take such foods, who gave birth as a result, and in other cases their children bore the imprint of some of the things which had been the object of

73. One of a number of cases where Guillemeau gives an erroneous reference, perhaps indicating he was writing from memory rather than with the classical texts before him.
74. Aristotle, *History of Animals*, VII. 5; Pliny, *Natural History*, VII. 6. 42.
75. Juice husbanded from unripe (green) grapes and used as a condiment in cooking.

an excessive desire.[76] Furthermore, although such foods are often the worst, because of the mother's craving for them often they are digested without doing her any harm. Hippocrates says that it is better to eat and drink things which are a little worse rather than something which is better yet less agreeable.

For drinks to accompany her meals, she should choose a clear, mellowed wine, not too strong, which she should water down well. Such wine has the power to calm the stomach and all the parts that assist digestion and generation. If a woman cannot drink wine, she should use hydromel and well boiled barley water, or a well prepared tisane,[77] so that her stomach is not weakened or chilled from drinking freshly drawn water, for we must remember the heat of the stomach and of the organs surrounding it are required to cook the foods. Experience shows us that pregnant women always have weaker and less well heated stomachs than other women, since the womb draws most of the heat from all the entrails, as a result of which the stomach is deprived of heat.

Her sleep should be taken at night so that she can properly digest the food that she has consumed, for fits of wakefulness can bring about indigestion and illnesses that cause early births rather than large, fine children. She should especially avoid sleeping after dinner, but in the morning she may indeed keep to her bed if she so wishes, without (like great ladies) making day into night and night into day. For as Hippocrates says, good sleep comes at night, not in the day. However, she may rest until nine o'clock — at other times, sleep may be harmful.

She may take moderate exercise, for violent exercise causes the cotyledons, by means of which the child is fed, to slacken. Even carriages or carts should be avoided, especially during the first three months, for just as we see that flowers and fruits fall from the trees for little reason when a breeze rustles the tree, so it is equally common for pregnant women who for some trivial reason move or stir, or even miss a step, to give birth prematurely.

It was not without good reason that the Romans forbad their wives to travel in carriages, and the same rule should be followed today,

---

76. Cf. 109, n. 139; 266-7.

77. The remainder of the paragraph ('so that her stomach.... heat') was added in 1620.

particularly in the case of women who are prone to injuries, and they should walk slowly, with no haste, taking the greatest possible care of themselves during the first three months.

And in this respect the pregnant woman should be like someone who wishes to carry a heavy load suspended on a small string — if you take good care to carry it gently without jolting it roughly, it will be possible to convey it easily to the desired place, but if the string is jolted and jerked, roughly shaking the load attached to it, its weight will increase and it will be bound to break the string since it cannot bear the shifting weight.[78]

She should avoid loud noises and sounds, like thunder, gunshots and heavy bells. In his book *On Theriac*, Galen says that some pregnant women have died from the fear thunder caused them. If the woman is frightened of injury or of giving birth, she should be carried in a litter or a chair by strong men, especially for the two hours before she eats, for just as women can easily miscarry in the first months since the child (although small) is not firmly attached to the womb, so when it is big and heavy, its weight can cause it to fall down and be born. Thus all violent exercise and all heavy work should be avoided, as should anger, shouting and immoderate laughter.[79]

The fourth, fifth and sixth months, she will be able to use more liberty; the seventh and eighth, she will contain herself quietly; and when she is in her ninth month, she may exercise more. Thus, in his *Politics*,[80] Aristotle orders that pregnant women should not be sedentary, and that they should not follow too inactive a way of life; and when they have the honor of carrying a child, every day they should visit the temples of the gods by way of exercise. Plato expressly orders this in his *Republic*, out of both devotion and religious piety.[81] But Aristotle speaks on this subject as a physician, as he demonstrates in his book *On Generation*.[82] He says that in countries in which women are accustomed to work, they do not have nearly so much trouble in bearing children, and they give birth more easily. In brief,

---

78. This whole paragraph ('And in this respect... weight') was added in 1620.

79. Cf. Liebault (109), Duval (266) and de Serres (336, n. 140).

80. *Politics*, VII. 16.

81. The statement in fact occurs in Plato's *Laws*, not *The Republic* (*Laws*, 789e).

82. *Generation of Animals*, IV. 6.

when women take exercise, they give birth more swiftly, for exercise uses up the excrements that idle women gather.[83]

Similarly, in the first four months she should not indulge in amorous pursuits in case she damages the child she carries and causes her menses to flow, as also in the sixth and eighth months.[84] But in the seventh and ninth months she may partake in them, especially in the ninth month, and some think that this eases the delivery.

Aristotle is of the following opinion, which is completely in contradiction to Hippocrates: a pregnant woman, he says, should avoid the company of her husband. One can easily reconcile Aristotle and Hippocrates: the philosopher means that throughout pregnancy the woman should not have amorous relations, except only towards her time of giving birth, to stir the child and allow it to be born more easily. For after this act, when it comes into the world it is normally lubricated, as it were, and covered with mucus and slippery secretions which assist its birth.

It is also necessary for the pregnant woman to have a relaxed stomach, not constipated, and every day, if possible, she should empty her bowels. If this does not happen naturally, she should be assisted by taking some sweet prune juice every morning, like that from damsons, or well baked and sugared apples cooked with a little fresh butter. She may also take a broth cooked with borage, bugloss, lettuce, purslane, patience and a very little of the herb mercury. She may also take some suppositories which are not too sharp; enemas made from head of veal or mutton with a little aniseed or fennel, in which red sugar and oil of violets have been dissolved, will help her, if used sparingly; avoiding all drugs which can cause a loose stomach so that she avoids the risk of miscarriage, as Hippocrates says in his fifth book, aphorism 34.[85] However, Hippocrates also holds the view that pregnant women can be purged when necessary from the fourth to the seventh month. But before the fourth, or after the seventh, he does not advise it, and forbids it expressly. However, today physicians

83. Another example of the theory of bad humors building up if the woman is idle. Cf. 101, 183, 265.

84. Guillemeau here follows the traditional view that births in the seventh or ninth months are safer than in the eighth month.

85. 'When a pregnant woman has violent diarrhea, there is danger of her miscarrying.'

ignore this when necessary, especially since medicines which we use for this, like rhubarb, cassia, manna and tamarinds are not as strong as those used by the Ancients, such as hellebore, scammony, turbith, colocynth and others. Special care should be taken to avoid giving her any stimulating drinks that provoke urination or the menses. For, as the same author says, it is impossible for the child to be healthy and born at full term if women have their flow.

Bleeding them is forbidden unless it is absolutely necessary, especially when the child is already quite large, since it needs more nourishment and food than at the start when it is small.[86] For if you remove its food, it becomes thin and weak, often being forced to attempt to leave the womb in order to obtain food. However, there are some women who have so much blood that one is obliged to draw some out, since too much could suffocate the child — or if they are very ill, bleeding is essential. The most suitable time, although bleeding is not necessary, is from the fourth to the seventh month. I saw one pregnant woman who was bled eleven times on account of pleurisy, and she bore her child to full term and was safely delivered of it.

As far as troubles of the mind are concerned, the pregnant woman should be cheerful and happy, avoiding all melancholic moods and worrying thoughts that might cross her mind. For, as Aristotle says, a pregnant woman should have a mind at peace, and Avicenna says the same. When women have conceived, they should be kept free from all fears, distress and troubles of the mind, and they should not be told anything which might cause them to be sad or afraid. Indeed, sensible women who wish to have children will avoid listening to sad and frightening histories; they will never look at an ugly or deformed picture or person, for fear lest the imagination impress on the child the image of this picture or person.[87] If they do this, women will be confident of being delivered safely and joyfully, and they will know that with the help of God they will bear their fruit to its full term, and it will be born into the world without great difficulty, assuring them of a prompt and safe delivery.

Finally, they should remove their corsets as soon as they realize they are pregnant, not crushing themselves for fear lest the child

86. C.f. the advice given by Jean Liebault (113).
87. See discussion above (175, n. 76).

be deformed or unable to grow naturally. They should dress lightly rather than heavily. They should wear a mantle rather than a dress that constrains and constricts them too greatly.

Chapter 6: How the Pregnant Woman Should Conduct Herself during the Nine Months of Her Pregnancy

Now that I have prescribed the regimen a pregnant woman should follow throughout her pregnancy, she should also follow, if she judges it good, the recommendations I shall set out, which are not entirely necessary, but useful and helpful to preserve her beauty and also her health.[88]

As soon as she knows that she is pregnant (probably the second or third month) she should wear a gold chain around her neck, in order that after her delivery her breasts do not become excessively swollen and large and droop like sacks,[89] and to avoid the possible risk of too much blood being turned into milk, which may curdle, and then suppurate and putrefy. Some prefer a steel chain, or a little bar of steel placed between her breasts, or also putting a piece of cork there and two other small pieces, one under each armpit. This treatment is strongly recommended.

Take leaves of fresh sage, periwinkle and ground-ivy, a handful of each, a small half-handful of hemlock; boil all these in water and wine, and when the liquid has been removed from the fire, add a dash of rose vinegar. For between five and ten minutes in the morning, place on the breasts a cloth soaked in this warm infusion, then wipe them with fairly warm cloths. You may do the same thing with the juices extracted from these same herbs. When she has reached the third or fourth month of pregnancy, and has felt her child moving and stirring, which is the time when her stomach starts to become large and swollen, she should use a well-chosen swathe to support her womb. First she should anoint it with some salve or pomade, and she should continue

88. Writers of vernacular manuals are aware of the importance of advising pregnant women on how to safeguard or regain their physical charms. Cf. Liebault's translation of Marinelli's treatise on women's beauty (see 67).

89. The French word for sacks (*'bezasses'*) calls to mind the fourth line of Clément Marot's celebrated humorous poem 'On the ugly breast', c. 1535: 'Breast, or should I say sack?' [*'Tetin, doy je dire bezasse?'*]

to do this until she reaches her ninth month, for fear lest her abdomen become covered with varicose or broken veins, furrowed, and full of wrinkles, which will leave her with a deformed, ugly, ruined abdomen, hanging down like tripe. This occurs because of the great weight of the child that expands and stretches the skin — it causes the pregnant woman great pain and tension in the abdomen and the groin.

Here are salves or a pomade:

Take kid and sow caul,[90] three ounces of each; fat from a capon and a goose, one and a half ounces of each; cut these into small pieces, melt them in an earthenware or leaded pot, adding as much water as necessary, taking care that it does not burn. Then it should be strained through a cloth and afterwards washed in water until it is white and has lost its smell. Once this is done, it should then be melted again in a double vessel, adding to it an ounce of deer's marrow, and then it should immediately be washed in rose or orange-blossom water, or some other sweet-scented water, if you wish adding to it two or three grains of musk or civet, if they do not harm the womb.

Others use this salve: take the fat of a dog and the fat of a sheep from around the kidneys, two ounces of each, one ounce of spermaceti,[91] an ounce and a half of oil of sweet almonds. These fats should be prepared and washed as above, then melted with the rest and then washed in rose or sweet-scented water.

Others take many sheeps' feet, some 35 or 40, the bones of them having been shattered, and they are boiled in plenty of water. Then they extract the fat and marrow which floats on the top, which is thoroughly washed in ordinary water, and of this they take two ounces, and the same amount of duck fat, one ounce of spermaceti and six drams of white wax. Then all of this is melted together in a double vessel, and washed with these waters.

Some women who do not want to rub their stomachs every morning with one of these salves put on their abdomen the pelt of a dog or another pelt, which should be carefully prepared as follows, and they change it more or less every two weeks when it is spoiled, and they only have it removed after two or three days if it is creased and wrinkled.

90. Caul is a thin fatty membrane lining the abdominal cavity.
91. Wax obtained from the head of the sperm whale.

Take the skin of a dog or other animal dressed for making gloves; wash it several times in ordinary water, then in rose water; dry it in the shade. When it is prepared and dried in this way, soak it in the following oils and fats.

Take an ounce and a half of white Mesve ointment of roses, one ounce each of oil of St John's wort and of sweet almonds, half an ounce each of fresh butter and spermaceti. When all this has melted in a double vessel, the skin should be soaked in it for three or four days, and every day pressed, then replaced in the oils. Then it should be removed and hung out in the air for two or three days so that the moisture drips out and it dries. Then it should be cut to fit the size and shape of the abdomen.

Those who are most exacting use both these salves and the skin as well. Those women who do not have the good fortune to do one or other should take just a quarter of fresh butter, well rinsed in fresh water and rose water, and an ounce of sweet almond oil, and half an ounce of spermaceti, and they should melt all this together before smearing it on the abdomen.

It should be noted that these salves must be kept in a varnished earthenware pot, covered by more than a finger's depth of rose water to prevent them smelling rancid.

When the woman has reached the ninth month of pregnancy, if she has remained in good health, she should continue to use these salves, and start to take more exercise than previously. She should take a gentle walk before her meals the first 12 to 15 days, then she should exercise more strenuously. Even for the first eight or ten days of her ninth month, it will be very useful to have her sit in the morning in the decoction I shall describe, in a half-bath, for a quarter or half an hour. Then she should be well dried and placed on her bed, and smeared and daubed with such a salve on her back, all along the sacrum bone and the buttocks, and at the front from her navel downward, especially over her pubic bone and groin.

Take mauves and mallows with their roots, and motherwort, two handfuls of each; three ounces of lily roots; a good handful each of camomile flowers and of sweet clover; seeds of flax, quince and fenugreek, an ounce of each. Boil all these in river water in order to obtain a decoction, and half a bath.

Take three ounces of the fat of a hen, an ounce and a half of duck fat, two ounces of fresh butter, an ounce and a half of linseed oil. All of these should be melted together, and then well washed in water of pellitory and artemisia, adding two ounces of mallow mucilage.

Throughout this time, every day before eating she should take an ounce of good, sweet almond oil extracted without heat, together with half an ounce of white wine, and one ounce of pellitory water.

Some women have profited from taking the yolk of an egg, and then drinking a small quantity of spiced, good-quality wine. Others take a little wine and water, and in it dissolve a dram of linseed.[92]

It may happen that the woman does not feel her child at all during the pregnancy, or only very little; in this case, she should wear something on her navel which will give the child strength, like the following sachet. Prescription:[93] powder of rose, blackberry and of both coral and clove, of each half an ounce; of angelica seed, two drams; of mastic, half a dram; of ambergris, two grains; of musk, one grain; enclose all in a pouch lined with fine cotton.

She may use tablets such as these. Prescription:[94] bark of aloes, cinnamon, prepared coriander, clove and nutmeg, of each one scruple; deer heart's bone, sandalwood, burned elephant bones, bark of aloes, of each one scruple; shavings of ivory and sapphire and prepared pearl, prepare of each two scruples; gold shavings and finely cut silk, of each half a scruple; of ambergris, six grains; of musk, two grains; dissolve in eight ounces of sweetened rose water; make tablets of two drams in weight.

It is possible to make an opiate with syrup of apples and bugloss and borage, or even with the same powders and wax, laudanum and a little jasmine oil to make a plaster to put on the navel.

This regimen should be followed for a pregnant woman who has a good disposition, and has not suffered any misfortune or anything other than trivial incidents in her pregnancy, and who bears children well and painlessly. But since there are many women who are afflicted by various misfortunes during their pregnancy, it has seems right to me to deal briefly with these here before moving on to childbirth.

92. The next three paragraphs ('It may happen... navel') were added in 1620.
93. In the French text, this prescription is given in Latin.
94. In the French text, this prescription is given in Latin.

Chapter 7: On Various Accidents That May Befall Women during Their Pregnancies

It is very appropriate for a woman at any time at all, and especially during her pregnancy and after her delivery, to take the best care possible of her beauty, for there is nothing that obliterates and diminishes a woman's beauty more than frequent childbearing. But since health is even more precious and to be prized above beauty, and a pregnant woman can be afflicted with various accidents and misfortunes, it is essential to look at the ways to preserve and deliver her from them during the nine months she is bearing her child. For if the mother is lost, the child's life is put at risk. In his book *On the Generation of Animals*, Aristotle believes that when other animals bear offspring, they are not subject to any illness, whereas on the contrary women during their pregnancies are often ill.[95] Hippocrates says that they are normally pale and look poorly in order to show that they are subject to various ailments.[96]

In ancient times, when men and women were sold as slaves, if a woman was found to be pregnant, she was not handed over or guaranteed to be in full health by the vendor, according to Vitruvius in book 2,[97] because by nature she would be subject to various maladies, and especially during the first three or four months of pregnancy. Such ailments occur for various reasons. First, because, as Aristotle says,[98] they live for the most part an idle life, and they eat bad foods which turn into excrements which cause various obstructions, the source and origin of all their sufferings. The second cause is that the blood which they had been accustomed to purge every month when they were not pregnant is retained and suppressed in large quantity; it runs to the womb to be purged and expelled as usual, and being unable to be shed, and even less to be consumed and digested by the child which is still small, it flows back copiously into the veins, especially those near the stomach. Remaining there a long time it is corrupted and becomes of a bad quality, causing the unnatural appetite which the Romans

95. *Generation of Animals*, IV. 6.
96. *Diseases of Women*, I. 34.
97. *On Architecture*, II. 9. 1.
98. *Generation of Animals*, IV. 6.

called '*pica*' or '*malacia*': a loss of appetite, hiccups, vomiting, pains in the stomach, side and lower abdomen, and in the back, hips and groin, difficulty in urinating, palpitations and fluttering of the heart with faintness, coughing, a tightened stomach and diarrhea, swollen thighs and feet, and sometimes miscarriage as they cannot carry their child to full term. It also causes other accidents which we shall discuss shortly, starting with that which affects them most frequently and for the longest time, that is '*pica*' or an unnatural appetite.

BOOK II

Chapter 1: On the Position of the Child in the Mother's Womb and on Its Birth

[This chapter was added in its entirety, in 1620, by Charles Guillemeau. The translation below omits the first part of the chapter, devoted to a lengthy account of the position of the foetus in the womb. I start with Charles Guillemeau's description of the birth itself.]

Thus it is easy to see that there are three things which cause natural childbirth to occur. The first is the child's lack of respiration and air, especially since once the heat of the heart has increased, it needs to be better ventilated, and cannot live without more cooling and ventilation. The second is the lack of food; not being able to derive and take enough to sustain itself from the mother, it is obliged to seek it elsewhere. The third is the restricted space in which it is enclosed, in which it can no longer contain itself, so it is obliged to stretch and seek a larger, more suitable space, and this causes it to break the membranes in which it is contained, together with the waters, in this way pressing the mother and stimulating her by the bitterness of the waters to do her duty to deliver it.

Now, as Hippocrates says at the end of his *On the Nature of the Child*, there are three ways for the child to be born.[99] The first is head first, and in this case the woman gives birth easily. The second is with the side presenting or a transverse lie, or feet first, and then the mother has a difficult delivery, for some die in the process, or their children, or both mother and child do. In his book *On an Eight-Month Birth*,[100] Hippocrates lists only two ways, head first or feet first. In his book *On Superfetation* he lists three:[101] head, feet or side; under side, he includes the hands presenting.

Aristotle, in chapter 8 of Book VII of *The History of Animals,* says birth happens in two ways, one natural, the other unnatural. The natural way, common to all animals, and almost the ordinary and universal, is to present head first. The other, which is not natural (and

99. *On the Nature of the Child*, XXX. 10.
100. *On an Eight-Month Birth*, X. 2.
101. *On Superfetation*, 4.

which is seen almost only in women and not in other animals, and which occurs only uncommonly, as Galen writes in Book VII chapter 15 of *On the Usefulness of the Parts of the Body*),[102] consists of several other kinds of presentation, and we shall look at each separately in its proper place, and at the means of dealing with them.

In such a struggle,[103] the mother and child feel great pains, indeed greater than all other animals. That is because of her sin, God having willed that women should give birth in pain for having been the cause of death.[104] But natural reasons can be adduced. First that woman is most delicate and frail, more predisposed to fear and possessed of less stamina than the females of all other animals, which are more sturdy, braver and stronger. Now to give birth requires great determination and strength, as Hippocrates says. Secondly, pregnant women lead a sedentary life and pamper themselves greatly. When it is then time to give birth, they find it very strange, and are not so ready and fit to suffer the pain and hard work, since they are not accustomed to them. Apart from their indolence and sedentary life, they eat many bad foods, and such a way of life causes an accumulation of many excrements and excess humors, and the quantity of excess humors makes them short of breath, which is the most damaging thing in giving birth. For, to give birth easily and effortlessly, the woman must hold her breath. This is the reason for the pain and long labor that women suffer in most deliveries. The third is that the child has a head which is larger in proportion to the rest of its body than in other animals, as Albertus Magnus says,[105] which is why Aristotle calls small children 'dwarves'.[106] Since the head comes first, it causes a great opening and dilation, and thus great pain.

Now among all the women who suffer the most pain are those who have not given birth previously, because they have not previously experienced this labor, as Hippocrates writes in his book *On the*

---

102. Modern obstetricians reckon that 96–97% of full-term births are cephalic presentation; in other words, breech presentations account for approximately 1 in 30 births at full term.

103. Guillemeau uses the word '*combat*', designating the birth as a battle.

104. Genesis 3:16.

105. Guillemeau may be recalling the statement by [pseudo-] Albertus Magnus that a large foetal head impedes delivery: see H. Rodnite Lemay, *A Translation of pseudo-Albertus Magnus's 'De Secretis Mulierum' with Commentaries*, 108.

106. *On the Progression of Animals*, 710b.

Nature of the Child,[107] and those who are older, especially since the pubic bone and the hip bone and sacrum cannot so easily be shifted and as it were parted, as the coccyx does from the sacrum,[108] as in the case of young women, for the ligaments and joints are harder, stronger and less yielding.

I know that many great persons have debated this question, and among others in our time Monsieur du Laurens[109] and Monsieur Pineau,[110] who take opposing sides, which I invite the reader to consult. But for my part, I believe what experience has shown me, having witnessed the labor of more than 500 women over 40 years,[111] in the delivery of some of whom I clearly heard the cracking and moving apart of these bones, and I put a finger between the two bones, feeling a clear gap. And all women who experience a painful labor complain of the pain they feel in this place. Furthermore, having placed a hand beneath their buttocks, I could feel the separation of these bones. In addition when, shortly after the mothers' deaths, in order to save the children I opened up several women who had been in labor, and carried out a cesarean, I found these bones to be separated and drawn apart, and the ligaments which joined them were very soft and had expanded, for this is the area where the greater part of the womb rests and presses down.

Now such a dilation and expansion does not come about, in my view, all of a sudden, nor at the very time the woman is delivering. My opinion is that the bones begin to expand while the child is still

107. *On the Nature of the Child,* XXX. 11.

108. Guillemeau is describing the slight separation of the pubic bones during childbirth, which allows the passage of the child. The following paragraph is another demonstration of the heated debates among practitioners and theorists in the period over whether or not the bones actually parted. See also Rousset (32) and Liebault (119).

109. André Du Laurens (1558–1609), Professor of Medicine and then Chancellor of Montpellier, and first physician to Henri IV and Marie de Medici. His *Works of Anatomy* [*Opera Anatomica*] were published in 1593, with a posthumous French translation of his *Works* [*Œuvres*] by Théophile Gelée, appearing in 1613.

110. Séverin Pineau (c. 1550–1619), anatomist and surgeon in Paris; published a famous and controversial Latin treatise, *Physiologial and Anatomical Treatise* [*Opusculum physiologicum et anatomicum*, Paris, 1597] on determining signs of virginity. It was republished in 1639 as *On the Signs of Intact and Despoiled Virgins* [*De integritatis et corruptionis virginum notis*].

111. This useful statistic (relating to Jacques Guillemeau's career rather than Charles Guillemeau's to date) gives an indication of the practical experience of a general surgeon who had particular expertise in childbirth. In contrast, Bourgeois reported having conducted some 2,000 deliveries over a rather shorter career.

growing in the mother's womb, nature having the forethought to create such an opening little by little, which is achieved by the heat and dampness in this area. For the idea that they suddenly dilate in this act of childbirth is hard to believe, not that I wish to deny that part, even the majority of the dilation is accomplished during delivery, since the ligaments which support and link these bones are very moist and softened and very dilated. Indeed, you will see that women reaching the end of their pregnancy have wider hips and their pubic bones are broader than when they were not pregnant.

Now in the child's efforts to be born naturally, it presents with the head down, which happens, as Hippocrates says,[112] because of the weight of the head, which is heavier than all the other parts. For as it is attached to the walls of the uterus by the navel, which is the center of the body, having its head above and the two thumbs against the eyes, swimming in its waters and turning around as necessary (as though on a scale), that which is heaviest tips downwards and brings with it the lighter part, and the head brings with it (as it is said) the buttocks and the legs, the head presenting at the moment of crowning. Indeed, it must be thought that the great Creator ordained it thus, so that the child would be born safe, healthy and alive from the mother's womb without causing her any injury, for fear that if the feet, arms or other parts presented first, the child would become impacted on account of one of these. It is not without reason that Pliny said, 'man is born by the head, the dead are carried away by the feet' ['*humanum esse capite nasci, mortuos pedibus efferi*'],[113] for death is the opposite of life.

Moreover, you should believe that whether the child is male or female, if it comes out head first, it will have its face turned downwards and its head up. It is an old error to claim that girls are born with their heads up and boys with their heads down, kissing just their mothers' behinds. Both boys and girls are normally born in the same way. This also facilitates the birth since the nose and chin are more easily hidden and able to slide into the cavity near the coccyx than if they had to slide towards the pubic bone. It is also safer for the child, for, in most births, blood and other excrements come out of the womb and might

112. *On the Nature of the Child*, XXX. 10.
113. *Natural History*, VII. 8. 46.

fall into the eyes, nose and mouth of the child, which would harm it and make it choke if it had its face upward.

Chapter 3: On Midwives[114]

Daily experience demonstrates to us that some women give birth without the help of any midwife. However, Antiquity shows us that midwives have always existed, even that certain women practiced medicine.[115]

Hippocrates swore by Apollo and Asclepius, and by Hygieia and Panacea as gods and goddesses of medicine;[116] Ovid mentions Ocyrrhoe, daughter of the great physician Chiron, who practiced medicine because of her curiosity.[117] Origen in his [2nd] *Homily on the Exodus* speaks of two midwives, most learned in medicine, who were from Egypt, and he names them Sephora and Phua.[118]

Apart from such curiosity, Necessity, the mistress of arts, constrained women to learn and practice medicine together, for when they suffered various illnesses afflicting their private parts and were without any remedy, without which some would languish and die wretchedly, they did not dare to uncover and reveal their illness except to other women, believing that to do so would be shameful.

This is reported to us by Hyginus,[119] who tells how the Athenians had passed laws forbidding women to study medicine. At this time there was a certain girl called Agnodice,[120] who strongly wished to

114. In 1609 this was the first chapter of Book II.

115. On the status and roles of midwives and other women health practitioners in Antiquity, including the issue of their degree of literacy, see R. Flemming, 'Women, Writing and Medicine in the Classical World', *Classical Quarterly* 57 1 (2007), 257–279.

116. Apollo, the Greek god of medicine, was the father of Asclepius, the god of healing, and Hygieia (Health) and Panacea (Universal Remedy) were among the latter's children.

117. Ocyrrhoe the seeress was the daughter of the centaur Chiron, a renowned physician: see Ovid, *Metamorphoses*, 2. 638–9.

118. The midwives Sephora and Phua are named in Exodus I:15; Origen proposed an elaborate allegorical reading of this chapter, in his second homily, mistakenly listed as the 'Homelie xi' in the French text.

119. Gaius Julius Hyginus (c. 64 BC–AD 17), Latin author of a collection of *Fables*.

120. On the classical myth of Agnodice (or Agnodike in Greek), see H. King, *Hippocrates' Woman*, 181–187. The significance of Agnodice as an emblematic figure for Renaissance women is demonstrated by the poetess Catherine des Roches who cites her to advocate women's right to education: see Madeleine and Catherine des Roches, *From Mother and*

study medicine, and in order to achieve her aim more easily she had her hair cut and dressed up as a man. Thus disguised, she began to study under the physician Herophilus.[121] But when she had learned medicine, having been advised that there was a woman who was afflicted in her private parts, she went to her to offer her services. The sick woman refused, believing this was a man, but when she had proved to her, by lifting up her tunic, that she was a woman, the patient entrusted herself to Agnodice, who treated her and fully cured her. And, with the same skill, she treated and cured others. When the physicians learned this, since they were no longer called upon by women to treat them, they accused Agnodice of having had her beard shaved off in order to take advantage of women who pretended to be ill. Then she took off her robe and showed them that she was a woman. This made the physicians accuse her of a greater crime, that of having broken the law which forbad women to study and practice medicine. When this came to the ears of the most respected women, they immediately rushed to the magistrates of the Areopagus[122] to tell them that they did not consider them to be their husbands and friends, but rather their enemies for wanting to condemn the woman who restored them to health. This caused the Athenians to withdraw this law, giving leave to gentlewomen to learn and practice medicine.

Now as the greatest illness that women can have is that which lasts nine months, which reaches its peak and is cured by childbirth, it should not be doubted that such women undertook these studies and practiced delivery of women, and there have been midwives in all ages. In his treatise *On Flesh* [*De carnibus*], Hippocrates speaks of birth at seven months and directs the reader to midwives who attend such births to learn the truth thereof.[123]

Daughter, ed. and trans. Anne Larsen (Chicago: Chicago Press, 2006), 83. (I am grateful to Gianna Pomata for drawing this parallel to my attention.)

121. A famous Alexandrian physician (c. 335–280 BC).

122. Hill in Athens where councils were held.

123. Although Hippocrates speaks of birth at seven — as opposed to eight –. months in *De Carnibus* (section 19), he does not refer to midwives' testimonies. This is probably an instance of Guillemeau half-remembering a passage, and mistakenly conflating it with another. In the preceding passage, Hippocrates has claimed that all he knows about women's experience of the moment of conception is what he has learned from women themselves: Hippocrate, *Œuvres complètes*, ed. E. Littré, VIII, 610–613.

In the third book of Galen's *On Natural Faculties*, he says midwives do not tell women in labor to get up nor to sit in the chair before the neck of the womb is open for the child to be born, which they can know by feeling with their hand.[124] In his book *On the Causes of Diseases,* he also speaks of the errors committed by midwives when they deliver children, and also in the book *On Prognosis,* he tells the story of a woman from Boethina who had a flow of blood; she developed a swollen abdomen, which the midwives took to mean she was pregnant. This is definite proof that there were midwives in the times of Hippocrates and Galen. Diogenes Laertius[125] and Valerius Maximus[126] report that Phaenarete, the mother of Socrates, was a midwife. It is even the case that in Antiquity judges ordered a salary to be paid to those women who practiced medicine and were midwives, as confirmed by Ulpian[127] book 1, section 1, *Of Extraordinary Jurisdiction* [*De extraordinaria cognitio*]; just as they were punished if they had been bad practitioners and unworthy of their profession, as we see in the law 'If a midwife…' ['*Item si obstetrix*'].[128]

Amongst those women who practiced medicine, there were some who took a special interest in delivering women in childbirth, and to distinguish them they were called 'wise women' or midwives,[129] or maybe they chose to be known by the term themselves, for by their nature women wish to be superior to men. In any case, it is easy to establish that there were women who practiced medicine and others dedicated to delivering women in childbirth. The latter used to have three duties in ancient times, as recorded by the lawyers, and by Plato in his *Theaetetus*,[130] and Galen in his commentary on the 62nd aphorism of Book V of Hippocrates.

124. *On Natural Faculties*, III. 3.

125. Diogenes Laertius, historian of philosophy, makes this statement at the opening of his life of Socrates in *The Lives of Eminent Philosophers* (c. 225 AD).

126. Valerius Maximus, Roman moralist and collector of historical anecdotes, in his *Nine Books of Memorable Sayings and Deeds* (c. 31 AD) 3. III. 4, exemplum externum 1.

127. Ulpian (c. 170–228), a jurist, wrote an extensive commentary on various aspects of Roman law.

128. See Ulpian's commentary on this edict: VIII. 10 on *Lex Aquilia*.

129. The rest of the sentence plays on the French word for midwife, '*sage-femme*', literally meaning '*wise* woman'.

130. In the *Theaetetus*, a dialogue about knowledge, Plato draws an extended analogy between the tasks of midwives and his own role as a philosopher.

The first duty was to accomplish the union of the husband with the wife, including knowing how to judge whether they were able and fit, or unable and unfit to continue their line and have children — this is difficult to establish. For this reason, today there is no woman wise enough to be able to declare this. The second was to attend the delivery and birth of children, either furnishing remedies (as is reported by Terence, who says: 'Give her the drink which I ordered and the amount which I ordered'),[131] or by using their hands. Only those who had had children were allowed to do this; as Plato says, a person is not as fit and experienced to accomplish an unfamiliar task as a person who has full knowledge and experience of it.[132] But the midwife was not permitted to start to exercise her profession until she was past bearing her own children, particularly because Diana,[133] who is the goddess who presides over childbirth, is sterile, and a woman who is still bearing children was thought to be greatly handicapped and less suited to the work and the effort. The third was to know and declare whether or not women were pregnant. For this reason, the Roman law laid down by the deified brothers[134] stipulates that three midwives, who are well versed and experienced in their art, should inspect and examine the abdomen and judge whether the woman is pregnant.

Subsequently, in addition to these three duties, midwives have taken it upon themselves to judge a girl's virginity. However, all the famous universities of Italy have rejected and condemned the judgment of midwives who say they can determine girls' virginity. In his *Observations* (for the French) on the same subject, Monsieur Cujas follows them, declaring that it is very difficult, if not impossible, to know whether or not a girl is a virgin, and that the civil law has never recognized the authority of midwives to determine this.

131. The words of the midwife Lesbia (known for her tippling) in Terence's *Andria*, Act III, sc. 3.

132. Plato's argument is expounded in *Theaetetus*.

133. In Roman culture, childbirth was associated with the Lucina-Diana aspect.

134. The 'deified brothers', a phrase given in Latin in Guillemeau's French text, refers to the reign of the co-Emperors, Marcus Aurelius and Lucius Verus (161–9). Ulpian, *Justinian's Digest* 25.4.1, gives a detailed account of the background to the law requiring three midwives to inspect a woman suspected of pregnancy. (I am very grateful to Peter Brown for locating this reference for me.)

Chapter 4: What the Midwife Should be Like

Various things are necessary and to be looked for in a midwife; these concern her person, disposition and intelligence.[135] As far as her person is concerned, first she should be of the right age, neither too young nor too old; of a good physical disposition, not prone to any illnesses, nor deformed in any part of her body; clean in her habits and person, especially having hands which are small and clean rather than large, and her nails pared low and evenly, and during deliveries she should wear no rings on her fingers or bracelets on her wrists. She should be agreeable, cheerful, strong, powerful, industrious and accustomed to hard work, so that she does not fall asleep while sitting with the woman, for this can sometimes take one or even two nights.

As far as her disposition is concerned, she should be gentle, courteous, patient, sober, chaste, not argumentative, nor easy to anger, not arrogant, avaricious or inclined to gossip about what she may see or hear in private relating to the household or the lady she has delivered. For, as Terence says, it is not right to entrust to the hands of a drunken, careless person a woman who is in labor with her firstborn.[136]

As to her intelligence, she should be prudent, wise and clever, so that she may sometimes use fine words to flatter. This was done by midwives in antiquity, as Plato says,[137] for no other reason than to humor and beguile poor women who were scared. This is a proper use of deceipt, permitted to surgeons; it is done for the good of the patient. For, as Terence again says, often deception can be a great healer in serious illnesses.

Now, above all else, the midwife must know that Nature, the handmaiden of this great God, in all things has ordained a beginning, increase, state, perfection and decline. It is demonstrated clearly and above all, as Galen says, in the birth of a child, when the mother brings it into the world. For Nature existed before and is earlier than time, and in what she does she is wiser than art, or than any midwife can

135. In this chapter (II. 2 in 1609), Guillemeau echoes many common classical and Renaissance observations on what constituted the ideal midwife. Soranus, for example, devotes two early chapters of his *Gynaecology* (I. i and ii) to the topic, but Guillemeau's account is independent of any single source, probably largely reflecting his own experience.

136. See 192.

137. See 192, n. 132.

be, and wiser even than the best and most excellent craftsman who can be found, as Galen declares.[138] For it is Nature which determined the day of the conception and the hour of the birth of the child, and indeed it is something worthy of astonishment that in so little time, and as it were in the twinkling of an eye, the neck of the womb, which has been so tightly closed for nine months that not even the point of a needle could penetrate it, suddenly starts to stretch and dilate to allow a passage and exit for the child. This cannot be understood, Galen says,[139] but only wondered at. And even in book XV[140] of *On the Usefulness of Parts of the Body*, when he wanted to show the providence of Nature, he said that mistakes in Nature are rare, and that the normal course of Nature always proceeds with such measure and order that out of a thousand births, scarcely one will go awry.[141]

Thus the midwife, the relatives and those others in attendance should not be in any haste; they should let Nature proceed — while providing, however, such assistance as necessary. This will be described shortly, and the labor will be divided into three stages.

Chapter 5: What Should be Done When the Pregnant Woman Thinks She is Close to Giving Birth[142]

When the hour of delivery has come, the pregnant woman must prepare herself in the following manner. She should have the midwife and the nurse[143] summoned immediately, it being necessary that she should have them with her sooner rather than later. For there are some women who give birth very quickly, and without the help of

---

138. Throughout the treatise *On the Usefulness of the Parts of the Body*, Galen exalts Nature's excellence. For example, in XV. 5, he lauds Nature's ingenuity in providing amniotic fluid to ease the passage of the foetus at birth, an action which midwives can only imitate by soaking the neck of the uterus with fluid.

139. *On the Usefulness of the Parts of the Body*, XIV. 3.

140. In 1609, the reference to Book XV was given correctly; in 1620, it is erroneously given as Book V.

141. *On the Usefulness of the Parts of the Body*, XV. 7.

142. In 1609, this was chapter 3 of Book II.

143. The word used in French ('*garde*') designates the attendant who will stay with the mother after the delivery; this woman does not have the training or knowledge of the midwife.

anyone, even though they may have been in labor a long time with their first child.

Meanwhile, a small bed should be prepared, a small couch of moderate size, very firm and solid, of medium height, for the comfort of both the mother and of the midwife and others who will be near her and attend her in her labor. The bed should be positioned in a convenient place for coming and going around it, away from doors, and fairly near the fire. It should be provided with mattresses, and well covered with sheets and undersheets, in order that they may be changed as necessary. At the foot of the bed, between the two mattresses, a wooden log should be laid horizontally, so that the woman can flex her feet on it and have more strength by bending her legs, as we shall discuss later.

As soon as she feels herself to be experiencing the goads of contractions and pains, which are those of true labor, it is good for her to walk around the room a little. Then she may lie down again to be warm, and later get back up and walk about, waiting for the waters to gather and the opening of the womb to be prepared. For it is painful and very difficult for her to bear remaining in bed for a long time; although it is true that when in bed, even if previously she had some contractions, she may be able to rest and sleep if she feels tired. For in this way the mother and child will regain their strength and the child will be ready to be born at the hour ordained by God, and the waters will gather the better. If the labor is long, the mother may be given some clear soup or the yolk of an egg, with a little bread, and she may drink a little wine and water, However, care must be taken not to fill and overload her with too much to eat or drink.[144]

It is quite certain that women do not all give birth in the same fashion, for some give birth in their beds; others sitting in their chairs; others standing, being held and supported by several people, or even leaning on the edge of a bed, a table or a chair; others kneeling; others supported under the armpits. But the best and safest way for them to give birth is in bed (this is what I advise).[145] And to ensure a good,

144. The last recommendation ('care must be taken… drink') was added in 1620.
145. Cf. the similar advice given by Bourgeois for normal deliveries that are not protracted, although she favors the woman sitting or standing if the child is not descending. or if the labor is long and painful: *Diverse Observations,* I. 10.

straightforward delivery, the midwife and those present, such as relatives and friends and nurses, must do as follows.

First the woman in labor should be placed on her back, her head raised a little on a cushion, with a good pillow under the small of her back, so that her back is not out of alignment. Under her buttocks and the sacrum should be placed a small, but fairly wide pillow so that she is slightly raised, with these parts somewhat higher, for if she sinks down, a woman never has such an easy birth, and her position plays a significant role in this. Her buttocks and thighs should be wide apart, and her legs should be pulled up towards her buttocks, the sole and heel of each foot flexed firmly against the log which is positioned at the end of the bed precisely for this purpose.

For some women, it helps to run a sheet under the lower back and buttocks, doubled over four times. The sheet should be a good foot wide or more, and long enough that it may be held by two women or servants, one on each side, in order to lift the woman up a little as she labors, applying gentle counterforce — this should be done when she has contractions. Raising her up in this way brings her much relief, and allows her contractions to pass more easily.

Apart from the two women, or servants, who lift the bandages, there should be two other female friends or relatives whose hands she can squeeze and press when she has contractions. And each of these will put her other hand on one of the mother's shoulders to prevent her lifting herself up too much, so that she bears down better. For often, as she presses her feet hard against the log that is placed horizontally at the bottom of the bed, she lifts her upper body. Sometimes I have instructed one of these women to press very gently with the palm of their hand on her upper abdomen, encouraging the child, little by little, to descend. Such moderate pressure eased the labor and allowed the contractions to be borne more easily.

The woman in labor, having been positioned thus, must remain resolute and bear down as much as possible when her contractions come, letting them grow as strong as possible, holding her breath, shutting her mouth, and straining as though she wanted to empty her bowels, rather than wailing and crying.

In his book *On the Generation of Animals*, Aristotle made the very accurate observation that women who draw their breath upwards have

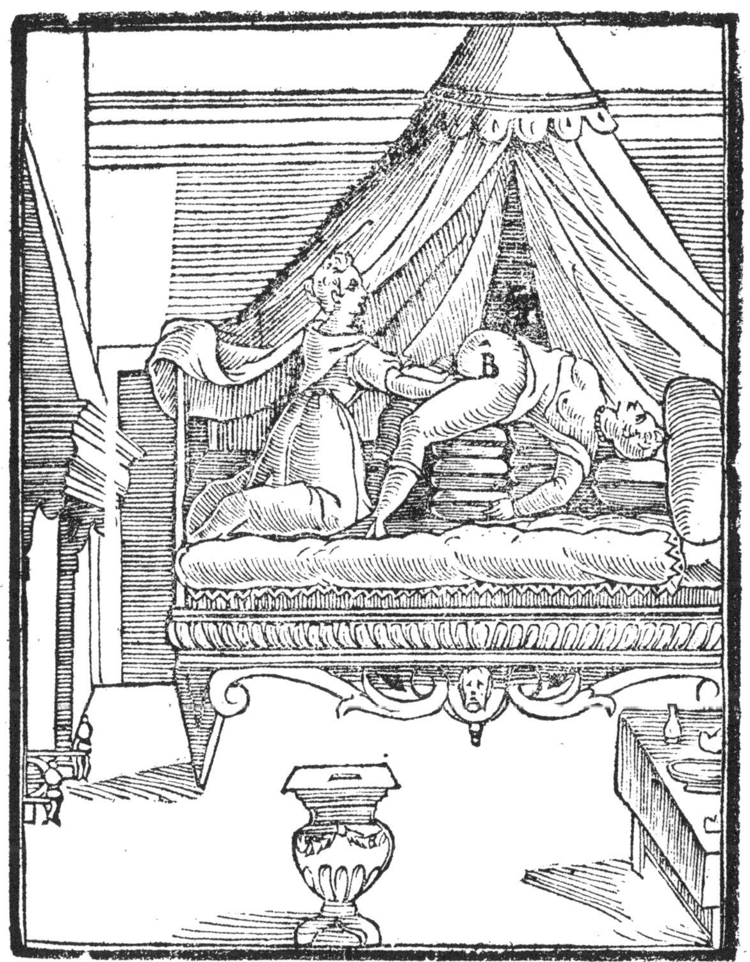

16) Supine delivery

Scipio Mercurio, *La Commare*, Venice, 1601
(Wellcome Library, London)

difficult labors, because they cause the diaphragm to rise, whereas in such an act it should fall and push down. It is true that the woman must take rests without pushing too hard when she experiences several small contractions; she should gather them together into a single one so that she can use them fully at the right moment. If she is wearing around her neck an eaglestone,[146] loadstone, the skin of a urus,[147] or other pendant, which might hold the child back, they should be removed and fastened on her thigh. Above all, she should do as she is instructed by both her relatives and friends and the midwife. Equally, she should endure her suffering with patience, calling upon God for help, since both her own life and that of her child are at stake. And she should remember that God Himself said: 'Let woman give birth in pain and sorrow',[148] for it would be rare to see a woman delivered without pain. Euripides made Medea say that she would rather die twice in war than give birth once.[149]

But in histories we read that there are certain countries where women give birth without pain. In his wonderful narrations, Aristotle says that the women of Liguria give birth without pain,[150] and that as soon as they are delivered, they return to their work. Those who have written the history of America say the same about women from that continent.[151] That is to say, they get back up without delay, and are so kind to their husband who has gone to the trouble of making the child that immediately after the delivery they give their place over to their husband, who is looked after and indulged like a newly delivered mother; and in this way, he is visited by all their friends and relations who bring them gifts.

146. Traditionally believed to promote a safe pregnancy and to shorten labor.

147. A type of wild cattle surviving in Europe until the seventeenth century.

148. Genesis 3:16.

149. *Medea,* line 250.

150. From what is now recognized as a pseudo-Aristotelian work, *Of Wondrous Things Overheard* [*De Mirabilibus Auscultationibus*], ch. 91.

151. See, for example, Jean de Léry, *Account of a journey to the land of Brazil* [*Histoire d'un voyage faict en la terre du Brésil*, 1578], ch. XVII.

Chapter 6: On the Duty and Role of the Midwife, concerning What She Must Do in the First Stage of the Delivery[152]

When the woman who is about to give birth is lying in her bed in the position described, with the midwife near her, the midwife should first ask the woman if she is at the end of her pregnancy and ready to give birth, and she should find out when the woman conceived. Then she should feel her abdomen and, looking closely at it, she should reckon whether the upper parts are almost empty and fallen, and the lower ones very full and large, which will indicate that the child has descended. In addition, she should ask the woman if she is having pains, and what they are like, where they start and finish, and whether they are small, strong and frequent; whether they start in the lower back, running around the abdomen without stopping at the navel, and even whether they run along the groin and finish internally at the bottom of the abdomen, which corresponds to the inner neck of the womb. This is a sign that her labor is starting. In addition, the woman may have a slight fever, and sometimes will shiver all over because of the effort that nature demands as it wishes the child to be delivered.[153]

To be quite sure, the midwife may put her hand inside, having first greased it with fresh butter, or pig fat or another unguent that we shall describe. If she observes that the inner neck is straight and dilating and gaping, as it does when the woman is on the point of conceiving, it is a definite sign that the woman is soon to give birth, for right throughout pregnancy it is rounded and shut, both to hold the child in and to prevent anything from entering the womb, as Galen writes in Book XIV of *On the Usefulness of the Parts of the Body*.[154] It may be that some mucus or waters will escape and run out of the neck, these being indications that the labor is imminent, as Hippocrates says: 'if they are pale, they usually denote that it will be a girl, and if they are reddish, a boy'.

152. In 1609, this was chapter 4 of Book II.

153. This last sentence ('In addition… be delivered') was added in 1620.

154. This sentence was an elaboration in 1620; the reference to Galen (*On the Usefulness of the Parts of the Body*, XIV. 3) is also a later addition.

This mucus comes from the dilation of the inner neck and from the membranes surrounding the child, which start to want to break, and also because of the cotyledons and the threads, which break away from the walls of the womb. This will also be evident from the waters that start to gather and bulge, resembling a bottle, or rather a bladder that protrudes and is full of water. Once the waters start to do this, it is only a question of waiting until the woman is in labor for the birth to take place. Hippocrates observes three damp secretions during labor: the first is mucousy, the second reddish, and the third is the waters in which the child floats.

This is the end of the first stage that the midwife must watch for.

Chapter 7: On What the Midwife Must Do in the Second Stage[155]

As the waters are gathering in this way, bulging under the pressure of the contractions that build up little by little, the midwife should station herself near the mother, sitting in a chair lower than the bed. She should position herself in such a way that she can easily slip her hand (which she must keep lubricated) in the mother's lower parts when necessary. In this way, she will be able to determine whether the child is coming naturally or not: for by gentle touch, through the membrane which contains the waters, she will be able to recognize the round shape of the baby's head or something uneven. If when she touches she recognizes something round, hard and even, it is likely to be the head of the child, and it will be coming in a natural position. If she feels something uneven, the opposite is likely to be true.

Once she has established that everything is proceeding well, according to nature, when the woman's contractions increase and the child struggles and thrusts in its attempts to be born, and the womb contracts and tightens to be delivered of this burden, the midwife and all those present must encourage the mother, for fear lest she put herself and her child at risk.[156] They should exhort and beg her to hold

---

155. In 1609 this was chapter 5 of Book II.

156. The 1620 edition added the reference 'and all those present' (in 1609 Jacques Guillemeau specified only the midwife) and the observation 'for fear lest she put herself and her child at risk'.

her breath, closing her mouth and pushing downwards, as though she wished to empty her bowels, and they should reassure her that she will soon be free of her pain, and that her child is only trying to come into the world. She should be encouraged to be patient, and told that soon she will have a fine son or fine daughter, according to which she has said she would prefer.

And above all at this time, the midwife's duty is not to rush or hurry anything; she should refrain from forcibly widening the passage for the birth, and should certainly not break the waters or strip the membranes that contain them; she should wait patiently until the waters break of their own accord.

Either because of ignorance, or impatience, or because they are in a rush to go to deliver other women, some midwives tear the membranes with their nails and break the waters. This presents a great danger and is to the detriment of the poor woman and child, which is left high and dry because the waters have drained away and emptied before the time for the child to come into the world, indeed often before the child has fully turned, and this has caused the death of various women and numerous children. But, when the waters have freshly broken through the efforts of the mother and child, then both the midwife and the friends and those present[157] must continue to encourage the mother, especially when her contractions increase, begging her in the name of God to make use of them and let them intensify as much as she can. Meanwhile, the midwife should continue to lubricate all the mother's lower parts with butter, or another salve or grease. And when the head appears ready for delivery, the midwife should cradle it gently between her hands, and when it is delivered and the mother's contractions increase, she should pull the shoulders out neatly, slipping her fingers under the armpits, choosing the opportunity and moment when the contractions are intensifying and she can gently grasp the child. For the child's body is tender, delicate and soft, and if it is treated roughly, its whole body or some part of it may be deformed.[158] It should be noted that the contractions do not stop, or only slightly, when the child's head and shoulders come out. However, the poor woman needs some time to recover her breath,

157. The friends and those present are, at this point, mentioned in the 1609 text.
158. This sentence ('For the child's body… deformed') is added in 1620.

and should be exhorted to remain of good courage. Once these things have been accomplished, after pulling out the shoulders, the midwife will easily pull out the rest of the body, and she should do this without haste or precipitation.

But since in a natural birth the child emerges with its face and stomach facing backwards, once it is totally out, it must be swiftly turned to lie on its back so that it does not suffocate or choke because it cannot breathe and take in air or breath. If it has the umbilical cord twisted around its neck, as sometimes happens, it should be unlooped. Often the child is also so pale and faint that it appears to have no life and be unable to breathe; in this case, a little wine should be blown into its mouth, nose and ears, as much as is necessary.[159] When it has come to and starts to cry, the midwife should feel the cord, jostling and shaking it so that she can gently extract the placenta to which it is attached, instructing the mother to cough and to hold some salt in her hands, and, keeping them closed, blow into it.[160]

If the placenta does not come out quickly, the midwife should keep the outer mouth of the womb as dilated as possible with her hand, pulling and loosening the cord as gently as possible.[161]

Meanwhile, the midwife or another person should place their other hand lightly on the top of the womb of the mother, pressing it gently down. When the placenta has been delivered, it should be placed on the child's stomach; then the child and the placenta should be immediately wrapped in a cover and sheet, and brought to the fire. The child's head should be covered with a sheet folded over five or six times, but it should not be suddenly exposed to the light of a

159. This is what Bourgeois did in 1601, with the permission of Henri IV, in order to revive the dauphin (the future Louis XIV) after Marie de Medici's long labor: see *A True Account of the Births of my Lords and Ladies the Children of France* in *Diverse Observations*. See also my analysis in 'La théâtralisation de la naissance du dauphin'.

160. The movement of controlled exhalation is intended to loosen the placenta from the womb.

161. This sentence ('If... possible') is added in 1620. Treatises of this period expect the midwife to take responsibility for delivering the placenta, and in reports of births it was often portrayed as the most dangerous and controversial stage. Whereas onlookers could understand a midwife's difficulties in extracting a badly positioned foetus, they were less forgiving of any failure to deliver the placenta, or of any injuries the woman sustained in the process. The post-partum death of 'Madame' (sister-in-law of Louis XIII) in 1627 was imputed to Bourgeois's rough delivery of the placenta (although it is now thought probable that the death was caused by peritonitis).

strong fire or of the candle or daylight, for fear that such a change may damage its sight.[162] But, its eyes should be covered so that it can open them little by little and grow accustomed to the light, for all sudden changes are disagreeable to nature.

Although we said above that the woman needs to be encouraged when the waters have broken, and must make every effort to give birth so that her child follows the waters, it must be established whether the pains are those of labor or not, and whether the waters which ran out are the actual waters in which the child floats. For there are some women whose waters break and flow out copiously a long time in advance, even though they are not ready to give birth so soon.[163]

I have seen this happen to a number of women, and recently to Mademoiselle Arnaut, who was six to seven months pregnant and suffered from a bad colic for nearly two months, with stomach pains every day at certain times. While she was at her residence in Andilly,[164] she asked me to go and see her. She wanted to know whether I thought she should come to Paris, and I advised her she should, on account both of the great pains she was suffering and of the size of her pregnancy, for I thought she might be carrying two children as she had done just one year before. When she reached Paris, her colic subsided to a degree, then, shortly after, she released a bucket of waters without any pain, feeling as though she was no longer pregnant. Five days later she gave birth most happily to a fine daughter, with little pain, and losing only a very small additional quantity of waters.

I saw another lady who lost waters in abundance more than ten days before she gave birth. She did not take to her bed, but continued about her daily business. This should be carefully noted, so that we do not hasten the birth if pains do not follow of the kind which we have described as appropriate to childbirth.

162. It should be noted that Jacques Guillemeau had published a *Treatise on Diseases of the Eye* [*Traité des maladies de l'œil*, Paris: Charles Massé, 1585] more than 20 years earlier.

163. Guillemeau shares the concern of modern obstetricians that a delay between the rupture of the membranes, with the resulting loss of waters, and the onset of labor may lead to infections of the womb.

164. About 20 km north of Paris.

Chapter 8: On What the Midwife Must Do in the Third Stage of the Delivery[165]

As soon as the child is born and the mother has been delivered of the placenta, the midwife will gently lower the mother's legs, having the log removed from her feet, and she will place a cloth (or a very clean sponge, which has first been washed in warm water, and squeezed out) between her thighs and close to her nether parts, so that they are not left open for fear that cold air might enter. Then she will pick up the child and the placenta and take them close to the fire, as has been described.

If the placenta took a long time to come out or be extracted, so that the child does not remain between the mother's thighs for too long, running the risk of suffocating and dying because it is often so weak, the midwife should tie and then cut the cord to separate the child from the placenta. She will do this as follows.

She should have a length of doubled thread and a pair of well sharpened scissors, and she should tie the cord with the thread a good inch away from the child's navel, using a double knot and then knotting it once more. The knot should be neither too tight nor too loose. If it is too tight, it will cause great pain and it will drop off too soon, before the scar has closed between the living and the dead flesh; and if it is too loose, it often causes some hemorrhaging from the umbilical vessels which are not properly compressed and checked by this ligature. So a medium-tight knot is to be favored. Then, when it is tied, the cord needs to be cut with scissors, one inch below the tie. And so that the knot does not come undone, and the thread does not slip and come loose, the midwife should take a little band of cloth, unwound and soaked in rose oil, and what remains of the cord should be wrapped in this and placed on the stomach with a little cotton also soaked in this oil so that it is not crushed when the baby is wrapped up and swaddled. If the knot is tied in this way, the piece which has been tied will wither and dry, and four or five days later the dead flesh will separate from the living. This should not be hurried and it should not be pulled away.

---

165. In 1609 this was chapter 6 of Book II.

Some believe that the cord should be tied to a shorter or longer length according to the sex of the child. For males, it is left longer, and its length is believed to make the tongue and the male member longer, and this allows them to speak more eloquently and serve the ladies. And if it is cut short, almost touching the abdomen, for females, their tongues and their nether passages will be narrower and tighter. And indeed, commonly when it is a boy, ladies laugh and say to the midwife, 'Make it a good length for him', and for girls, 'tie it short'.

Hippocrates instructs that when the knot is tied, it should be done as follows. If a woman has had a painful birth, and the child has remained in the womb for a long time, not being delivered easily, but with effort and pain, and perhaps even needing a surgeon's instruments, he believes such children will not live long, and their cord should not be cut until they have urinated or sneezed or cried.[166]

As soon as the midwife has tied the knot, she must clean the child's face and its whole body, including under the armpits, the top of the legs, the buttocks and joints, either with freshly melted butter, or with sweet almond oil; others use rose oil, or walnut oil so that the skin is tougher, and to stop up the pores of the skin so that the air cannot harm it, as well as strengthening all the parts of its body.

Avicenna[167] says that roses and sage should be boiled in wine, and the decoction used to wash the child using a small, soft sponge, and this should be repeated for three or four mornings when the child is stirred and unswaddled.[168]

As soon as the child was born, the Ancients used to wash the whole body except the head. And so that its skin would become firmer and tougher, and so it would withstand external threats, it was rubbed with finely ground and powdered salt, mixed with a little virgin olive oil. If the child was very damp, plump and stout, they repeated this for seven or eight days.[169]

When the child has been stimulated, rubbed and then dried, and wrapped up by the midwife or others in this way, it may immediately

---

166. *On Superfetation*, 15.

167. The works of the Arab philosopher and physician Avicenna (c. 980–1037) remained highly influential throughout the Renaissance. See his chapter on the care of the newborn infant: *Canon*, Liber I, Fen 1, doctrina I, ch. 1.

168. 'and unswaddled' was added in 1620.

169. This whole paragraph ('As soon as … eight days') was added in 1620.

be given a little wine with sugar on a spoon, or one dose of theriac[170] dissolved in a little wine in winter or in summer (because of the heat) in a little blessed thistle water[171] or other cordial water.

Avicenna recommends just giving it a little honey and rubbing some on the top and bottom of the tongue with the finger which one has dipped into the honey; and this allows one to see if there is a strand binding the tongue, and if necessary, to cut it.

Chapter 9: On the Care She Must Take of the Woman Once Delivered[172]

While the midwife cuts the umbilical cord, and cleans the child, the mother's nurse, or other people who are with her, should take care of two things.

The first is to give the mother this drink:

Take two ounces of almond oil; an ounce of syrup of maidenhair; half an ounce each of blessed thistle water, pellitory and white wine. Mix all these together, and beat it in two glasses.

This should be given to the mother to drink. It is a remedy that soothes and relieves the throat and the trachea, which will have been over-heated and expanded through the mother's cries and lamentations. It will also serve to bring on her lochia and prevent the contractions being too strong.

The second thing is to skin a fresh sheep, and take its fleece while still warm to wrap around the lower back and abdomen of the woman. This will comfort her and firm up her limbs, which have been, as it were, torn apart from each other in the great effort of childbirth.

Avicenna recommends just skinning a live hare and taking its skin to put on the mother's abdomen.

---

170. Theriac was a widespread antidote to many illnesses, often containing over 60 ingredients, including viper's flesh, opium, cinnamon, and many herbs. It was given, for example, by the physician Héroard to the newborn Louis XIV after the hard labor Marie de Medici had endured. (See my analysis in 'La théâtralisation de la naissance du dauphin'.)
171. Carduus benedictus, made by distilling thistles and herbs, and believed to purge thick, slimy humors, and to be an antidote to venomous bites.
172. In 1609 this was chapter 7 of Book II.

Then either the midwife, if she is not occupied with the child, or another woman who is tending the mother, will apply to all the lower lips and the lower abdomen this remedy:

Take two ounces of oil of hypericum, one ounce of rose oil, two whole eggs; mix these all together and warm it a little.

This should be immediately applied with a very clean, unfolded cloth or fabric, as I have said. Also, under her calves you should place a rolled-up pillow to keep her knees up so that her thighs and legs do not slump out of alignment. She should be neither sitting nor lying, but in a midway position, with her head and body more upright than reclining, to allow her lochia to flow more easily. Then, when the midwife or nurse has taken off the sheep's skin, which should have been left in place for two or three hours, they should bind the mother's abdomen after first rubbing in oil of hypericum, sweet almond and roses (all blended together). This bandage will keep the womb in place and also help gently express the lochia without letting any air enter, for this could cause great contractions.

The bandage should be of cloth, folded double four times, and wide enough to cover the whole abdomen; it should be placed, with no folds or wrinkles, below the small of the back and the womb. While this is done, it is essential above all that the mother should feel no cold, and that air cannot enter the womb, for since the womb is now empty this can easily happen. It would cause her to swell and it would block the opening of the veins from which the lochia flow, and if these are suppressed it causes pain, contractions, suffocation,[173] fever and other such problems.

I saw this happen to a wellborn lady who got up on only the second day after giving birth. Cold air entered her womb and caused her to swell and die in appalling pain. This is why in *On the Usefulness of the Parts of the Body,* Galen instructs women to avoid cold air when they have their flow.[174]

---

173. I.e. suffocation of the womb, a common supposed ailment of the nursing mother.

174. This case history and the reference to Galen ('I saw... flow') were added in 1620. The advice needs to be understood within the broader context of *On the Usefulness of the Parts of the Body*, in which Galen attributes the imperfection of the female to the fact that she is colder than the male, as a result of which her reproductive organs are internal rather than external (XIV. 6).

Now when the mother has been cared for as described, much though she may want to sleep, she must be forbidden to. She should be kept awake with encouraging words and her nurse will tend her breasts, as will be described in the third book in its proper place.[175]

When the mother has spent three or four hours without sleeping, she can be given a broth made of knuckle of veal and poultry, or if this is not available, a couple of egg yolks. She should rest and if now she wants to sleep, she may be allowed to, since this will be some four hours after her delivery. The windows of the room and the doors should be firmly shut, without making any noise.

All this concerns natural childbirth in which there has not been any problem, the woman not having had an over-long labor, or great pain, just what is normal, and as was foretold to her for her sins, that is to say that she would give birth by the sweat of her brow.[176]

Chapter 16: The Way to Deliver the Mother When the Child has Died in the Womb[177]

When it has been carefully established that the child has died, the mother should be positioned in the same way that has been described when speaking of extracting the child in the case of a hemorrhage.

If the child presents an arm, shoulder, the back, stomach, or other parts of the body, without delay it should be rotated as gently as possible, and pulled by the feet, as we shall explain in detail for all births in which the child presents in various positions, whether alive or dead.

But, if it is dead at delivery and comes head first, and there is little or no hope of delivering the mother without assistance, and if her strength is visibly fading, the safest thing is to intervene manually. So the surgeon should gently slip his left hand (stretched full length but keeping his fingers together in the shape of a spoon as though he wanted to keep some liquid in them) into the neck of the womb, either into the lower part facing the rectum, or at the side between the head

175. See Book III, chapter 2.
176. Again, cf. Genesis III:16.
177. In 1609 this was chapter 13 of Book II.

of the child and the neck of the womb.[178] When his hand is far enough in, with his right hand he should slide in his hook, as shown here.

Below his left hand, between the head of the child and the base of his left hand, he should direct the hook immediately to the side of the child's head, towards the ear and the petrous bone, if possible, or another place such as in the eye socket or the occipital bone, always keeping his left hand in the place where he has put the hook. Then he should rock the head gently with his left hand, and at the same time, with his right hand in which he is holding the hook which has been stuck into some part of the head, he should pull on the hook and withdraw it, instructing the woman to bear down and push as though she were giving birth on her own. And it is important to note that the surgeon should take his cue to pull the hook when the woman is experiencing contractions, for at the time of the contractions the child will come out more easily.

Sometimes it happens that the hook cannot be inserted high enough inside the woman for it to be possible to pull the complete head out in a single movement, and having pulled the head some way forward, the surgeon is forced to remove the hook from the first place where it was stuck in the head, and to insert it into a second place higher up than the first one. The surgeon should be able to do this skillfully, as we described above. Equally, if the first time the hook was not so securely and well positioned, so that it slips and loses its original hold, he will need to reinsert it more securely in another place.

Once the child's head is extracted, the hook should be removed from it, and then as skillfully as possible, the surgeon should slip his fingers under the child's armpits to pull out the shoulders and the rest of the body. He will extract the child more securely in this way than by pulling on the head, and he should not be in any hurry, but instead give the mother the chance to regain her strength, waiting until she experiences some contractions.

While the surgeon is carrying out this operation, the poor woman should be given a spoon of wine, or she should be allowed to suck a crust of fresh or fried bread soaked in wine or spiced wine, and

178. The 1620 edition gives more precise detail than the 1609 version, which reads, 'So the surgeon should gently slip his left hand, stretched flat between the head of the child and the neck of the womb.'

Illustration of the hook for extracting a dead child from the mother's womb when it presents head first, and when the head is wedged between the sacrum and the pubis so that it cannot be dislodged and pushed back up in order to rotate the child and pull it out by the feet,without causing great suffering and sometimes the death of the mother. It can also be used to extract the head if this is the only part remaining in the womb. It should be 10 to 12 inches in length, sufficiently strong and thick, and broad enough at the cupped end.

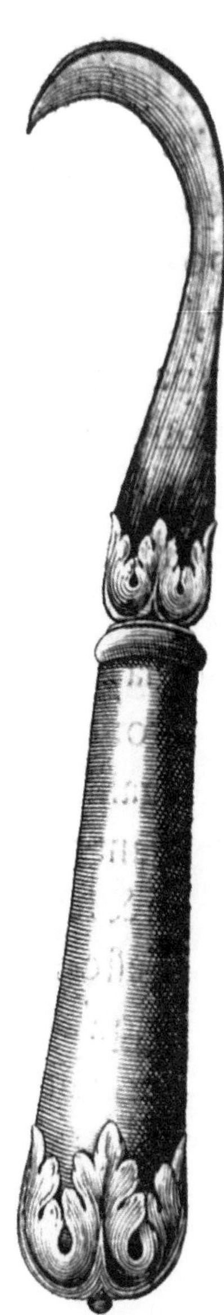

17) Surgeon's hook

Jacques Guillemeau, *De la grossesse et accouchement des femmes*, Paris, 1620
(Library of Royal College of Obstetricians and Gynaecologists, London)

she should be encouraged further by being told that she will soon be delivered.

This art of extracting the dead child from the mother's womb is safer and speedier than that of trying to push it back in with the aim of rotating it until the feet present so that they can be used to pull it out. For whenever the child's head is lodged right down between the pubic bones, it is impossible to push it back up and rotate it without grave risk to the mother, and without causing severe bruising of the womb, which brings various repercussions and sometimes death, as I have seen happen. And if the child should be alive before being rotated, it is suffocated before the rotation can be accomplished.

I know that some people will assert that some children have been extracted with the hook while living although they had been judged dead in the mother's womb, and because of the blow of the hook they had suddenly died. And in truth such an action is cruel. I would say in reply that great care must be taken to establish whether the child is alive or dead before introducing the hook, and if there are signs that it is alive, you should delay as long as possible before extracting it with the hook. But if it is dead, there is no basis for refusing to extract it by means of the hook, for the reasons I have explained above. However, if it is alive, it is most debatable whether it should be extracted with the hook in a case in which we suppose the mother to be close to death and having no more strength without this operation, it being more expedient to lose the child than the mother. Both would die if we delayed any longer. It is debatable whether in order to save the mother (who is more precious than the child) one must risk such an operation. Yet, in carrying out such an act, all those who conduct such an operation feel the weight upon their consciences. It is a theological point that I leave up to those who know more than I do about such matters.

Chapter 28: The Way to Pull the Child from the Mother's Womb by Cesarean Section[179]

We now need to treat the last kind of delivery, which needs to be carried out when the mother has died, in order to save the child and to allow it to be baptized. This is called cesarean delivery from '*a caeso matris utero*' ['from the cut womb of the mother '], after Caesar who was pulled from his mother's womb at the very moment she died.[180] The same thing[181] happened to a king of Navarre called Sancho: his mother was out hunting when she was attacked by Saracens; she was wounded in the abdomen and the child's arm protruded from the wound, and a nobleman called Guevara noticed this and pulled the child out of this wound and cared for it in secret. But when there was a disagreement about the election of a king, Guevara displayed him to the princes, and thus brought a peaceful resolution to their quarrels. And for this remarkable theft, the house of Guevara acquired the name Thief.[182]

This incision and extraction of the child after the mother's death should always be carried out in a well-ordered state, for 'lawyers judge a man worthy of death who buries a pregnant woman without first taking out the foetus, because it seems that the hope of its life has been destroyed together with the mother's.' ['*Iurisconsulti eum necis damnant qui gravidam sepelierit, non prius extracto foetu, quod spem animantis cum gravida peremisse videatur, de mortuo,*[183] *inferendo et sepulchro aedificando.*'][184]

I carried out such an operation on a number of women with great success, among them on Madame Le Maire, in the presence of my uncle, Monsieur Philippes, and on Madame Pasquier, immediately

179. In 1609, this was chapter 25 of Book II.

180. For the tradition ascribing the term 'cesarean' to the supposed method of delivery of Julius Caesar, see 17, n. 43.

181. The rest of this paragraph ('The same thing… Thief') is added in 1620.

182. According to legend, this occurred in 885, when Sancho de Guevara was fighting the Moors who had just killed the king and his wife in battle. For saving his king, Sancho was named Niño Ladron de Guevara, 'the little boy thief'.

183. Incorrectly given as *mortuor* in French text.

184. In the *Digests* of the Roman jurist Salvius Julianus (c. 100–170).

after her death, in the presence of Monsieur Paré[185] and the priest of St André des Arts.[186]

But first, before undertaking such an operation, the surgeon should look very closely and assure himself that the woman is dead, and her relatives, friends and others present should all acknowledge and judge that her soul has passed into the afterlife. Then the operation should be commenced immediately, for to delay it would bring the death of the child and the operation would be in vain.

While the woman is approaching death, the midwife or another attendant should leave her hand in the neck of the womb to keep it as open as possible, even though we know that the child, being in the mother's womb, breathes only through her arteries. Nonetheless, the outside air that can flow into it cannot harm the child, and may be beneficial. Now to be sure and to verify that the mother has drawn her last breath, some light feathers or a piece of wool should be placed on her lips and near her nose, for if she is breathing even slightly, she will cause them to move and fly away.

When he is convinced she is dead, the surgeon should uncover her abdomen completely, and without delay make a vertical incision of four finger-lengths on one side of the epigastrium, quite near the straight muscles, cutting through the skin and the three muscles of the epigastrium and the peritoneum, right into the cavity. Then he should slip his two fingers into the cavity, using them to raise the skin and muscles and peritoneum, and he should make a sufficient incision between them to disclose the womb and the child within it — the womb will be uncovered very easily. Then, at the same time, he should make an incision directly in the side of the womb, which he will find about two fingers thick, or more, without fear of hurting the child, since I have always observed that the placenta is situated in this place and the child is behind it. However, if there are signs that the placenta is detached and in another place, the surgeon should proceed more cautiously. In this case, with the two fingers of each hand, which he has put in the womb, the incision should be torn and enlarged rather than cut, as he sees it necessary to create an opening which is suitable

185. Guillemeau had been a student of Ambroise Paré, even in 1599 saving Paré's daughter from a life-threatening hemorrhage at the onset of her labor.

186. Parish in Paris, on the left bank of the Seine, now in the 5th arrondissement.

and large enough to pull out the child. When he has removed the child from the womb, he should take the placenta and place it on the child's stomach, and he should get someone to warm wine in their mouth and blow some into the nose, ears and mouth of the child several times, as we described above.[187]

Some believe that such a cesarean section can, and should, be practiced while the woman is still alive, in case of a difficult delivery. I cannot advise this since I witnessed it twice, in the presence of Monsieur Paré, and saw it performed by Monsieur Viart, Monsieur Bruner and Monsieur Charbonnet, all most experienced surgeons, who carried everything out with due skill and method. Yet of the five women on whom this operation was performed, none survived. I know that it may be argued that there are some cases in which women have been saved,[188] but if this is indeed so, it must be judged a cause of wonder rather than something which should be practiced or imitated. One swallow does not make a spring, and one experience is not sufficient foundation for a science.

After Monsieur Paré had demonstrated it to us, and seeing that it was not successful, he stopped performing the operation and rejected it, together with our College of Surgeons registered in Paris, and the soundest among the physicians who are Regents in the Faculty of Medicine in Paris. This question was fully addressed by the late Monsieur Marchand in two speeches, which he gave when he had the honor to be sworn in as a surgeon in Paris.[189]

187. See 202.

188. Guillemeau is clearly alluding to Rousset's writings, which had circulated widely in Latin as well as French by this time. See 7-10.

189. Jacques Marchand, the son-in-law of Guillemeau (see 6, n. 10). Bourgeois also considered Marchand an expert in deliveries.

BOOK III

Chapter 1: On the Regimen of the Mother after Delivery

Until now we have spoken of the care of the mother immediately after giving birth and delivering the placenta. Now we shall treat the regimen she must follow throughout her lying-in and the problems which may befall her at this time.

She must be kept moderately warm, for excess heat weakens and saps strength. But above all she must not suffer cold air, which is an enemy of the spermatical[190] parts, for, since cold air penetrates easily, it could enter the womb which is completely empty, and cause great pains and contractions, which would make the womb swell, together with the whole abdomen. So the doors and windows should be kept tightly closed.

Here is the regimen she should follow. First, she should live soberly, not partaking of a large quantity of food, for it is not good to fill oneself up again straight after a great emptying of the body, as Hippocrates and Galen remark in the book *On Acute Diseases*.[191] She should eat like those who have suffered an injury, and indeed for some women this is the case, and they suffer not only from an injury but from bruising, for in the great effort involved in the birth of the child, some membranes have been not only battered and bruised, but even broken and torn apart, as we see in women who are young or very old and who have not previously had children. Sometimes in their cases the passage from the womb and the rectal passage form a single opening. Others suffer substantial excoriations and injuries in all their parts, and if these are overlooked they can cause some to begin to fester and become gangrenous. Mothers should not heed what those nursing them say; they keep telling the mother that it is necessary to indulge herself. They say that she should fill her stomach that has just shed its burden; they remonstrate with her that she has lost a lot of blood, that she is continuing to lose some and that in the end she will become so weak that she will not be able to get up.

---

190. The French uses the term '*spermatiques*', designating the male and female 'seed-producing' parts (i.e. what we now recognize as ovaries and testicles).

191. Hippocrates, *On Regimen in Acute Diseases*, 5 and 11.

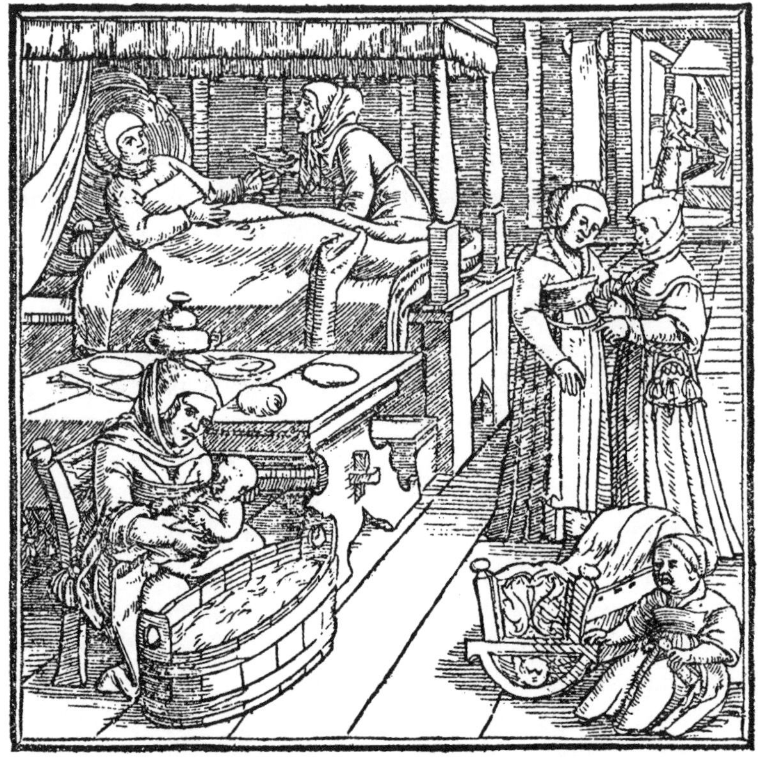

18) Woman in bed after delivery

Jakob Rueff, *De conceptu et generatione hominis*, Zurich, 1554
(Bibliothèque de Strasbourg)

Such reasons are quite unfounded, for most of the blood that she
has lost and which she is now losing during her lying-in is nothing
but excess blood, which serves no purpose. It has been retained for a
long time already, over nine months, and it is necessary for her health
that it should be shed from the uterus so that, instead of being swollen
and engorged as it now is, and full of blood like a sponge which has
soaked up water, it can be discharged and compressed so that it reverts
to its normal state. Furthermore, for the sake of her health, the newly-
delivered mother should not be as well fed for the first days, as popular
opinion would have it. This is to prevent the fever, which can befall
her, and the amount of blood that would flow back up to the breasts
to be turned into milk, for it may curdle and then produce an abscess.

Therefore, for the first five days, she should be fed on stocks, clear soups, panades,[192] fresh eggs and jelly. She should not gorge herself on meats, pearl barley, or almonds as she usually might do. In the morning, she should have a clear soup, at dinner another clear soup with two fresh eggs and some panade paste, and at supper she should have the same again together with some jelly to finish her meal. It is true that if she wishes to breastfeed her child, she can be fed a little more amply, drinking herbal teas to which has been added a grain of coriander or some cinnamon. Fine ladies in Italy use stock from a rooster as follows:

Take two roosters; pluck them well and remove the innards; boil them with a good amount of water in an earthenware pot until they are half cooked. Then take them out of the pot together with the stock, and cut the meat into cubes, which should be put into an alembic glass vessel, as follows.

Take two good handfuls of each of bugloss, borage and balm, and make a bottom layer of these in your alembic. Then put a layer of rooster flesh and a layer of gold leaf, together with a dram of powdered pearls, and then the stock on top. When it is all arranged in this way, it should be distilled using a double vessel, and you should get a pint or five-eighths of a quart from it. You should repeat this process as many times as necessary to give you sufficient distilled broth to feed the mother for 10 to 12 days. However, such a special dish is for princesses. The water for it should be drawn six weeks or two months before it is needed, and put in the sun in summer, or in the oven of a cake-maker in winter, in order to remove any rawness which might otherwise remain.

For my part, provided the mother has no fever, I allow her to take a little white wine, or thin claret diluted with twice the quantity of boiled water. There are some women who cannot endure wine; they should drink honeyed water or boiled water. If they want to drink during the day and between meals, or at night, they should be given a little syrup of maidenhair fern in boiled water, or some other syrup that is not astringent (because of their discharges). Once their pains, slight fever and the burning in their breasts have passed, they may be allowed to

---

192. A savoury soup, the thick consistency of which comes from the addition of one or more of the following: breadcrumbs, rice, flour, milk, butter or egg yolks.

eat rather more food. They may be given a little meat with their broth, such as rooster, chicken or pigeon, or a piece of boiled veal, mutton or poultry, or some other good meat.[193] After the eighth day, which is usually the time when the womb has been well purged and relieved, it would be wise to feed her better; she should be given solid food in larger quantities so that she can return to her normal condition.

During this time, she should still rest, not moving about or stirring greatly, nor even going into the outside air. She should speak little, if she can, and should not be made to make any noise, and she should converse with and be visited by only her closest friends and relatives, who will not tell her anything which might upset or sadden her.[194] She should sleep at night, not in the day. If she has indeed not slept at night because of some pain, she may sleep during the day at the time she feels the need. Since most women have slightly hard abdomens, and do not open their bowels, it would be very appropriate to give her a small enema, such as this one. Prescription:[195] leaves of mallow, pellitory and of a whole marshmallow, of each one minim; one flower of camomile and of clover of each by weight; seed of aniseed and of fennel, two drams of each. Cook in a decoction of head of castrated ram, from which remove three gills. In this, dissolve red sugar and common honey, of each two ounces; of fresh butter, three ounces. Make a clyster.

Sometimes one may also add to this an ounce of catholicon.[196] If the mother refuses an enema, she may be given a small broth of senna.[197]

I believe that, during their lying-in, Athenian women used to drink a broth of cabbage every day in order to relax their stomach, not

193. The advice in 1609 was slightly different: 'They may be given a little meat with their broth, such as rooster, chicken or pigeon, or a piece of boiled veal for dinner; and for dinner with the broth a little minced veal, mutton or poultry, or some other good meat.'

194. Guillemeau's advice runs counter to the tradition of many women attending the new mother, and amusing her for hours with their gossip. The 'gossip of the newly delivered mother' ['*caquets de l'accouchée*'] is regularly attested in literature of this period — being the subject of protests from moralists and impoverished husbands!

195. In the French text, this prescription is given in Latin.

196. A common panacea containing a large range of ingredients, usually including senna, rhubarb, cassia and tamarinds.

197. A well-known purgative and laxative.

(as Athenaeus says)[198] to drive away curses. For previously cabbages were the medicine of Cato and all his family. In fact, when the Romans drove doctors away, Cato said that a cabbage sufficed to cure all ills, and he even wrote a short commentary on it.[199]

The woman should cast aside all worries and sadness, and take care only of her health, and she should rejoice and give thanks to God for having accorded her the blessing of being delivered.

198. Athenaeus of Naucratis, Greek rhetorician and grammarian of the second/third centuries AD.

199. Cato the Elder (234–149 BC), *On Agriculture*, sections 156–157.

JACQUES DUVAL

On Hermaphrodites, Deliveries of Women,
and the Treatment Which is Required after Childbirth
(1612)

DES
HERMAPHRODITS,
ACCOVCHEMENS DES
FEMMES, ET TRAITEMENT
qui eſt requis pour les releuer en ſanté,
& bien éleuer leurs enfans.

*Où ſont expliquez la figure des laboureur, & verger du genre
humain, ſignes de pucelage, defloration, conception, & la belle
induſtrie dont vſe nature en la promotion du concept & plante
prolifique.*

Par Maiſtre Iacques Duval, Eſcuyer, Seigneur d'Eŝtomare
& du Houuel, Doŝteur & Profeſſeur en Medecine,
natif d'Eureux, demeurant à Rouen.

A ROVEN,

De l'imprimerie de DAVID GEVFFROY,
demeurant à la ruë des Cordeliers, ioignant
ſainŝt Pierre.

M. DC. XII.
Auec Priuilege du Roy.

19) Title page: Jacques Duval, *Des Hermaphrodits*, Rouen, 1612

(Library of Royal College of Obstetricians and Gynaecologists, London)

INTRODUCTION

TRANSLATION OF EXCERPTS FROM *ON HERMAPHRODITES, DELIVERIES OF WOMEN* (1612)

Preliminary texts:

Main chapters:

INTRODUCTION

Jacques Duval's treatise stands apart from the others translated in this volume because of the indirect angle from which he approaches the topic of childbirth. His work acquired most notoriety for its thorough discussion of hermaphroditism and of the particular case of Marie/ Marin Le Marcis. However, the first third of the book treats the more conventional subjects of procreation and childbirth, and on this basis merits inclusion in this volume. Duval's views on the delivery of women are shaped by his experience as a doctor in a provincial town; hence, he is above all concerned to prevent what he believes to be so many unnecessary deaths of mothers and infants.

Life and Works of Jacques Duval

Duval followed in the footsteps of his father as a physician in Normandy, settling in Rouen and marrying the daughter of a local apothecary.[1] The most notable detail concerning this marriage is the death in childbirth of his first wife, Anne Le Marchant, in 1581, a tragedy which goes far to explain his interest, two decades later, in educating midwives and surgeons in order to ensure better care in deliveries.

His career does not appear to have departed from that of most doctors in large provincial towns: there is, for example, no evidence of his serving at court or spending time teaching in Paris. His first two published works (both in French) were also unexceptional, an account of the discovery of local medicinal springs[2] and a treatise on curing catarrhal infections.[3] However, his subsequent volume, *On Hermaphrodites, deliveries of women, and the treatment that is required after childbirth,* provoked a legal controversy.

1. The only biography of Jacques Duval to date is that by K. Albaric, *Un Médecin ébroïcien, Jacques Duval. Son traité des hermaphrodites (1555?–1615?),* (Paris: Librairie Le François, 1934).

2. *Hydrotherapuetic Qualities of Medicinal Fountains Recently Discovered near Rouen* [*Hydrothérapeutique des fontaines medicinales nouvellement decouvertes aux environs de Rouen,* Rouen, 1603].

3. *New Way to Cure Catarrh and all Diseases Caused by it* [*Methode nouvelle de guerir les catarrhes et toutes les maladies qui en dependent,* Rouen, 1611].

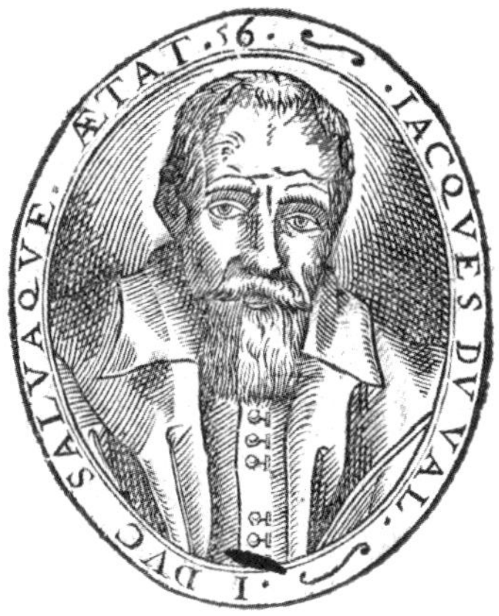

20) Portrait of Jacques Duval

Jacques Duval, *Des Hermaphrodits*, Rouen, 1612
(Library of Royal College of Obstetricians and Gynaecologists, London)

To deal with hermaphroditism, even within a medical work, was necessarily to approach the taboo subjects of homosexual and lesbian relationships.[4] Duval's account is centered upon his personal involvement in the case of Marie/Marin Le Marcis, a hermaphrodite who had started life as a female but subsequently developed male characteristics. Le Marcis had been tried and sentenced to execution in 1601; he was saved only when Duval, as one of the physicians required to provide expert advice, demonstrated that Le Marcis possessed a penis capable of ejaculation, and had thus not been guilty of a lesbian relationship with the woman he planned to marry. The publication of Duval's treatise may have been prudently held over for more than a decade after the trial,[5] but nonetheless, as Joe Harris has argued, the description in print of Duval's role (which had included manual

4. See the discussion of the problematic status of the work in my article, 'The definition of obscene material 1570–1615: three medical treatises held to account', *EMF: Studies in Early Modern France*, 14 (2010), 148–167. For a detailed overview of Renaissance attitudes towards hermaphroditism, see K. Long, *Hermaphrodites in Renaissance Europe* (Aldershot: Ashgate, 2006). She also provides a succinct analysis of Duval's treatise in the chapter 'Jacques Duval on hermaphrodites' in *High Anxiety: masculinity in crisis in early modern France*, ed. K. Long (Truman State University Press, 2002).

5. 'But when I was ready to deliver the present work to be printed, I reflected that it was not without good cause that the court had fixed a period of time during which this poor creature should not use his genital parts, male or female, in any sexual or procreative act [...].

stimulation of Le Marcis's penis) situates a complex eroticization of the hermaphrodite body within an otherwise conservative moral and social discourse.[6]

The actual printing of the treatise was itself delayed, or even stopped, in 1612. According to the nineteenth-century bibliophile Edouard Frère, the Parlement of Rouen issued an edict banning the book in April 1612.[7] It has proved impossible to trace any historical record of this edict — perhaps because a large part of the Rouen archives of this period were destroyed by fire in 1944 — and there are no documents corroborating it. However, in his response in 1615 to a treatise published the previous year by Jean Riolan (condemning Duval's account of hermaphroditism), Duval furnishes further details of the controversy surrounding his book's appearance, which provide important contextual information on the sensitivities the treatise aroused. He explains that when the title of his volume had come before the Chancellor of France to be approved for a privilege, it had — exceptionally — been referred for further enquiries to be made on account of 'the pleasurable and delightful subjects debated in it'.[8] However, the two expert physicians called upon to judge it had passed it with a clean bill of health.[9] From this evidence it seems likely that Frère's comment refers to the temporary suspension of the publication and sale of the volume, which was then reversed after the favorable report from the medical experts.

After the publication of his response to Riolan in 1615, we have no other surviving trace of Duval — either as a physician or an author. His biographers have assumed that he died in 1615, at the age of sixty,

---

I believed it to be my duty to delay the printing of my work until the will of the court had been accomplished.' (Letter to the Reader, 245)

6. '"La force du tact": representing the taboo body in Jacques Duval's *Traité des hermaphrodits* (1612)', *French Studies* 57 (2003), 311–322.

7. *Manuel du bibliographe normand* (Rouen: A. Le Brument, 1858), 415.

8. Jean Riolan (1580–1657), a noted conservative, was Royal Professor of Anatomy from 1613 and also First Physician to Marie de Medici. His *Discourse on Hermaphrodites* [*Discours sur les hermaphrodits*, 1614] was hostile to Duval, who responded to him in a *Response to the Discourse by Monsieur Riolan against the Account of the Hermaphrodite of Rouen* [*Responce au discours fait par le sieur Riolan contre l'histoire de l'hermaphrodit de Rouen*, Rouen, 1615].

9. See the 'Approval' signed by Jean and Charles de L'Orme (Ordinary Physicians of the King) that appeared in the 1612 treatise (238).

but it is possible that he simply lived on uneventfully for a while after the initial furore provoked by his treatise had died down.

Circulation and Afterlife of 'On Hermaphrodites'

Rather surprisingly, the original 1612 edition of *On Hermaphrodites* is the only one known before the nineteenth century,[10] yet the number of copies of this edition that survive in public libraries throughout France and abroad suggests that it achieved a fairly wide initial circulation. It is cited quite extensively, for example, by the mid-seventeenth-century physician Louis Meyssonnier in *The Care of Newly Delivered Women* [*Regime des femmes accouchées*].[11] There is, however, no evidence that it was translated into any other languages, certainly not into Latin, which would have ensured its international circulation. How could we account for the fact that, unlike Liebault's or Guillemeau's treatises on childbirth, Duval's was not republished in the seventeenth century, when childbirth was receiving increasing attention? It is likely that Duval's treatment of hermaphroditism was eclipsed, within two years, by Riolan's *Discourse on Hermaphrodites* [*Discours sur les hermaphrodits*] of 1614. Although Riolan took the contrary view to Duval, asserting that true hermaphroditism did not exist, his status as professor in the Faculty of Medicine in Paris lent authority to his work. Yet, this would not explain why at least the opening sections of Duval's treatise, devoted to reproduction and childbirth, were not reprinted. I suspect that the reason lies in Duval's position as a provincial physician, without patrons in Paris or at court. Publications which enjoyed long circulation and sustained popularity were usually those printed in the capital, often supported by patrons in positions of influence. The contrast is evident, for example, in the fact that Duval dedicates his work to Laurens Restaut, a councillor of the Parlement of Rouen since 1586, whereas the dedication to Guillemeau's volume,

---

10. It was republished by Isidore Liseux, in 1880, in an edition prepared by Alcide Bonneau, a defrocked monk with a taste for erotic literature, who claimed that bibliophiles had long wished to own and read the volume.

11. This short work appeared in Lyons in 1646: it cites both ancient and modern sources, with Duval's name appearing a number of times, alongside those of Liebault and Guillemeau. Meyssonnier refers to Duval as a 'famous doctor from Rouen'.

appearing several years earlier, allied Guillemeau's name with André Du Laurens, First Physician to the King.

More explicitly than Liebault's or Guillemeau's works, Duval's is also complicated by his wish to address both lay and professional readers. His 'Message to the Reader' makes it clear that much of the detail on reproduction was included as a frame for the episode of Le Marcis:

> I had the opportunity to write a history of this in a book, adding also an explanation of the genital parts of both sexes [...]. I know this to be necessary for an understanding of the subject.[12]

He justifies his opening sections by an additional reference to the commonplace argument that a better understanding of sexual or reproductive health will be helpful if readers consult doctors about their problems or conditions. Yet in the prefatory Message he moves immediately from these lay readers to the second group of readers whom he envisaged, 'young surgeons and midwives', arguing they will find information to allow them to act more competently both when called as expert witnesses in legal cases (like that of Le Marcis) and in the normal execution of their duties. The value of his work to these professional groups is underlined in his defence of the work's legitimacy, with reference to another familiar theme:

> ... the ignorance of the midwives who are not able to read or understand more serious and important books explaining the nature, aspects and form of all the parts of the human body.[13]

Duval is unique in putting a figure on the number of infant deaths in childbirth, which he attributes to the ignorance of some midwives: 500 newborns a year in Rouen. The number is surprisingly high,[14]

---

12. See 244.

13. See 247.

14. According to P. Benedict, there were on average c. 3,000 baptisms a year in Rouen in the period 1600–1620 (*The Huguenot Population of France*, 1991, vol. II, 13). If this figure

and may well represent an over-estimation. However, given Duval's personal experience of the death of his first wife in childbirth, it is clear that he had taken a keen interest in the subject, and his reforming zeal is no mere rhetorical trope.

Structure of 'On Hermaphrodites' and Selection of Chapters for Translation

Unlike Liebault or Guillemeau, Duval does not divide his work into separate books, but his discussion of childbirth, with which the book opens, effectively falls into three parts:

Chapters 1–18 on conception and pregnancy;

Chapters 19–24 on delivery;

Chapters 25–26 on care of the mother and child after the birth.

However, in the second and longer section of the book (chapters 27–81), Duval moves rapidly from an outline of the female reproductive system to a lengthy discussion of hermaphrodites and a detailed report of the specific case of Le Marcis. Within the context of the whole volume, therefore, the discussion of reproduction and childbirth serves as a preliminary frame, valuable in itself, but leading to an exceptional case history, which Duval believes merits pride of place. Interesting though the sections on hermaphroditism and Le Marcis are in their own right, they are too lengthy and too far removed from the main subject matter of this present volume to permit inclusion here.[15]

---

is accurate, Duval would be asserting that approximately one birth in six resulted in infant death due directly to the incompetence of midwives (rather than other causes), which would seem unlikely.

15. A full critical edition of the French text and / or an English translation of it, a major scholarly undertaking, would be most welcome, given the significance of the topic of hermaphroditism in medical and lay writings of the late-sixteenth and early-seventeenth centuries. One aspect that would merit particular attention, as is evident from my translation of the table of chapters (251-2), is Duval's keen interest in the relationship between astronomy and medicine (chs. 44–46, 52), with the final chapter (ch. 81) holding the configuration of the heavens partly responsible for Le Marcis's hermaphrodite form. Pomata has demonstrated that the term '*observatio*', which gave rise from the mid-sixteenth century to a new epistemic genre of medical writing, the *Obervationes*, re-emerged in the Renaissance precisely in the astral sciences ('Sharing Cases: the *Observationes* in early modern medicine', 201). This

Given the length of Duval's treatise, I have had to restrict my translation even within the first section to some key chapters that illustrate the nature of the writing and give a representative flavor of his lively style. I start with chapter 15, the point at which Duval moves from a detailed account of the anatomy of the male and female reproductive organs (the subject of chapters 2–15) to the process of conception and the ensuing pregnancy. My translation commences with the second half of this long chapter, in which Duval indicates external signs of pregnancy, and cautions midwives on the need to conduct internal examinations with great delicacy. Chapter 18, likewise, is primarily addressed to midwives, since it concentrates on the practical care of the mother just before the birth (diet, salves, baths, etc.). Chapters 19–20 present first normal and then difficult deliveries, still from the midwife's perspective, but insisting (in chapter 20) on the need for the midwife to summon a doctor to prescribe stronger remedies if the labor is protracted. I omit (for reasons of length) chapter 21 on advice if the mother is dying, and conclude the translation with chapters 22 and 23, in which Duval now addresses the surgeon, looking at cases of obstructed delivery, which must be resolved by manipulation, or by use of a speculum and manipulation combined. The chapters selected demonstrate that Duval's advice to both midwives and surgeons is couched in a style that makes the treatise accessible to both these groups, and even to lay readers.

Duval's Arguments and Style

At first sight, Duval's treatment of pregnancy and birth shares some obvious similarities with Guillemeau's treatise. Both organize a large part of their framework around the sequence of care in late pregnancy, and during and after delivery. Equally, both regularly cite classical and contemporary authorities as the sources of their recommendations. However, differences between the two authors are notable. Duval draws far more heavily than Guillemeau upon anatomists, commencing his treatise with 14 chapters devoted to a detailed explanation of the male and female genitals, and returning throughout to authors such

---

makes the intersection of medicine and astronomy particularly arresting in a work which prioritizes a single case history.

as Sevérin Pineau (c. 1550–1619), an anatomist and surgeon in Paris who had published a controversial Latin treatise on determining signs of virginity.[16] What most distinguishes Duval is his perception of anatomy as fundamental to an understanding of human nature and of the organization of the body. Like Guillemeau, he appeals to Nature, the handmaiden of God, as the highest organizing principle, but Duval is far more attentive to the excesses and deficiencies that he believes Nature can, on occasion, produce, leading to such exceptional cases as true hermaphrodites.[17] Thus, he justifies his potentially aberrant interest in the case of Le Marcis as an example of how, by means of natural prodigies, the human mind will be prompted to search for fuller understanding, leading it 'fittingly [to] praise and exalt the supreme power of the sovereign creator'.[18]

Religious faith underpins Duval's approach on several levels. From the repeated references to God, we may assume it was more than convention which made him assure his patron, Laurens Restaut, that 'I shall pray to God to keep you safe',[19] or remind the laboring mother that 'the sovereign Creator ... said to our common mother that she would give birth in pain, and she should arm herself with a strong heart',[20] or advise the midwife that if she summons the physician in case of protracted labor, he may be able to help her deliver the child 'with the help of God'.[21] These are all fairly commonplace invocations of God; more audacious is his association of God, albeit under the cloak of Nature, with sexual pleasures, licit or illicit. An early reference in his 'Letter to the Reader' situates this view safely within the context of Christian marriage, which Duval claims has safeguarded him from the temptations of impropriety, 'for God in His grace has taken this from me, removing the occasion for impure love by the long years and happy offspring which He has given and still vouchsafes to me in marriage'.[22] Yet, he also acknowledges — in a manner reminiscent of

16. See 187, n. 110.

17. See 241.

18. See 231.

19. See 242.

20. See 243.

21. See 275.

22. See 246.

Liebault and his continuer Pena[23] — that Nature uses sexual desires to ensure the perpetuation of the human race. For Duval, this leads to the additional and rather uncomfortable recognition that nature has not contained such desires within marriage, or even confined them to the sexual act itself, but 'through some mysterious instinct, granted such a sensual excitement and sexual stimulation when the mind thinks of it, by naming it or just alluding to it'. Duval thus acknowledges that the sexual matter of his treatise may excite his readers — a comment the more disturbing given the book's troubled printing history. It is noteworthy that he offers no answer to this moral dilemma (nor, as will be discussed below, does he attenuate his language), asserting only, as a counterweight, the belief that by saving children from death before or at birth, he is ultimately saving souls.

What motivates Duval in his account of childbirth is above all the wish to save the lives of mothers and their children. Prompted in part by the loss of his own child and first wife after an obstructed labor, which had continued for four days, he movingly commits himself to the better education of young surgeons:

> … so that women of all stations may receive their good support, and so that their cruellest mortal sufferings may be reduced, alleviated and ended; their illnesses cured; their lives saved and preserved; and their children, who would otherwise perish at birth, may be delivered more easily and safely while they enjoy good health and recovery.[24]

Following in the footsteps of Rousset, he is a firm supporter of cesareans on living women as a last resort, both because he had seen some successfully practiced in his youth, and because he believed a cesarean alone might have saved his first wife. Perhaps on account of having witnessed her distressing labor, he is also concerned that midwives should do everything possible to prepare women for an easier labor. Hence his interest in diet, salves and baths before labor, as well as in the most comfortable and efficacious positions for women

23. See 71-74.
24. See 247-8.

to adopt during labor. He is sympathetic to the mother's need for rest, cushions and support during the labor,[25] and mindful that different women may have very different needs and temperaments, which the midwife must recognize.[26]

As to the midwives, Duval's attitude is divided. On the one hand, as we have seen, he blames the high number of deaths of newborns in Rouen on incompetent midwives, and roundly lambasts newly pregnant women who risk miscarrying by allowing 'ignorant' midwives to perform internal examinations.[27] It is probably a sign of his concern about the lack of education in a provincial town that he feels it necessary to explain exactly how midwives should perform these examinations (e.g. first asking the woman to pass urine, applying an enema). In his assessment, the number of skilled midwives able to manage the most difficult deliveries is distressingly low:

> In this case, the poor mother needs not a mere servant, an attendant or an ignorant midwife, but one who is really wise and careful, and these are very few in number.[28]

Yet he does acknowledge that a few midwives can be excellent practitioners, citing in particular Bourgeois, the Queen's midwife, because she had claimed (in the first volume of her *Diverse Observations* of 1609)[29] only on two occasions in her whole career to have had to insert a hand into the uterus to remove a placenta. Despite his reservations, and his repetition of the familiar injunction to midwives to call upon physicians or surgeons sooner than they were wont to do, we might note in conclusion that Duval had thought it worth consulting midwives and female birth attendants before writing his treatise, having 'specific discussions on precise matters with midwives or those women who attend births'. If his treatise is not

25. See 272.

26. 'the midwife should first consider whether the woman she is called upon to help and care for is strong and in good health, or weak, frail and fragile' (262); 'She should also take care to guard against the problems which can arise because of different mothers' natures' (274).

27. 'for they allow midwives, some of whom are indeed ignorant, to examine them without due care' (256).

28. See 277.

29. *Diverse Observations*, O'Hara and Klairmont Lingo, I. 14.

flattering to their profession as a whole, it nonetheless recognizes the need for male physicians to consult with them and to contribute to their better education.

The pedagogic function of Duval's treatise invites a further comparison with Guillemeau's work on the level of style, not least because there are some striking differences. It is not surprising that as a physician rather than a surgeon Duval cannot resist, from time to time, displaying his humanist learning, with a casual allusion to Horace,[30] or several choice classical anecdotes. Yet he is aware that his readership might include two groups of practitioners who would shun more weighty Latin volumes: first, the midwives,[31] and secondly 'the barbers and also … some surgeons who have not worked sufficiently at perfecting their skills, so that when they are called to assist women who are ready to give birth, often they do them far more harm than good'.[32] Confident that his teachings could improve this situation,[33] and aware that he is addressing primarily the lower ranks of practitioners (as well as lay readers), Duval sometimes adopts a style which contrasts with his humanist elegance.

In providing a detailed account of anatomy and of the nature of conception and pregnancy in the first section of his treatise, he not only values clarity above the dictates of decorum, but positively delights in popular, and on occasions vulgar, expressions. This is clear from the subtitle of the work, which speaks of the 'laborer' and 'field', commonplace vernacular metaphors for the male and female sexual organs. Similarly, in the chapter headings, the penis is designated as the 'male rod or genital member' (chapter 6), and the chapter devoted to the clitoris also uses its popular name, 'On the clitoris or *"gaudemihi"*' (chapter 10). In part, such vivid language or images might be designed to help midwives, surgeons and perhaps lay readers follow Duval's explanations, as for example when he describes the triangular shape of the cervix after conception comparing it to 'the rear end of a chicken,

30. See 247.

31 See 245.

32. See 247.

33. 'God willing, they will no longer do so in the future if they take care to follow the teachings of this present book.' (ibid.)

as we say'.[34] Yet how far does he convince us by his protestations that his explicit sexual language serves only justifiable pedagogic ends? In the same chapter, when listing the signs of conception, he is himself aware that while freedom to speak of sexuality may be legitimate within marriage, in other contexts the same freedom may be a sign of shamelessness:

> If the woman is able to speak freely to her husband (I speak here of the type of women who are chaste, leaving for later the question of unchaste and shameless women), he will say that when he withdrew his male member it was dry and lacking in moisture at its tip.[35]

Quite frequently, Duval appears to enjoy a style that strays beyond the mere dictates of clarity. Some of his extended metaphors treat uncontroversial subjects, such as his comparison of the conjunction between pain and pleasure to the tiles on either side of a roof;[36] others are humorous, like the comparison between conception and a full fishing net.[37] But at times, he is clearly playing with sexually explicit metaphors which have a long literary history, as when he speaks of 'the riches of their [women's] secret treasure-stores, and of the hinges, doors, locks and keys to open them'.[38] It is notable that the majority of the colorful metaphors are used in the earlier chapters, concerned with the anatomy of the reproductive parts, whereas the style in the chapters on pregnancy and delivery becomes much more factual: the nature of generation lends itself to more playful suggestiveness than does the relief of pain and the saving of mothers' and infants' lives.

We should also remember that Duval's treatise builds up to the dramatic episode of his proof of Le Marcis's true sexual nature. I suggest that the tone of the earlier chapters on anatomy needs to be appreciated as a preliminary to this. In his prefatory 'Letter to the

34. See 257.

35. See ibid.

36. See 261.

37. 'the woman should be assured that she has fished most well, given her net has remained full of her catch' (259).

38. See 261.

Reader', he has already revealed this pivotal moment, and it is striking that here he makes Le Marcis's 'male member' the active subject of a series of verbs (my italics):

> 'But by means of the marvelous skill of this great creator, the male member *reached* such a state that it *could show* itself and actually *come out* for the purpose for which it is meant, to release both urine and reproductive seed. Often it *would also retract* itself and *remain hidden* away inside.'[39]

For Duval, the actions of the genital parts and the act of procreation are a source of wonder, to be observed almost like a drama, and recorded in evocative, even performative language. It is no accident that at the start of the 'Letter to the Reader' he draws an explicit parallel between the court's final decision and the ending of a play:

> Just as it was a well-accepted convention in ancient theaters to hear the voice of Jupiter coming from a special machine to unravel the most difficult problems, so I have been delighted to hear the final decision of the court when Nature pleased herself in the creation of Marin Le Marcis, making him of uncertain sex.[40]

The reader, whether a medical professional or a layperson, will witness the trial 'acted out' in Duval's account of it. He has prepared us for the drama of the latter sensational chapters by his vigorous account of the anatomy of generation. The daily dramas of pregnancy and childbirth may not, in contrast, merit quite such a distinctive style, but Duval nonetheless clearly conveys his pity for women's suffering in labor and his grave concern at the mortal risks facing them and their offspring.

39. See 243.
40. See 241.

TITLE PAGE [1612]

ON HERMAPHRODITES, DELIVERIES OF WOMEN, AND THE TREATMENT WHICH IS REQUIRED AFTER CHILDBIRTH FOR WOMEN TO RECOVER THEIR HEALTH AND RAISE THEIR CHILDREN WELL.

In which are explained the form of the laborer and the orchard of humankind,[42] signs of virginity, deflowering, conception and Nature's fine work to promote conception and prolific growth.

By Monsieur Jacques Duval, squire, Lord of Hectomare[43] and Houvel, Doctor and Professor of medicine, born in Evreux,[44] residing in Rouen.

IN ROUEN,
From the press of David Geuffroy,[45]
in the rue des Cordeliers,
beside St Peter's.

M.DC.XII.

With the King's Privilege.

---

41. The metaphors of the laborer ('*laboureur*') and field or orchard ('*verger*') were commonly used in vernacular French to denote the male and female sexual organs.

42. Small town, approximately 40 km south of Rouen.

43. Town some 55 km south of Rouen.

44. A Protestant printer and bookseller working in Rouen from c. 1598 to 1629.

APPROVAL[45]

Approval Given by the Ordinary Physicians of the King

We, Jean and Charles de l'Orme, the undersigned, Councillors and Ordinary Physicians of the King, father and son, certify to whom it may concern that the book entitled *On Hermaphrodites*, printed under the name of Monsieur Jacques Duval, doctor in medicine, residing in Rouen, deserves to be published on account of the remarkable nature of its subject. Delivered by us on this 12th day of March, 1612.

Signed, De L'Orme.

De L'Orme.

With their initials.

45. Placed at the end of the volume, between the Table of Contents and the Privilege.

PRIVILEGE

Extract from the King's Privilege

Louis, by the grace of God King of France and Navarre, to our dear and faithful councillors, those conducting the courts of our Parlements in Paris and Rouen,[46] the provost and bailiff of these places, or their lieutenants and all other officers of justice whom it may concern. Our dear and well loved Monsieur Jacques Duval, doctor in medicine, lord of Hectomare and Le Houvel, residing in our said town of Rouen, explained to us that he recently wrote a certain book entitled *On Hermaphrodites or male concubines, in which is demonstrated the way of delivering all pregnant women*, etc.[47] He had been advised by his friends to publish it for the public good. He wished to do so, but feared that the booksellers to whom it was entrusted would be frustrated in their task, or that others would wish to take the task of printing and selling it, which would deprive them of their expectations and of the fruits of their investment and labors. For this reason, he asked us to grant the necessary letters. On this account, by these present letters, we have allowed, agreed and granted, and we do now allow, agree and grant to Duval that he may have the book printed, sold and distributed throughout all our kingdoms, by such booksellers or printers as he may wish, and none but those whom he has charged with it, and who have received permission from him, may print it, have it printed, sold or distributed for a period of six years from the day when the book shall first have been printed. And the penalty would be the confiscation of the copies and a fine of a thousand pounds. Thus we instruct you and entrust to each of you the order that, according to this present authorization, you leave and suffer to be left to Duval the right and opportunity to enjoy and use fully and peacefully this privilege, and you should oblige all those concerned to respect it, by

---

46. There were nine Parlements (acting as sovereign courts) in France at this time, one in Paris, eight in the provinces.

47. It is strange that here the book is recorded with a rather different title from that which appears in the edition printed in 1612. This sentence of the French in the Privilege begins '*Des Hermaphrodits ou concubins*', '*concubins*' alluding to the hermaphrodite's role as a (male) sexual partner.

all due and reasonable means, and we wish that a brief statement of these letters should be put at the start or end of the book, so that they may be seen to have been respected, and sold in the full knowledge of all. For such is our will.

Issued in Paris, the last day of February, the year of Our Lord 1612, and the second of our reign.

By the King in his Council.

De Canonne.

And sealed with the yellow wax, under the seal of the Great Chancellery of France.

LETTER TO LAURENT RESTAUT

To Monsieur Laurens Restaut, Councillor of Our
King in the Court of His Parlement of Rouen,
Lord, Baron, and Chatelain of Fort-Moville[48]

Sir,

Just as it was a well-accepted convention in ancient theaters to hear the voice of Jupiter coming from a special machine to unravel the most difficult problems, so I have been delighted to hear the final decision of the court when Nature pleased herself in the creation of Marin Le Marcis, making him of uncertain sex.[49] Because he took qualities from both sexes, he proved his virility with a woman to whom he was engaged, and whom he hoped to marry. The judges of this place had considered it a great crime on his part. This makes me believe that lawyers wish, through their prudence, to conserve the human body in the condition in which Nature created it, rather than, like the Ancient Roman soothsayers, destroy and ruin it. This is a very reasonable position, given that at any time this great handmaiden[50] produces some remarkable excesses, and that she also often offers a marked insufficiency. So, from what we perceive, it is necessary that the noble science of the law legislate in matters which human providence has not been able to resolve adequately. Finding that you greatly excel in this, because of the various great forms of learning which you ably bring together with your professional skills, such that one can scarcely find a subject of debate with which to confront you without both extremes being instantly clear to you, and without you then wisely finding a middle way composed of equity and justice, rather than following an excessive path, either rigorously severe or overly clement; and being aware, in addition, of the favor of your friendship, I have addressed the present treatise to you, so that it may travel freely around the

---

48. Fort-Moville fell within the area of Beuzeville (Normandy). 'Chatelain' was a feudal title, approximately equal to viscount.

49. On Duval's role in the case of Le Marcis, see 225-6.

50. I.e. Nature.

world shielded by your protection. I beg you to accept it as kindly as you would were it more deserving. In the hope that you will grant this, I shall pray to God to keep you safe. From he who desires always to remain, Monsieur, your most affectionate servant,

Duval.

LETTER TO THE READER

Knowing, dear Reader, the rare and unusual effects of Nature — which we may rightly call by the name of miracles, as coming from the power of Him who is not in any way constrained by the rules and laws which He established from the first creation of all things — I believe these should serve as spurs to awaken man's over-stupid mind so that he may seek causes which are concealed from the senses. Then, finally, having dissipated this shadowy cloud of ignorance, he may, together with the royal prophet David, fittingly praise and exalt the supreme power of the sovereign creator. And I was strongly moved by such a burning desire when the case of a girl was brought to my attention.[51] She had been baptized, named, cared for, brought up and always dressed like the other girls of her kind until the age of twenty, when she was finally shown to be a man, and proved to be such on several different occasions, by way of sexual intercourse with a woman to whom he[52] presently became engaged by exchange of vows, and by the promise of marriage.

In his case, one could not recognize the particular marks characteristic of the two sexes which are normally seen in hermaphrodites, both in those who are complete and in those who have some trace of imperfection, as most often happens. Or the female characteristics may have been totally obliterated, giving way to the masculine ones without any trace of the feminine ones remaining, as is seen in women possessing a male member or in female-men.[53]

But by means of the marvelous skill of this great creator, the male member reached such a state that it could show itself and actually come out for the purpose for which it is meant, to release both urine and reproductive seed. Often it would also retract itself and remain hidden away inside.

51. This paragraph provides a very good example of Duval's ornate style. I have broken into three sentences in English the single, intricate opening sentence he uses in French. Throughout the translation I have also tended to use a single English word in place of pairs of synonyms in French.

52. I have imitated in English the shift to the masculine pronoun; in French the transition is less surprising because 'as such' (*'comme tel'*) also used a masculine inflection.

53. The Renaissance, like Antiquity, normally assumed that women might change into men, not vice versa, as an example of nature moving towards the more perfect (male) form.

This caused me to fall into deep reflection upon the case. When I was summoned to the medical and judicial inspection, together with other physicians, surgeons and midwives,[54] in order to confirm this fact and to pronounce on it as an expert witness, I thereafter undertook detailed research into a number of fine histories and serious authorities. These furnished ample discussion of the various causes and reasons which could contribute to a complete understanding of such a rare case. I succeeded in organizing and presenting these so clearly that, with the help of the Almighty who deigned to dispel my ignorance and remove my blindfold, I explained things most plainly and unmistakably in my report to the court, when we were asked to enter the room and give the reasons for the differences in our reports, which were quite contradictory. As a result, this poor hermaphrodite,[55] who had been condemned to make honorable amends, walking naked, bearing a torch, through the town of Monstierville, and then to be led to the gibbet to be hanged, strangled, and finally have his body burned to ashes, obtained, notwithstanding all this, that the sentence of shameful death was lifted and annulled, and he was released from prison with permission to return to his home town. This was despite the unfavorable verdict which could have been reached from the contradictory reports of 15 or 16 physicians, surgeons and midwives, who all unanimously reported that he had nothing other than a woman's body, from which it could have been inferred that he had used the promise of marriage to abuse the other woman with his clitoris, like a tribade.[56]

I had the opportunity to write a history of this in a book, adding also an explanation of the genital parts[57] of both sexes, not only because I know this to be necessary for an understanding of the subject, but with the intention that by this same means (killing two birds with one stone) readers interested in this treatise might be informed about them, and that those needing to consult doctors about conception, procreation of children, or the causes and cures for infirmities which

54. The three groups usually called upon in legal issues concerning sexuality.

55. Duval uses the term *'gunanthrope'*, a neologism, literally meaning woman-man, to convey the intersexuality of Le Marcis.

56. I.e. like a lesbian taking the active sexual role.

57. Here and throughout the translation I employ the English adjective 'genital' as the cognate for Duval's use of *'genital(e)'* in French.

often affect these parts, should be able to respond competently to questions, and thus help doctors to gain the knowledge required, so that their patients might have their wishes satisfied.

It should also allow young surgeons and midwives to be more confident in compiling and making their judicial reports on questions concerning the different sexes, virginity, deflowering, conception in women, signs of secret abortion or childbirth, and other things affecting the genital parts, for they are often consulted about them by those in legal positions.

It should also provide good and necessary instruction for midwives about what they must arrange and undertake when women who are giving birth call upon them.

And finally, it should inform surgeons about all the ways they must master in order to deliver pregnant women skillfully when a midwife cannot accomplish a natural delivery as she would wish.

Thus, in this way giving a brief, ordered account of what must be done before, during and after deliveries for both the mother and the infant, I am doing what is in my power to reduce the causes of the death of a great number of babies. Some are forced to meet death as soon as they have come into the light of the world; others, without even having passed from the somber cavern of the mother's womb, travel from one form of darkness to another, sometimes taking their sad, exhausted mothers with them to the same tomb, as though swept away by a virulent disease. But when I was ready to deliver the present work to be printed, I reflected that it was not without good cause that the court had fixed a period of time during which this poor creature should not use his genital parts, male or female, in any sexual or procreative act; and he should wait until he had more fully demonstrated towards which of the two natures he inclined the more. Given that God is present in the company of those who, for a good reason, have gathered together in His name, and that He presides among judges who love fairness, and who favor justice without hesitation, like those from whom the present decision came, I believed it to be my duty to delay the printing of my work until the will of the court had been accomplished.

Then being duly informed that the hermaphrodite is now in a better state of manhood than he was previously, and that bearing the name of Le Marcis the younger he practices his trade as a tailor, and fulfils all the functions proper to men, has a beard, and the means to satisfy a woman and make her pregnant, I judged that there was no longer a reason to delay publishing this work.

If in this history I use expressions which may appear coarse, or somewhat ribald,[58] which may, however slightly, offend the ears and thoughts of those who, being engaged in more serious contemplations, would wish for words and descriptions suited to their disposition and desires, I would beg them not to hold it against me, and to believe that it is not because of any natural lewdness on my part. For God in His grace has taken this from me, removing the occasion for impure love by the long years and happy offspring which He has given and still vouchsafes to me in marriage. In addition, my calling and the philosophy to which He has called me (as Socrates was wont to say) would have sufficed to dispel any such juvenile, foolish thoughts.

It is, rather, the consequence of the things I am treating here, which concern what is most delightful and sensual in man, that is genital seed, which is so abundant that the learned Fernel did not hesitate to say 'man is totally seed' ['*homo totus semen est*'].[59] So I must mention this, and the parts intended for the act of procreation which this excellent worker, Nature, greatly wishes to favor in order always, and ever more to encourage men to continue their race. She did not just arouse a great pleasure when one comes to this activity, but she also, through some mysterious instinct, granted such a sensual excitement and sexual stimulation when the mind thinks of it, by naming it or just alluding to it, that even if I used the hieroglyphs of the Ancient Egyptians, or just the gestures of the Englishman Thaumaste[60] to indicate them without otherwise naming them, I still could not block out that simple pleasure which Nature has chosen to decorate the allusion to them.

58. On the rich variety of terms for describing the female anatomy in particular in the sixteenth and early-seventeenth centuries, see Klarimont Lingo's article, 'The Fate of Popular Terms for Female Anatomy in the Age of Print', *French Historical Studies* 22–3 (1999), 335–349.

59. Jean Fernel, first physician to Henri II, devoted Book VII of his *Universal Medicine* [*Universa Medicina,*] published posthumously in 1567, to procreation, the first few chapters dealing in detail with human seed.

60. Reference to the comic episode in which Thaumaste communicates by sign language in Rabelais's *Pantagruel* (1532), chs. 18–20.

As against this, they should weigh up closely the manner in which, if this work is clearly understood, I shall prevent a large number of inaccurate reports, and the loss of an almost infinite number of souls which, without their having the opportunity to enjoy the light of this world, are obliged immediately to follow the same path back as that which the sovereign Creator held out to them.[61] This is because of the ignorance of the midwives who are not able to read or understand more serious books explaining the nature, aspects and form of all the parts of the human body.[62] The same is indeed true of the barbers and also of some surgeons who have not worked sufficiently at perfecting their skills, so that when they are called to assist women who are ready to give birth, often they do them far more harm than good. God willing, they will no longer do so in the future if they take care to follow the teachings of this present book, in which they will find that I have achieved what the Roman orator sought,[63] and what Horace praised greatly in his *Art of Poetry* [*Ars Poetica*]:[64]

> He avoids all risk of censure it seems to me
> Who mixes and unites the useful with the sweet.

I thus refresh and delight the minds of men (although this is not my main purpose) by the display of virile riches and of the exhibition of the hidden tools in women's most secret treasure houses, in the use of which both find great delight. I also elevate the minds of those who call themselves midwives (although often falsely and without justification) that they may truly be able to become wise in their profession,[65] of which the world has such need. I also instruct barbers and address the minds (which guide the skilled hands) of young surgeons, to whose education I again this year devote myself, so that

61. Duval subscribes to the Catholic belief that a physician has a duty to ensure newborns survive long enough for their souls to be saved through the sacrament of baptism, rather than being condemned (unborn and thus unbaptized) to the Limbo of Infants.

62. Compare the comments in 1609 by Bourgeois who also commented upon the number of midwives lacking the anatomical knowledge she considers essential to their profession. She argues that this would be remedied if physicians allowed midwives to attend public dissections of female cadavers: *Diverse Observations*, I. 36.

63. An elliptical reference to Cicero.

64. Horace, *Ars poetica*, l. 343.

65. A play in French on the word *'sage-femme'*. See 191, n. 129.

women of all stations may receive their good support, and so that their cruellest mortal sufferings may be reduced, alleviated and ended; their illnesses cured; their lives saved and preserved; and their children, who would otherwise perish at birth, may be delivered more easily and safely while they enjoy good health and recovery. For I believe that the ignorance of some midwives (it is these that I condemn, not the good ones) is the reason why 500 children[66] die every year in this town of Rouen before they can receive the sacrament of baptism, as I know from the laments which I hear daily. I believe there are no people so lacking in understanding that they will not praise God for his wish to favor the delivery of my work, given that:

> It is an excellent art to preserve safely
> The life of a child worthy of succeeding.

66. See 228.

TABLE OF THE CHAPTERS
CONTAINED IN THIS BOOK[67]

67. The numbering of chapters in the table of contents contains quite a few slips. I have corrected these, indicating cases where the sequence in both the table and the treatise is broken.

68. Duval uses the image 'the inner place of shame' (i.e. pudendum) of the woman'.

69. I.e. the inner lips or labia minora.

70. The shaft of the clitoris.

71. The Latin term meaning 'pleasure me', used in popular French.

72. I.e. cervix.

73. Unlike some of his contemporaries, Duval does not doubt the existence of the hymen.

74. On Liebault, see 66-74.

75. 'Gynandres' (singular: 'gynaner'), a neologism formed by analogy with 'androgynes', is employed by Duval to indicate cases of intersexuality in which those previously designated as women are later recognized to be men.

76. The French uses a surprising expression, which literally means 'in the mother's vagina', to indicate from the moment the male seed entered the mother's body.

77. Duval uses the word 'vulve' in French, referring to the clitoris and surrounding tissues.

78. See above, n. 75.

79. The chapter number LIX does not appear in either the treatise or the table of contents.

80. See above, n. 75.

Chapter XV: On the Body of the Womb, Its Opening, Praise of It, and the Signs of Conception

[The first half of this long chapter — not translated here — is devoted to a general anatomical discussion of the vagina, cervix and womb, with particular attention to the changes once a woman becomes sexually active. Like many Renaissance writers, Duval eulogizes the womb as the recipient bearing new life. My translation starts from Duval's account of the physical examinations which reveal pregnancy.]

The midwife should feel inside, right up to the neck of the womb, when the woman wants to know if she has conceived, and not just be content with placing her hand on the abdomen. For on introducing her middle finger this far, if the area is compressed and squeezed, having a kind of triangular shape, so narrow that it seems nothing can be pushed further inside without doing violence to it, it is the most certain sign of conception that a woman could wish for.

However, all the following signs are often misleading: just feeling the abdomen from outside, even in the region of the womb a little above the pubic bone; or putting a clove of garlic, or something strongly scented and well wrapped, like musk, in the passage in order to observe whether the smell then comes back up the nostrils;[81] or giving the woman hydromel prepared with rainwater to drink when she is going to bed in order to find out whether the fumes from these smells rise up; or whether after drinking honey mixed with water she feels abdominal cramps, and saying if she does she is pregnant, and if not she is not. For, from the first days, the womb is covered by the bladder to such an extent that it cannot be felt. When a woman's flesh is too substantial, which the wise Fernel[82] calls a material flaw, the smell of anything put in the passage will not rise up, even if bitter and sulphurous, and if the woman is accustomed to drink hydromel, or some sweet drink, she will not feel any cramps.

In this respect, moreover, urine is of no use at all. Thus from all these signs you cannot draw any definite knowledge which can be relied upon.

81. On this method of detecting pregnancy, cf. 31, n. 70.
82. See 246, n. 59.

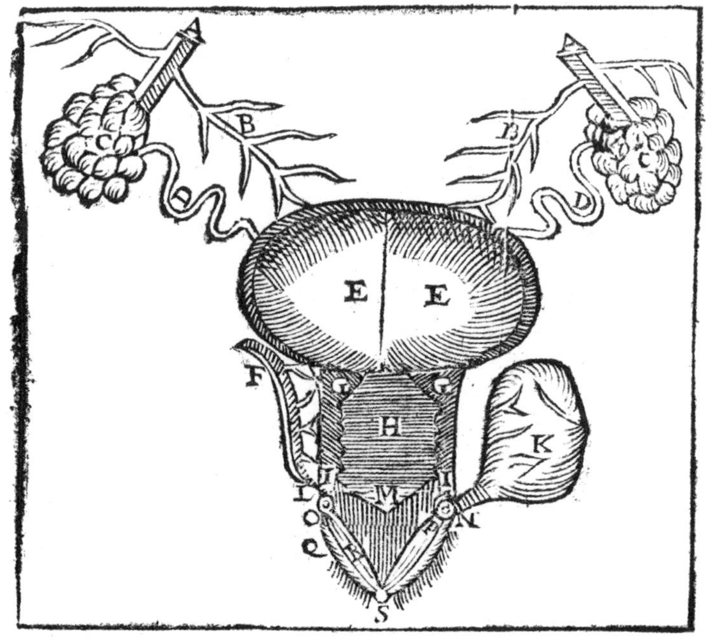

21) Anatomy of the womb

Jacques Duval, *Des Hermaphrodits*, Rouen, 1612
(Library of Royal College of Obstetricians and Gynaecologists, London)

Indeed, I see women who are so concerned to know if they have conceived that often their curiosity is so great that they cannot wait until the appropriate time to gain true knowledge, and this causes them to lose the fruit of their conception, for they allow midwives, some of whom are indeed ignorant, to examine them without due care. Instead of gently feeling the pregnancy and the neck of the womb to compare it with the tightening of the opening, they proceed so clumsily and with so little care that they kill the child, or they make an opening for it to come forth prematurely. I shall explain here the signs for which they should look in order to establish whether the women have conceived or not, doing the best I am able in this respect.

It occurs that after pleasurable relations with her husband, indeed even more delightful than usual (for conception is not accomplished without pleasure),[83] soon afterwards the woman comes to feel a

83. It was commonly believed that female as well as male orgasm (with the discharge of female and male seed) was essential to conception.

constriction of the neck of the womb, which contracts in order to retain and preserve the seed it holds. This gives her a sensation not only in the lower abdomen but also radiating out to her hips, with a small, slight shudder, almost like that one may experience when, in perfectly good health, one has urinated. It causes a small, momentary feeling of discomfort around the navel and lower abdomen.

This is followed by a slight chill in the neck, and a heaviness of the tongue such that the woman may stumble in speaking, and there may be some irritation and heaviness, which make her wish to sleep. If the woman is able to speak freely to her husband (I speak here of the type of women who are chaste, leaving for later the question of unchaste, shameless women), he will say that when he withdrew his male member it was dry and lacking in moisture at its tip. In addition she will not feel the male seed flow back down a little later as she is usually accustomed to do.

To be more certain, if the woman puts her finger into the passage, she will find that the neck of the womb has tightened and closed up so that she would not be able to insert the shaft of a needle into it, and it is made so narrow through this compression that it acquires a somewhat triangular shape, like the rear end of a chicken, as we say.

At the end of the month, instead of having her regular menses, or because of the lack of these, instead of feeling a tiredness and heaviness in her limbs, the woman may find herself more lively, active and thinner than usual, so that she will feel as though her clothes are dropping off her, as though they are too big and ill-fitting for her body, and she may experience some pain. Yet she will feel her breasts to be firmer, harder and more swollen than usual and darker in colour, especially around the nipples. In pale women, both breasts will be redder than usual, and in dark women they become reddish-brown and higher than usual.

Then there also occurs an untypical kind of lassitude, apathy and heat, and she does not wish for, or accept, the company of her husband.

Her face takes on freckled marks of various reddish hues because of the climaxing and stirring of the blood, which finds its normal path blocked and so rises higher. This causes heaviness, sluggishness and sleepiness after eating, and her eyes become duller and more sunken than usual.

Next, women may go off their food, experience nausea and feel they will be sick in the morning, and some indeed are sick, or at least often bring up a very watery saliva, which is called 'spitting on the embers'; they may want the strangest things to eat, with such a burning desire that often their children bear the marks of this when they are born if the desires have not been satisfied, because of the illness known as *pica*.[84] According to Galen, this happens principally when the child starts to grow hair, in the second month, in his view. This is also the time, according to Pliny,[85] when women suffer most from headaches with dizziness, vertigo and a greater distaste for food, their natural menses being retained without an obvious cause.

Their abdomen is larger, firmer and harder on one side than on the other. Their pulse is irregular, first fast, then slow.

And in truth when a woman experiences further loss of appetite together with such weakness and torpor that she believes herself to be suffering from some other illness, she may consult doctors without explaining to them everything detailed above, and obtain from them prescriptions for purges and bleeding which will do her harm because they lead to an elimination of substances, often causing serious harm. And this is because she lacked the patience to wait for the appropriate time to gain full knowledge, that is to say the third or fourth months, when women feel their children quicken; some say they feel this at six weeks.

This contradicts the opinion of Aristotle who claims in Book II chapter 3 of *The History of Animals* that the soul does not enter the child's body until the third or fourth month. For even if we assume, as is most often the case, that the movement is not felt until three months, the child is nonetheless completely formed, and it remains only for it to have the strength in its limbs to demonstrate this. If it happened that the child were late in quickening, and the desired movement did not occur at this point, if the mother has a very strong wish to incite it to prove its presence by some movement, she may follow the advice of

---

84. On *pica* or unnatural appetites in early preganancy, cf. the comments of Liebault (109, n. 139) and Guillemeau (184).

85. *Natural History*, VII. 6. 41–42.

Cardano,[86] which is to place a cloth soaked in cold water on the most swollen part of the abdomen. For when the child feels this discomfort, it will shift and move away. The application of the cloth should be repeated two or three times. Cardano reports that it is more reliable to use water than wine, which attracts the head.

If the majority of all these signs are present, and especially those which are attributed to the first and second month, the woman should be assured that she has fished most well, given her net has remained full of her catch, and when its timely movement comes, she will be fully reassured.

Before this, if the midwife is inopportunely called upon to examine the woman to give her opinion on whether she has conceived, she will do well to ask her to pass her urine before introducing her hand so that this urine does not prevent her from feeling the womb which lies behind the bladder. In addition, she should ensure that she has emptied her bowels, either naturally or by means of an enema, so that the midwife is not misled by the fecal matter which remains in the right intestine and can cause the womb, that is above it, to ride up too high, and give a false impression that conception has taken place. When this has been done and the woman is well positioned on her back, the midwife should palpate the bottom of the abdomen so gently that she cannot harm the small embryo, which is wonderfully soft and delicate. Then putting her finger into the passage in order to judge whether the mouth of the womb is opened or closed, she should act with such care that she spares no effort to avoid harming the woman.

As for those women who wish to know whether they have conceived a son or a daughter, they may be able to make a reasonable guess according to the various signs indicated below, which they will have felt more on one side than another.

For if there are more stirrings on the right side, and the face is redder; the eye brighter, more lively and alert on this side; the breast firmer, the nipple redder or darker and more raised than on the left; if the child has moved halfway through the third month; if the right side is fuller, harder and firmer than the other; and the whole abdomen rounder (to observe this, the woman should be laid on her back on a

86. Gerolamo Cardano, a sixteenth-century Italian physician whose most famous scientific and medical work *On the Subtlety of Things* [*De subtilitate rerum*, 1550] ran to 21 volumes.

mattress so that one is not misled by the position); if when she stands she is more inclined to put her right foot rather than her left forward first; and if when she is sitting down, she rests her right rather than her left hand on her knee in order to assist her in standing up when she needs to: all these things indicate that she has conceived a son. But when on the contrary they occur on the left, they indicate it is a daughter.

In general, a woman's whole body will feel more lively, bright and alert throughout her pregnancy; the colour of her face will be brighter and clearer; and her nipples will be more pronounced; her eyes more lively and animated when she is carrying a son than when it is a daughter. This is because conceiving a male produces more heat than a female, which is why all these signs appear.

Because it can occur, though rarely, that a woman has her natural menses during her pregnancy, the blood will flow at 30 days if she has conceived a son, and at 40 days if it is a daughter, according to Hippocrates in his book *On the Nature of the Child*.[87]

Chapter XVIII: How Women Should Conduct Themselves as Their Term Approaches

If there were women who said they felt no pain, no suffering when their child comes forth, as there are some who say they have no pleasure in the tilling of their field[88] (although this is contrary to the truth, begging their pardon, and especially in the case of that tilling which is done with so much energy that procreation results from it), I would not give myself the labor of adding the chapters which will follow.[89]

87. See *On the Nature of the Child* ch. XVIII, in which Hippocrates considers that the male embryo is formed in 30 days, the female in 42, periods corresponding (he believes) to the cessation of blood flow so that the embryo can be formed.

88. Compare the metaphor used in the book's title (see 237, n. 41).

89. Compare the treatment of the same topic in Liebault (115-126). Certain anecdotes and comments common to both authors indicate that Duval composed his chapter with an eye on Liebault's account.

But the fact is that, as the divine Plato says,[90] good and ill, joy and sadness, fortune and misfortune, pleasure and pain are so intertwined that they appear like a continuum, or like two joined, pegged planks which are meant to form the two slats or sides of the inner structure and roofing of a building, so that when you reach the top of one side you tip over onto the other one. One cannot have great, outstanding happiness without being about to encounter misfortune. In consequence, women cannot have such pleasure in the tilling and sowing of their natural field without running the risk of experiencing some terrible pain. Given the connection, in Plato's image, of the two slates at the top of the house, where on one side there lie sadness, grief and pain, they want to refuse the act and they say they will never use such a laborer. Yet if one speaks to them once they have crossed the ridgetile and are on the other side, they take a different approach. They say that the structures of buildings overlook different regions; that they are now on the side where a good wind blows, and the rain is softer and less stormy; and they thereupon forget their memory of pains and suffering in these circumstances. Thus they become very attentive towards men, by which I mean towards their husbands, and they show themselves to be ever willing.

I thought it my duty, since I had the occasion to give an account of the riches of their secret treasure-stores, and of the hinges, doors, locks and keys to open them, at the same time to teach how one should receive and remove what has tarried there a sufficiently long time. For I know well that in so doing I shall please them all, giving them very good means to help the midwives and nurses to care for them well, just as they will please and help their husbands so that they pay the midwives and nurses well, at the due time.

The care I dedicated to the study of excellent, famous authors in order to compose the present work, and my specific discussions on precise matters with midwives or those women who attend births,[91] and in addition the experience I have had in this sphere both in my own household and outside it, mean that I have thought it appropriate,

---

90. Plato proposes this theory (although he does not use the simile of the roof tiles) in *Phaedo* 60b-c.

91. Duval uses two terms in French, distinguishing between '*obstetrices*' (trained midwives) and '*matrones*' (women who attend births without having received training).

in order to provide good support and help to this gracious fair sex in their dreadful sufferings, to divide into three parts my account of the care which is needed in childbirth and delivery. I have done this in order to make it useful and suitable not only to a peasant woman but also to a great lady and princess, so that each may be appropriately helped, supported and served. These three sections will discuss what is required before, during and after the birth.[92]

On the subject of what must be done before a woman is ready to deliver her child into the world, the midwife should first consider whether the woman she is called upon to care for is strong and in good health, or weak, frail and fragile. These are the two points to which she must return in all considerations of temperament, nature, routines, habits, tendencies and personal ways. There is no other way of dealing with them without causing confusion.

Of those women who are strong and in good health, some are habitually so fortunate that, without requiring any further help, they easily deliver their children, and the midwife or woman overseeing the delivery has only to receive the child and take care of it as necessary. On this account, they do not deserve any further consideration.

But it can happen that some have a more masculine and virile tendency, and they are hard, dry and over-tight, as are many older women who have been brought up to work, and have either been married late, or God has not granted them offspring as soon as they would have wished; or they may have had children in their youth, but been filled with an excess of melancholic and freculent blood. In this case, it is necessary to avoid the excessively dry, hard nature of these parts impeding the dilation which is necessary for this purpose, or the heavy, viscous, thick blood, which is overly melancholic and cachectic,[93] being unable to flow freely after the birth in order to allow the purging of the necessary lochia after the delivery. This gives rise to very many long, serious illnesses which women say come from all their childbearing, but I would rather say it comes from the time they spend lying in bed, so that finally their deaths are brought about by this.

92. On the structure of Duval's treatise, see 229-230.
93. I.e. generally unhealthy and weak.

In such cases it is very advisable to feed them on foods with the power to cool and moisten, if not throughout all their pregnancy, at least one month before they are ready to give birth; we shall limit it to this time preceding the birth so that women are not misled in reading this advice, and take it to apply to other times. For their solid food, they should choose from the flesh of the following: veal, lamb, capons, chickens, partridges and other such kinds, preferably boiled and cooked with lettuce, sorrel, bugloss, borage, spinach, and other such herbs from the kitchen garden. They should often take clear soups made from these, and the meats will be better for them if prepared in this way rather than fried, grilled, roasted or cooked between two crusts. For those methods of cooking would make them harder to digest, and would cause heavy, viscous humors unlike those we desire. If by chance they are given meats roasted and cooked in their own juices, they should be chopped and mixed with a little water, verjus, sugar and cinnamon, the latter having the facility to achieve better, quicker deliveries. Easily digestible fish (like carp, trout, weaver, whiting, smelt and other such kinds) may also be good for them, prepared in sweetened butter and cinnamon. Grapes, prunes and other refreshing fruits, which contain much water, may also be useful to them in moderate quantities.

They should, on the other hand, avoid overly hot and dry foods, which can lead to melancholic, thick, dried-out blood. These include meats like beef, hares, cod, eels and other such things, especially when they are salted or spiced; pates of venison, saveloy sausages, jambon de mayence,[94] and other such things. Likewise, vegetables, cheeses, garlic, onions, quinces, walnuts, hazelnuts, medlars and hard-boiled eggs are not good for them. They should drink cider, beer, herbal drinks or mead, and white wine sometimes, or very thin claret, which is well watered, called '*oligophoron*'[95] by the Greeks, and they should avoid rough, coarse, strong, over-matured wines such as those out of the ordinary and from foreign places. They should be served as much to drink as they wish, and not refrain from drinking, for it helps greatly to keep them moist. It is better for them to eat a good number of meals rather than few, but they should take heed of the particular habits and

94. A salted ham that has matured for at least nine months.
95. Literally 'little-bearing'.

tolerance of their stomach, which should never be overloaded so that they do not vomit, for that is very bad for them. They should often take physical exercise, but without violence, and in warm, moist air rather than air which is cold and dry. They should ensure that their bowels are emptied promptly, every day. If they suffer from constipation, they should periodically take enemas to soften their movements, including the following in all the laxatives: dark honey, pellitory, pulp of cassia and diacassia, with butter or oil of lilies, violets and sweet almonds. From time to time, they should also take six drams of cassia pulp with an ounce and a half of syrup of violets or rose water; soon after, they should inhale a moist, cooling soup, not so much in order to prevent the cassia turning into solid food within them, as to dilute it in the stomach and keep the body as moist as possible. Or they may be given two ounces of good Calabrian manna in a capon stock.

In the month before the birth, it would be most appropriate to rub oil of lily or sweet almonds and duck or goose fat into their lower abdomen, groin, the inside of the thighs and the region of the sacrum. Or you can make the following liniment: take an ounce each of linseed oil and of sweet almond oil; half an ounce each of chicken and duck fat; mucilage from mallow roots and fenugreek seeds soaked in water; mix them all together and make the liniment and rub it into these parts morning and evening. A most excellent remedy for this condition is goose fat warmed over a low heat. If you wish to moisten the parts still further, take a very plump chicken and without larding it, roast it slowly over a low heat for a good two hours, then use the same recipe as above.

When the woman is close to her time, say six or seven days away, it is very good to prepare her a half-bath with a decoction of lettuce leaves, purple mallows, senna, pellitory and sweet clover, linseed, pumpkin and fenugreek. She should bathe in it twice a day, or even three times; the morning and at four or five in the evening, and sometimes at midday. She should not stay in it for long, just for half an hour at the most, so that she keeps easing the dilation of the iliac and pubic bones (otherwise known as the isles and barriers or Bertrand bones).[96] This is especially necessary since the isle bones sit

---

96. In his *Popular Errors* (Book V, ch. 4), Laurent Joubert also listed these terms, commenting that midwives often use a different nomenclature for the female genitals, leading to

more tightly against the sacrum in women who are already old, over-dry, hard and like men, than in women who are naturally soft, tender and delicate. Without this, it is impossible for natural childbirth to be accomplished as it should be. This is amply demonstrated by Séverin Pineau in his *Observations*.[97] He argues that the name sacrum was given to this posterior bone, situated towards the bottom of the loins, because it is by sacred and divine help that it moves apart, separating from the sacrum in order to allow the child free movement and passage — otherwise it could not safely be delivered into the world.

The water need not be very hot, just moderately warm, like milk from a cow's udder, or even less so. For it matters only that the warmth is sufficient that the chill of the water does not cause contractions. As the woman enters the bath, she should be given stock made from capon or chicken, together with the herbs mentioned above, and it is good to add the yolk of an egg, together with a little saffron and cinnamon. When she comes out of the bath, she should be put to bed and the parts already mentioned should be rubbed with the liniment, or one of the oils or greases and mucilages specified above. If the woman should have some infirmity on account of which she may not get into the bath, the seeds and herbs mentioned above can be prepared in sachets, boiled in water, and placed upon the lower abdomen, the area of the sacrum and the inside of the thighs for six mornings and evenings. Alternatively, sponges or felts may be dipped in the decoction in order to apply a compress. Once the sachets or sponges have been applied, oils and liniments should be used as described above. For in this way women will avoid long, painful labors, violent contractions and long, dangerous, life-threatening illnesses, for the purgations following the birth will flow well, as nature desires.

In the case of more delicate women, they should consume particularly fortifying foods, avoiding those which soften, which may do them more harm than good. For their weakness often comes from excessive physical rest, idleness and lack of occupation of the mind. Sometimes, indeed, they suffer from internal catarrh, which

---

confusion between them and physicians.

97. Duval cites Séverin Pineau a number of times in this treatise. The discussion of the anatomy of the pregnant woman occurs in Pineau's *Physiological and Anatomical Treatise in Two Separate Books* [*Opusculum physiologicum et anatomicum in duos libros distinctum*, 1597, 177–181].

flows down into the womb, causing it to be wetter and moister than it should be.[98] As a result, some of these women are obliged to keep to their room, to avoid even moderate exercise, and indeed sometimes to lie still in bed and subject themselves to sulphurous aromas in order to lift the womb somewhat and avoid a premature delivery. This is especially so if they have suffered premature births previously. For it often happens that a woman will be delivered at the same time and number of months and weeks as she was previously, unless she takes good measures to avoid this. In such a case, apart from what has been said above, she should wear a plaster called 'of the countess' [*comitissae*] or 'against rupture' [*contra rupturam*] on her lower back.

As for what must be observed by all pregnant women: they should avoid sitting with their feet hanging down or their legs crossed, for it deforms the child and makes the labor painful because it compresses the abdominal muscles, which does them great harm. They should also seek to avoid carriages, coaches and carts when being transported anywhere; instead, they should use sedan chairs or litters. They should avoid dances and balls, and they should especially not dance the flip[99] or '*courante*',[100] which are so dangerous that they would seem to have been invented by the enemy of the human race precisely for women who are too ready to whirl, and shamelessly abandon themselves to lewd men; these dances promote premature births. I have seen such sad and unfortunate accidents befall young women and respectable ladies that as a result just of this they have been unable to bear children or heirs. They should also avoid all things giving rise to vomiting, great losses of fluid, especially of blood, either through the nose, hemorrhoids or, worse still, from the womb.

They should also avoid all frights, anger, melancholy, and other violent passions of the mind which often cause miscarriages. They should also take care not to stare at representations of strange things and unusual forms, whether in paintings or sculptures. For this reason, I admire the wisdom of those women who remove tapestries and pictures which depict such images from their bedrooms, in order

---

98. Duval is following the widespread belief that catarrh circulates around the entire body. His interest in the subject is clear from his authorship of a treatise devoted to it. (See 224.)

99. A popular later-sixteenth-century dance involving whirling and twisting.

100. A lively dance.

to avoid the memory of them being too firmly imprinted on their minds. For although this does not have the same force as at the very beginning of their pregnancy, still something of it is always imprinted, which can damage the body of the child, either producing horrible marks, or perverse and unruly thoughts which bother the mind. Those who are with the mother should also avoid recounting sad and unpleasant news of the various problems, misfortunes, disasters and other unexpected things that may occur. However, if perchance any such thing does actually occur, or is imagined, wise women will obliterate this passion, using their reason, which is the only medicine against such disturbances.

Unfamiliar foods which do not correspond to the temperament of the human body can cause great harm, if not to the mother's body, certainly to that of the child, for the child is like a tender plant in a garden, obliged to draw its food from the sap. If this is alien to the nature of the plant, it soon causes it to die. So the child, which is a human plant (without a large area to spread its roots like the plant in a garden which can draw sustenance from all sides), is damaged more quickly because it is obliged to draw its food only from the mother, who can thus soon corrupt or damage it, even poisoning it if she does not exercise restraint by controlling her wayward, unbridled appetites. So she risks becoming the murderer of that which she should carefully protect as a mother. However, in case of necessity (for it can sometimes happen that, notwithstanding the strength of reason, a woman feels her desire exceeding her power of self-control), care should be taken that the strange and dangerous foods are tempered with suitable sauces, flavorings and condiments, so that the damage they might do is less serious. Her mind will thus be satisfied, her body harmed to a lesser degree and her child's body safely preserved.

Of the examples relating to this subject, I shall give two from the countless relevant ones. One concerns the news the woman receives; the other, wayward appetites. Marcus Aurelius[101] tells of Macrina, wife of the Roman consul Torquatus, who was pregnant. While her husband, for the sake of the republic, had gone away to fight the Volsci, her servants advised Macrina that an Egyptian man with a single eye in the middle of his forehead, was walking down the road,

---

101. The same episode, related by de Guevara, is also cited by Liebault (see 110).

and instantly she was overcome by a great desire to see him. She could not do so because of the great modesty in which she had lived up until then, never appearing in public, still less putting her face to the window to look out at a public road while her husband was away. Being overcome by this violent trouble of the mind, she suddenly died. The senate was so saddened because it knew the valour of her husband and the great modesty of the lady, that some time later it issued several edicts concerning Roman matrons who had shown themselves to be most generous when the Republic had been in dire necessity. Amongst other things it ordered that no one should dare to refuse a pregnant woman anything she requested honorably and legally.

As to the appetite for foods, I saw a woman who had an extreme desire to eat a turbot, and when she could not satisfy this desire she conceived a child whose mouth was shaped like a turbot's, and she explained this precisely by her desire to fill her stomach with what she desired. I held her child over the baptismal font — it did not live for long.

I know that such abnormal malformations do not come about within a month of delivery, which is what we are now speaking of, but, nonetheless, other problems may arise from them. There are reports of various other examples of this kind, like the woman who wanted to eat the flesh of the arm of a butcher when she saw it to be plump and tender.[102] Or of a woman who wanted to eat coal, or another who wanted plaster and similar things, and I shall leave these aside for the sake of brevity. In any case, women know how to express these desires so that they are quickly satisfied. And, moreover, they give rise to a popular proverb that a man who refuses anything to a pregnant woman will suffer a stye, like a grain of barley,[103] which grows on the eyelid. This stye can be referred to in French by words for drips of water or hail, because when the eyes are shut, those who suffer from a stye think they see a droplet or hailstone fall. This swelling is bothersome rather than dangerous. But if you ask them what it signifies, women will say that it is a great suffering that God has sent the person as a punishment for having cruelly denied what the woman

---

102. This anecdote, recounted by Levinus Lemnius, was also cited by Liebault (111).

103. The old French word for stye (*orgeol*) derives from the word for barley (*orge*).

had courteously asked him, a refusal which could have caused the death of the child.

Women who are more prone to miscarrying should avoid taking camomile either in the form of enemas or in bouquets that might be given to them to smell. They should also avoid saffron and cinnamon, which can provoke miscarriages. This must suffice on the subject of what must be done when a woman approaches the time of her confinement.

Chapter XIX: How a Woman Should Be Delivered

[In the first half of this lengthy chapter, Duval has discussed the much debated question of the length of pregnancy, citing a number of cases of pregnancies of more than nine or ten months. After an outline of the most common signs of the onset of childbirth, he now outlines the course of a normal labor.][104]

When the first waters have broken, we see that there are some women who do not give birth promptly if the efforts of nature[105] do not then follow. When this occurs, there may still be sufficient waters left in the amniotic sac to keep the passage moist in order to facilitate the birth.

However, this is rare and cannot be relied upon, especially since the amnion is fragile and easily broken, indeed more easily than the chorion.[106] For this reason, when the woman's waters break, care must be taken and she must be watched over, not being allowed to leave her chamber to go out into the air, even if she says that she is well and feels no pain, for one does not know whether or not the waters of perspiration are mixed with those of her urine. If this happens, and the waters have broken a long time before the birth, the labor will certainly be more difficult than normal.

This is when midwives need to grease their hands thoroughly with oils, liniments and soft mucilages which will lubricate and soften the opening of the womb, making it more supple, for it dries out and becomes constricted very quickly. This can put women's lives in danger, and the midwives should warn the family and friends who are

---

104. Compare the treatment of the same topic in ch. XLV of Liebault (see 115-126).

105. I.e. uterine contractions.

106. The chorion is the outer membrane surrounding the foetus, the amnion the inner one.

in attendance of the imminent danger, without perturbing the mother still further.

Apart from the oils we have already described to help women who are usually over-dry, so that they are properly prepared for a less tiring labor, the following liniment is very suitable. Take one ounce each of linseed oil and of sweet almond oil; six drams each of mucilage from mallow roots and from fenugreek; two grains of musk; one grain of civet; mix this all together to make a liniment. Chicken grease, obtained as described above, is also most excellent.

It is no bad thing either to give them two ounces of water with cinnamon, theriac or sweetened *eau-de-vie*. Or the following potion: take a pinch of gentian root, of juniper leaves and of ground cinnamon; four grains of saffron and of castoreum; one ounce of syrup of althea; dissolve all these in two ounces of hyssop water and give it to the woman to drink if she is in prolonged labor.

Then beat half a dram of root of white hellebore, a pinch of pepper and of sage, and blow the powder into her nostrils. Hold the nostrils tight to make her sneeze, the effort of which will cause her to bear down. Faced with this difficulty, the midwife would be well advised to ask one of the women present to press the lower abdomen of the woman with her hand, a little harder than she would do for a normal birth, as will be explained. This has been outlined as a warning, in passing, so that the woman does not exert herself before she is in true labor, and so that she does not run out of strength before the right time.

But when all the signs which have been mentioned above occur at the same time,[107] or a good number of them, and notably when you see that the woman is not relieved by being put in a warm bed, but that her pain continues and increases, the mouth of the womb is open, and following a contraction the midwife feels something pushing against her finger, so that what was soft at the top becomes firmer and somewhat harder, then there can be no doubt that this is true labor.

When this occurs, it is right that the woman should be mindful of the will of the sovereign Creator, who said to our common mother[108] that she would give birth in pain, and she should arm herself with a

---

107. The first part of the chapter listed the typical signs of impending labor.
108. I.e. Eve (Genesis 3:16).

strong heart. If she feels she has the strength, she should get up, put on some clothes or a mantle, according to her station, and walk around the room as much as she can, from time to time falling back on the bed to catch her breath, then getting back up to exercise her body, and she should even (if she has sufficient strength) walk briskly up and down the stairs to help nature all the more. For she will find her labor easy and light, or difficult and hard, according to the exercise and the movement she undertakes.

If she does not have the strength to walk unaided, she may be supported under her arms by two strong women, one holding her on each side, and she may lean on them as though her strength had deserted her; she should put no more weight on her legs than she can help.

When she feels a pain or contraction running down from the back to the lower abdomen, she should go up to a firm table on which there is a pillow to support her, and she should open her legs so the midwife (who has greased her hand with fresh butter, oil of lilies or sweet almonds) will put her index or middle finger in the birthing passage, reaching up to the mouth of the womb where the crown of the child is. The child will have descended from a high to a low position in order to push with its head and advance; and the womb will respond, and make its own effort with its lateral fibres in order to expel its burden. It will start to dilate to about the size of a penny, and it will be possible to feel the head through the membranes, for this is always the first part to present in any natural birth, which is why it is called crowning. When the midwife has reached this far, she should insert her index as well as her middle finger in order to dilate the opening, and in this way assist the efforts of nature as best she is able. Then if the waters flow out unprompted, she should simply wait to receive what Lady Nature will give her, for the child will soon appear.

If not, and if the chorionic membrane is too tough, as sometimes happens, in order to avoid the effort of nature — which alone can achieve anything at this stage — disappearing or becoming far less strong, she should break the membrane with her nails, or if necessary with scissors, then she should instruct the woman to hold her breath, and bear down. In order to assist it further, she should put her hand on the top of the abdomen, towards the navel, and gently push the bulge down, slightly easing it without applying any force. Or she can have the pressure applied by one of the women who is present, so that she herself can stand ready to receive the gift of nature, the delivery of the child.

Because it is rare that a woman in labor can remain on her feet throughout, she should be provided with a chair near the table, or something else of the same height, on which she can lean from time to time. This chair should be of medium height, say a foot and a half or two feet, open at the front and the back so that the midwife can examine her without problem, and so that the dilation is not hindered, and the sacrum is able to separate from the hip bones, and the coccyx or tailbone are not prevented from tipping back. These are the ways of nature without which the birth cannot proceed naturally, as is proved by an infinite number of reasons expounded by Séverin Pineau in the second book of his *Observations*,[109] which the reader who wishes to know more may consult. I shall leave this subject here in order to remain brief. Suffice it to say that the back of the chair should tilt backwards so that the woman can sit comfortably and rest in it when she is not experiencing a contraction. The chair should be upholstered on both sides or supplied with plenty of cushions to provide something soft on which the woman can sit, resting her thighs and buttocks on them.

In front of her she should have quite a broad cushion on which she should kneel when she feels a contraction developing, leaning with her hands on the table and gripping it firmly, holding her breath in order to make as much effort as she can to push her burden down. Or she may put her arms around another woman's neck while she is bearing down, and meanwhile one of the midwives will gently press the abdomen down, helping nature to achieve what it desires. The other midwife, having lubricated her hand with oil of lilies or melted fresh butter, will seek to dilate the opening, doing what she can to widen the birthing passage, as explained above.

And if it happens that a woman is so weak that she cannot remain in a sitting position, she may be placed on the bed, covered with enough sheets and blankets, and in such a position that her head and her whole body are raised so that she breathes more easily. Her buttocks

109. See 187, n. 110.

should be a little lower, but much higher than her feet, which should be resting on a bar so that she does not slip; she should bring them back up towards the buttocks, keeping her knees well raised and open.

Under her lower back a sheet should be spread, large enough that when it is folded over several times it is still a foot wide. When a contraction comes, two of the women who are with her should lift her up in the sheet, holding it on both sides, so that the effort of nature can run its full course and move the iliac bones and let the coccyx tip back. With the patient supported in this manner under her armpits, with her loins raised, a woman can push the child down quite gently, and the midwife, once her hand is lubricated, can dilate the mouth of the womb.

To help the delivery even more, she should say that everything is going well, that the child is well positioned for the birth, that the patient must make even more effort than before, and that it is a son or daughter depending on what she has recognized the mother's wish to be, and she should say that she is sure of this from her manual examination, so that the mother's spirits are kept up.

In order to accomplish everything described above, this midwife must be strong, neither young nor old, kind, patient and unassuming, so that she will suffer the mother's[110] laments with patience, giving her something to eat or drink in order to keep her strength up when the time is right. She should always keep her hands lubricated with oil of violets, lilies, sweet almonds, or grease of duck, chicken, pig, or at least unsalted butter. She should recommend that the mother turn her cries, moans and lamentations into efforts to help nature by holding her breath rather than shouting and moaning, especially when the efforts of nature[111] are present.

And if the mother should be very weak, she should give her a dram of confection of alchermes, dissolved in two ounces of water of artemisia, or in two ounces of water with cinnamon, or in one ounce of water of hyssop and one ounce of cinnamon water. Or it is also appropriate to use one crown's worth of sparrow-hawk dung dissolved

---

110. Note that Duval, who has been referring to the mother as the patient ('*la patiente*') in French now calls her 'the ill woman' ('*la malade*'), returning to the idea that pregnancy is an illness.

111. i.e contractions.

in hyssop water. All this is to be done if necessary in order to avoid causing a fever by the use of too many hot remedies.

An aetite or white magnetite stone should be tied on the inside of her thigh, very near the groin, the skin of a snake around her abdomen.[112] If she has a belt made from the skin of an animal called an elk, she should tie this also around her thigh; but, as soon as she is delivered, they should all be removed since such cures, which have the secret power to draw the womb down, could also cause harm by bringing about a prolapse.

If the midwife feels the child's head leaning more to one side than the other, being turned towards the groin as it were, she should position the woman on her opposite side, then insert a lubricated hand (as described above) and reposition it, touching this delicate creature so gently that she does no more than slide her hand over its face, knowing that it can easily be injured, so she will take care not to press down upon it or make any sharp movement.

She should also take care to guard against the problems which can arise because of different mothers' natures, for instance, if they are too fat, thin, young, old, tall or short, weak, feeble, fearful, or prone to give birth prematurely or very late. Or if they have eaten badly in some respect during their pregnancy; or if they suddenly suffer from intolerance of hunger, thirst or the use of smells which prevent the contractions moving down towards the womb, stopping short instead above the navel. Or if the iliac bones, sacrum and coccyx are badly shaped and too dry, or if the mouth or even the neck of the womb is hardened and narrow. A particular pain — ulcers, genital warts or rhagades — may sometimes bother them, and these may be a problem either in themselves, or for the neighboring parts, because they prevent the natural stretching and dilation required in childbirth.

To this must be added the questions of how tough the membranes are, the thickness of the placenta; the weakness of a child unable to help very much; the dryness of these parts which will have arisen if the waters have broken too soon; or the child having an over-large head or a monstrous body. In all of these cases, the midwife will use the specific remedy for the situation in so far as is in her power. Or in case of uncertainty, she should not be slow to summon the help

112. For all of these remedies, cf. Liebault ch. 45, on which Duval is partly drawing.

of a physician, who will overcome all these difficulties by the use of appropriate medicines, and with the help of God will allow her to deliver the child if it is in a good, natural position, with its head down. The face, however, may be turned to either side when the child comes out, for a boy will have its face turned towards the seat, a girl on the other hand will have her face turned towards the bladder and clitoris.[113]

If it chances that the umbilical cord, which is normally two cubits[114] in length, is wrapped around the child's neck when it is born, it may often happen to be looped two or three times, which puts the child's life in danger. The concern for the mother should be momentarily laid aside, and the cut made at the child's navel; the cord should then be tied to the mother's thigh, or otherwise given to another woman who is present to hold, or something may be attached to it to hold it down so that it does not disappear back into the womb. Then the child should be looked after as will be described hereafter, so that the mother may again be taken care of. If the mother has not eaten for a long time, or if she has been very weak, she should be given a little wine with a piece of fried bread dipped in it, or some hippocras, or cinnamon water, or spirits to give her a little more energy and restore her strength which will have been sapped by so great an exhaustion on account of the great contractions which may often be too violent. Women know well how to describe this.

Chapter XX: What Should Be Done in a Long and Difficult Delivery

After having given a sufficient explanation of what is required when a delivery is natural, easier, and as we would wish, it is now time to move on to an account of what is necessary when there is some difficulty.

Childbirth is made more painful and difficult, according to Baldvinus Ronsseus, on account of a mother's bad temperament and

113. Duval uses the French term '*clitoris*', a relative neologism at this date.
114. A cubit is approx. 46 cm.

disposition, or because of the child and its placenta, or otherwise because of some external factor.[115]

As far as the mother is concerned, this occurs when her body is squat and fat, or over-dry and hard, when the womb is small and compressed, and the woman unaccustomed to bear pain, and in addition is ashamed and unwilling to undress and expose her particular state, whether it be inflammation or an ulcer which is currently present in the womb, or an ulcer which was there previously and has left some scarring, or finally when she is so very weak that she cannot assist in the birth.

The difficulty resulting from the child occurs when it is unusually large, or has an oversized head or a monstrous body, which makes the birth what is called in popular parlance 'snatched'; or when there are several children who obstruct each other's exits, and especially if there is superfetation and a younger child lies in the way preventing the one who is struggling to be born at the right time.[116]

External factors include: when the woman has been beaten, injured or hurt, or troubled by the air outside being too cold; also, when she has been afflicted by sadness, fear or worried by some other unfortunate external event which has so disturbed the child that it cannot adopt the right position which it would wish to, presenting head first, as we have said above. Instead, it will be found to present a shoulder, an elbow, a hand, the buttocks, the stomach, one side, a knee or a foot. It is rare for the child to present with both hands or both feet, because of the natural position, which we described above. Such a position is only found after a woman has suffered most serious distress, cruel contractions and violent pains and the child has been able to move about during the course of them. This is most perilous, if the truth be told.

It is not as perilous, however, as the situations described above, and especially when the placenta has completely detached itself from the womb to which it had been fixed, and presents before the child.[117]

115. Baldvinus Ronsseus (Baudouin Ronsse, a Flemish physician, d. 1596), *Medical Treatises*, vol. II, *On the Diseases of Women* [*Opuscula medica*: vol. II, *De morbis muliebribus*].

116. Renaissance medical treatises abound with heated discussions of superfetation (the conception of a second pregnancy after a first is already established), a phenomenon common in animals, but now considered to be very rare in humans.

117. I.e. the condition of *placenta praevia*.

For then there is a danger that because of its bad position, the child may be unable to get its breath, which it does only by means of the iliac arteries, and these no longer function in such a situation, so that often the child suffocates.

In this case, the poor mother needs not a mere servant, an attendant or an ignorant midwife, but one who is really wise and careful, and these are very few in number. She should be quick to position the woman so that her head and shoulders are lower than her buttocks. Then she should hold the knees open with the heels close to the buttocks, keeping the area decently covered; and she should put a cloth soaked in cold water on the protruding arm or leg of the child, so that when it feels the cold it will withdraw them, or at least it will assist the midwife's efforts as she will do what is in her power, being as gentle as she possibly can, to push them back. For the child's limbs are so sensitive and fragile that there is a risk that the effort she makes on her own to push them back might only bruise and seriously damage them, without achieving anything much.

So, after she has pushed back and repositioned in the womb the presenting elbow, hand, knee or foot, doing this with the greatest care and dexterity that she can summon for the particular situation; or if without having felt any protruding limb, she finds the child presenting with its stomach, back or side, so that it comes doubled on itself, or with one or other shoulder presenting at an angle: she should instruct the woman to open her mouth and breathe out, rather than holding her breath and bearing down. The woman will be naturally inclined to do this because of the cries and wails she will be making on account of the cruel, terrible pains she suffers. Then, when she has lubricated her hands thoroughly as described above, she will try to lift the child over the obstacle of the bones, and by pushing it back she will position it so that, if possible, it presents head first, which is the best and natural position. If this cannot be done, and if she finds the child has taken a position so far from where it should naturally be that both its feet are at the mouth of the womb, she should pull them gently and deliver the child in this way. In the same way, if she finds both the hands are well positioned, she should do the same thing. When the placenta presents first, she should do what she can to push it back,[118] trying as she does

118. Cf. the advice of Bourgeois to midwives: *Diverse Observations,* I. 7.

this to bring the head forward, as has been said several times. If this fails and she cannot achieve what she wishes, it will be a wise action on her part to summon the doctor, who will prescribe a purging enema, containing among other things benedicta or ground-ivy with some diacassia, catholicon, red sugar and mercurial honey. By mouth he will administer water of calf's head, or shavings of ivory if she has a fever, or he may give her one or two ounces of water with cinnamon, or with strong alcohol or theriac. Or he may do as follows:

Take two drachms[119] of good rhubarb, and put them to soak with two pinches of cinnamon in two ounces of juice of parsley, or an equal quantity of cinnamon water in a solution of a pinch of castor oil and of root of dictaminus, and one ounce of syrup of mugwort. Make a potion of this and give it to the patient to drink.

Or alternatively, take half a drachm of some of the skin which is found in the gap between the two halves of the walnut, called 'nauci', and of some very fine cinnamon. Beat them well; take an ounce of some juice of parsley mixed with white wine or cinnamon water and of syrup of mugwort; mix them together and give them to her to drink.

The scents of labdanum, bedellium, alipta moscata, grey amber, musk and civet are necessary for the lower parts. But for the nostrils, the woman needs to smell stinking feathers from a partridge or old, burned slippers. If you repeat the enemas, they should be both bitter and softening at the same time. As for the poultices which are put on the lower abdomen and the inner thighs, they should use emollients, with roots of mauves and mallows, leaves from these plants and leaves of violets and senna, seeds of linseed, fenugreek and other similar ones.

After this emollient poultice, the following treatment should be applied. Take three ounces of the pulp of a gourd and of the leaves of maidenhair, two ounces of juice of rue, and as much lupin flour as is needed, and make a cataplasm to place on the abdomen; to this you may also add one ounce of coccus pills. And then, apart from the treatments indicated above, which work through their occult powers, it is also very helpful to attach to the right thigh some storax calami, green coriander, or polygonon and cyclamen roots. Root of henbane should also be bound and tied to the left thigh, and an emery stone

---

119. A drachm or dram is an eighth of an ounce.

should be held in the right hand. She should also be given one écu's[120] weight of ivory shavings to drink in cinnamon or theriac water.

Wearing coral around the neck helps greatly. Savory crushed and placed on the abdomen draws the child from the body, whether dead or alive. Having the woman drink ass's milk with a little salt water or rose water can also achieve this. Some people apply crushed mugwort and a woman's milk to the abdomen, with great success. Jean de Villeneuve and Jean de Saint-Armand[121] strongly recommend that over the region of the groin you should hold 12 or 13 coriander seeds tied up in a cloth held tightly by a child who is a virgin, whether a boy or a girl, and she should be given a drink of half a dram of borras stone in strong white wine, or in an ounce of cinnamon water. And Victorius Faventinus[122] strongly approves this remedy. Take an ounce of the peel of horse-radish and of leaves of herb mercury, three grains of saffron, two drams of well powdered cinnamon; mix these all together and put the mixture in a piece of red taffeta which you should hang around the patient's neck; and soon afterwards she will give birth. The smell of burned geest will also work, or of bitumen of Judea,[123] which is more suitable. Sneezing caused by powder of hellebore, pepper and a little euphorbia is very suitable.

While these medicines are being administered, the midwife should not relax, but rather keep a close watch, and at the onset of each new contraction she should try to reposition the child so that it presents head first, or if not so that she can grasp both the feet or both the hands to pull it out.

When she has delivered the child after such a long, hard labor, she should check whether the cord is swollen and filled with blood after being too roughly shaken. If it is, she should cut it and let a little blood run out to avoid the risk of it festering or becoming inflamed; then she should tie it two finger lengths from the abdomen. She should twist the thread around it twice, tying two knots if it is enlarged and

---

120. A gold or silver coin.

121. Jean de Villeneuve was a contemporary physician in Provence; Jean de Saint-Armand was a 13th-century physician from Tournay, celebrated for his translations and commentaries of works by Hippocrates and Galen.

122. Benedetto Vettori (Benedictus Victorius Faventinus), 1481–1561, physician, philosopher and Professor of Medicine at Padua.

123. An asphalt compound.

swollen. She should not tie it too tightly so that she does not cause great pain with the thread; nor should it be too loose, so that the blood does not run. Then she should hand the child over to the nurse or other women who are present, and now take care of the mother, delivering the placenta if it has not come out together with the child.

In order to deliver it, she should take in her hand the cord she has cut, and she should gently press and rub with her hand the area of the mother's abdomen which is swollen, in order to encourage the greatly dilated uterus to contract, return to its smaller size, and expel the afterbirth of the newborn child. However, she should avoid pulling or applying any force to the cord for fear lest it break, since it is very fragile. This would be a most serious thing, for if the mouth of the womb has no obstacle, it would quickly close up, and in this way make the delivery of the placenta much more difficult, and might even cause the mother's death.[124]

If it happens that this slight effort is not sufficient, she should advise the mother to hold her nose and close her mouth so that she bears down and tries to push out what is left. She may indeed also give her the sneezing powder spoken of above to make her sneeze, and at the same time the woman should hold her nose, close her mouth, and the violence of the sneeze will affect the lower regions to which it is directed rather than the upper ones. And should it occur that the delivery is not accomplished by this means, she should then properly be given an enema with a decoction of herbs which work on the uterus, and in which colewort,[125] ivy and mercurial honey or althea have been dissolved. While these remedies are being administered, the midwife should try all the gentler means she can think of to encourage nature to fulfil its duty. She can first shake the cord and apply a little traction, alternately dilating the mouth of the womb and holding it open, and sometimes also running her hand over the abdomen and thighs, and placing a hot cloth on the abdomen, and other such things. She should be mindful that this is a natural course of action which is not achieved in a single moment, and that often it requires some kinds of stimulation so that Nature, this sovereign princess, can recover

124. Several treatises warn of the serious dangers of a mismanaged delivery of the placenta. See 97; 145, n. 16; 170; 202, n. 161; 204.

125. Cabbage or kale.

her strength and be induced little by little to carry out the desired expulsion. This she will finally accomplish, given time. This is why one should not use force to achieve what can be done gently.

For as Madame Boursier, midwife to the present Queen, says in her *Observations*,[126] it is rare that it is necessary to have to extract the placenta from inside the uterus. She prides herself on having delivered more than 2,000 women, without being obliged to insert her hand to dislodge it from the uterus. She says she would never do so unless obliged by one of these three necessities. The first is if the mother suffered an extreme loss of blood; the next, if she were having convulsions;[127] and the third and last, if a high temperature had so dehydrated her body that the child's afterbirth remained fixed and could not be separated just by nature.

In order, however, to give nature even more help, it would be good to make the mother vomit by putting a finger at the back of her mouth, and using a fumigation to rise up into the womb. This fumigation should be made with mugwort, savory and dictaminus boiled in white wine. Smoked adana[128] and storax is also suitable, as indeed are other remedies used to bring on the menses. A dose of a dram of castor oil in cinnamon water is excellent for this purpose, as also when it is applied to the lower abdomen, blended with pennyroyal or leek, and some of this may even be introduced in the birthing passage. For this you may also use myrrh, savory, madder and parsnip roots whether in a drink, placed on the abdomen or given as a perfume.

Those who are unable to obtain the commodities found in towns, and who have to use what they find in the fields, make a fumigation with cats' or lambs' droppings and horses' nails, or apply a cow's afterbirth to the abdomen; or they administer some part of it which they have kept, and beaten and mixed with white wine.

While much must be entrusted to nature in this delivery, yet one must not think that, when an over-long and insurmountable delay is recognized, it would be wrong for a midwife to do her duty. She should grease her hand well with oils, liniments or animal fats as mentioned above, then put it into the womb, following the cord, and take hold of

---

126. Duval here refers to the first volume of Bourgeois's *Diverse Observations* (I. 14).

127. The condition that would now be recognized as eclampsia.

128. A large fish, similar to sturgeon.

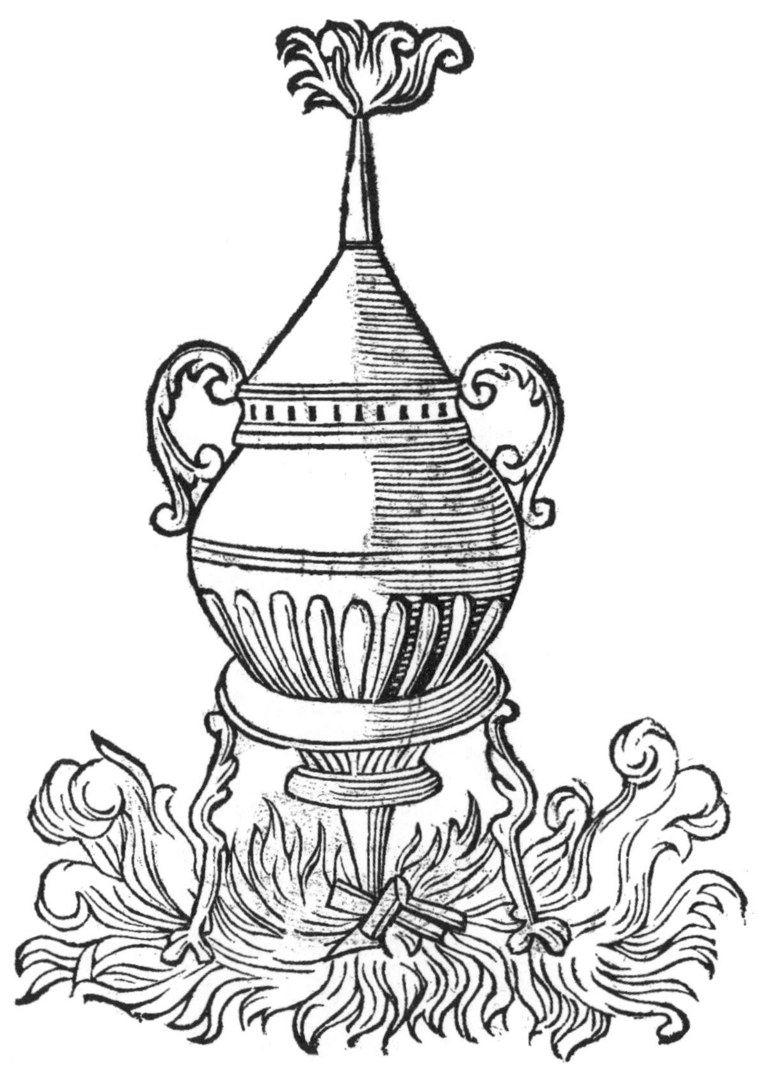

22) Instrument for fumigation of the womb

Scipio Mercurio, *La Commare*, Venice, 1601
(Wellcome Library, London)

the placenta with her finger. However, she should avoid pulling it out hastily lest she cause a prolapse of the uterus, which would be a very dangerous thing; rather, by gently moving the placenta from side to side, she should succeed in extracting it.

She should avoid what ignorant midwives do, who seize the placenta in the womb, and instead of delivering it, not only cause prolapses but also very dangerous ulcers of the womb.[129]

She should also ensure that what she has pulled out is complete, and that no part of the afterbirth remains inside, since the putrefaction that would occur would have serious consequences. Any part of the placenta which is not delivered immediately tends to decompose, infecting the whole body with bad vapors, but this we shall leave aside for the present, since it is not the midwife's area, and it is sufficient for us to warn her of what constitutes her duty.

Furthermore, if there chance to be two or more children, when she has received the first, she should wait for nature to deliver the others. She should try to deliver them as soon as possible, but without using any force, especially since most commonly twins have only a single placenta,[130] with the division between them separated by only a single membrane,[131] so that what is left from the sack of the first child dangles from the last child and is too great a burden. In this way, if one of the twins has remained in the uterus too long after the birth of the first, this often causes the mother's death because of the decomposition resulting from the remainder of the placenta. This is why you should try to deliver the whole placenta at the same time if there is only one, which can be established by whether the placenta is incomplete. If it is complete, it is important not to be rough with anything that might be left, even if one knows there is still something in the womb. It has happened that children have been conceived not as twins, but as a result of superfetation, or conception which happened after that of

129. Bourgeois's *Diverse Observations* of 1609 also give examples of careless or rough midwives who caused uterine prolapse after delivery by tugging on the womb: *Diverse Observations* I. 36.

130. This affirmation runs counter to modern obstetric statistics, which set the rate of monochorionic pregnancies (i.e. with a single placenta) at about 20% of all twin pregnancies. However, Duval and modern obstetricians are in agreement on the point that single-placenta twin pregnancies carry a higher associated risk than twin pregnancies in which each foetus has a separate placenta.

131. The chorion.

the first child, and these children have remained one or two months, indeed up to four months after the first was delivered, and then, after a period of time, they were nonetheless born without problem.

If in this way God does not, in his grace, allow the midwife to deliver a woman of the placenta, either because of the death of the child, or the extreme weakness of the mother who may be on the point of death, the doctors or surgeons must be summoned. After having tried all other remedies, they will need to have recourse to obtaining the placenta by extraction or by cesarean section.

Chapter XXII: First Type of Delivery by the Surgeon's Hand

In order to carry out the first of these kinds of assistance, before all else the surgeon who has been called to deliver the woman in labor must consider her state, and whether she can withstand the demands of a difficult labor. Should he find her to be weak, fading and dying, he should not attempt to deliver her by his hand, unless it be the case that losing one, one wished to save the other: that is to say, the child who might still be alive. For it is impossible to carry out this procedure unless nature, if not actually a collaborator, is at least prepared to submit to the necessary rigors.

He should also consider whether the child is alive or dead, and whether the midwife may have bruised or damaged the passage by some of her endeavors. This is important for him in preparing to do his duty according to the circumstances, and also for his prognosis.

In doing this, provided he judges that the passage is not too narrow (which would prevent him achieving what he wishes), if it happens that the woman's stomach is not relaxed, a purgative enema should be administered, and then she should be given two ounces of fortified water, cinnamon water or hippocras, or instead a dram of alchermes diluted in two ounces of hyssop water, or blessed thistle water, to which should be added a little mallow syrup; or at least she should swallow an egg, and drink one helping of wine with a little sugar warmed with a cube of fried bread.

In summer, when the weather is too hot, he should send out all the people he judges not to be essential, for they only overheat the room, and in the winter he should have the chill of the air tempered by a good fire. Then, with men to assist him, or strong women who are not too easily scared, he will order that the doors and windows should be firmly closed.

Once this is done, the woman should be positioned on a fairly firm square of tapestry or on a good pile of clothes which should be placed for this purpose on the edge of the bed, and she should lie back on the bed, but raised up so that she is not lying flat, nor even half-sitting, but in a position so that even though she is lying down, she can breathe very easily and the muscles of her epigaster are not too strained.

When she has been positioned thus,[132] he should fix around her a bandage which is half a foot wide, running from the shoulder (like a scarf) down to the legs, first round one side, then the other, coming back up to the other shoulder, and as it crosses over it will make the shape of the cross of St Andrew[133] both at the front and the back. He should do this as many times as necessary so that the feet and legs are securely brought up against the buttocks, and so that the knees are splayed open and the lower abdomen compressed against the inner thighs. The patient should be unable to move, in the manner of those who are prepared for the extraction of a stone from the bladder. Or she may be firmly held by two people, her heels pressing against the edge of the bed and her back flat on the bed, and they should be able to lift her up when the attempt is made to pull out the child.

A gown or other such item of clothing should be thrown over her body, and a warm sheet folded over twice should be placed over her thighs and knees, so that those who are present cannot see what is being done, for otherwise this would be a cause of shame both to them and to the mother.[134]

Then the surgeon, having removed the rings from his fingers, clipped his nails and removed anything which might injure the patient, should grease the inside of her thighs, her lower abdomen and private parts with oil of sweet almonds, linseed, lilies or butter, or some other such liniment, and he should also coat his hands well in the oil so that they slide and move more easily. He should put his right

132. Cf. the advice given by Guillemeau, II. 5 (208-211).

133. I.e like a letter X.

134. This sentence confirms that even in the early-seventeenth century, the professional duties of a surgeon or male midwife were performed under cover.

hand very gently into the womb, and once it is inside, he should clench his fist against the mouth of the womb to dilate it. Then he will be able to tell, using this natural probe, whether there is only one child, and whether it is well positioned.

If it is badly positioned, he should push the body back inside if it is turned with one side or its back or stomach presenting; and he should also push back in the arm, leg, knee, elbow or shoulder if he finds them protruding from the mouth of the womb, and maneuver the head in such a way that it crowns, allowing the most natural birth. Before he pushes a leg back in the womb, he should tie a ribbon around it, like the kind women use to tie back their hair.[135] Then, when he has put it inside, and if possible located the other leg, he will pull it with the ribbon so that he holds both of the legs together. If possible, he will try to ensure that the child has one arm raised as it comes out, as most commonly occurs because of its natural position, and if both arms present, he will push one back for fear that if both arms were by the sides, the mouth of the womb might contract again after the shoulders had passed through, which could cause the child to be strangled. Otherwise he should pull it out quickly, allowing no delay, instructing the mother to keep her mouth closed and to bear downwards with her breath and strength, doing all she can to assist the process by tightening the muscles of her lower abdomen, or even making her sneeze.

Then, if the last resort cannot be averted, it will be necessary to push a hook in, guided by the index finger, to secure and pull on the head of the child. If the hands present first, they should be pushed back for fear lest the head remain flexed against the back, which would make the birth too painful and difficult; and the surgeon should always ensure that the head presents first. Because it happens that some arrogant midwives call upon the surgeon only after the death of the child, whose arm will sometimes have protruded for a long time, already dead and chronically ulcerated, it is then appropriate to remove the flesh with a razor as far as possible, and to cut the bone with serrated pincers, so that this flesh which has been removed covers the end of the bone which is left, to prevent the bone from injuring the womb.

135. Guillemeau had described delivering a woman, using exactly this method (*De l'heureux accouchement des femmes*, 1609, 267).

Then, having pushed the rest of the body back in, the surgeon will try to maneuver the head round to the entrance, or the feet if they present first, in order to pull out the whole body.

If the head should be so large in the case of a dead child that it cannot be delivered, even though it presents first, the surgeon should try to pull it out with hooks. But if this does not suffice, it should be broken with the serrated pincers, and extracted in pieces. If the child's abdomen is swollen, as often occurs two or three days after it has remained dead in the mother's womb, because of the liquids and gases which build up, an incision must be made with a sharp hook in order to pull out the guts and then the other parts which present.

Care must be taken in the case of twins lest, if one foot presents, and a ribbon is tied as described above, then pushed back inside, a foot of the other twin is not pulled. In order to avoid this and to make the extraction easier, the foot which has been pushed back in should be grasped around the thigh, so that there is a way of distinguishing the other twin.

When the child has been delivered in this manner, it is important to be very careful to remove the whole placenta, not leaving any behind, and to do this it is better to put in a hand and gently loosen and pull it rather than using a hook, which risks lacerating the womb.

This is what happened in 1581 at the extraction of my first child, who was pulled dead from the body of Anne Le Marchant, my first wife, after she had endured a difficult, cruel labor over four whole days, having no respite either day or night. The child could not be delivered in any other way both because of the size of its head and because the mother had suffered an injury to her sacrum such that the iliac bones could not separate at all. Thus, although the mother was strong and the child vigorous, and the womb sufficiently opened, yet the child was unable to come out and died on the fourth day, followed by the mother a week later. This was because a cesarean operation was not performed. I had suggested this expedient to Guillaume Le Marchand, a former apothecary, aged 60, and his wife, the father and mother of my late wife, since I had seen this done twice in similar cases under the care of the physician Monsieur Duval, my father. He had been desirous of furthering my instruction, and made sure I attended operations which in his view were rare, even when as a young child I was engaged in my early studies. But they refused this operation for their daughter because they had not yet heard of it being carried out in Louviers, where I was living at the time. As a result, the child was pulled out, as I have described above, by the surgeon Guillaume Auber, living on the Bridge of the Arch, who was very skilled in this procedure.

Chapter XXIII: The Manner of Delivering the Woman with the Help of a Speculum

The art of surgery, which is ever progressing, continually strives to find something of use to the human race, and seeing that there may be some slight obstruction or join at the mouth of the womb which prevents it from dilating naturally, it has invented the use of a mirror for the womb (called a *speculum matricis*),[136] which allows the surgeon to pull the child from the mother's womb more easily, although with greater trepidation, since this instrument is made of steel which is appropriate for this purpose. So when the surgeon feels that the mouth of the womb continues to present strong resistance, he should first reassure the mother, make sure the temperature of the room is correct, place his patient on the edge of the bed, bound securely and entrusted to those who will have to hold and support her, as described above. She should be covered in such a way that her lower regions are hidden from the sight of those present, but that nonetheless the surgeon is able to adjust his mirror as he wishes. As described above, he should remove his rings, if he is wearing any, grease his hands with the oils we have cited above or similar ones, and also grease the inside of the woman's thighs, lower abdomen and her private parts.

Then he should take his instrument which allows him to see, warm it a little, and cover it with the oils so that it can be manipulated more easily. Some would recommend that it should be covered with leather at the end, but that only presents a hindrance. For this reason it is

---

136. The use of the speculum for the womb [*speculum matricis*] is described in various surgical and anatomical treatises, including a letter from Ailleboust to Rousset, cited in Rousset's *New Treatise on Hysterotomotoky*, 109; Guillemeau, *On the Safe Delivery of Women*, 1609, 195; Girault's 1610 revised and extended edition of Daleschamps's *French Surgery* [*Chirurgie françoise*], 320 and 663. Its use was favored, as demonstrated in the latter examples, by the Parisian surgeon Honoré, celebrated for his expertise in difficult deliveries.

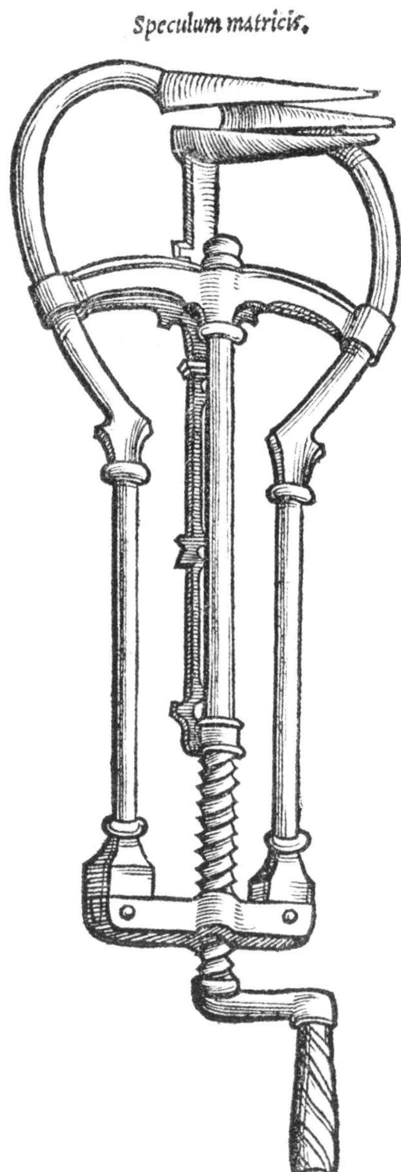

23) Uterine speculum

Jakob Rueff, *De conceptu et generatione hominis*, Zurich, 1554
(Bibliothèque de Strasbourg)

sufficient to keep it well polished and covered with oils or butters, which prevent it being too rough, so that when it is put inside it does not hurt or damage the parts of the body we described. It should have a beak of about 12 '*doigts*' in length,[137] so that it can be inserted right into the mouth of the womb,[138] for otherwise it would be of no use. For this passage is 12 '*doigts*' in length, and the instrument needs to reach the very end of it, and even be pushed further in, so that it reaches as far as the mouth of the womb or the inner part of this organ.

In inserting it, care must be taken that the end that is pushed inside does not harm the child. This could easily occur if unintentionally it were pushed too precipitously against the head or another limb of the child, which might happen to be crowning at the opening, since the full womb at this stage descends significantly towards the birthing passage.

When the speculum has been inserted as far as this orifice, it should gradually be opened by turning the handle towards the woman's abdomen, and when it is dilated far enough that one can put a hand in it, the hand should be moved up to ease the dilation. Then, when it is open sufficiently that an arm can easily pass through it, a man who is present should be asked to hold the handle of the speculum so that it does not close up under the pressure exerted by the mouth of the womb. Then the surgeon should stretch his hand, suitably greased as has been described, into the womb itself and reposition the child so that it is well placed for delivery, with the head facing downward. He should take care not to injure the head on the beak of the speculum. If it proves impossible to turn the child's head down, the two feet may be grasped and pulled into the speculum so that they can be held more easily.

However, if it happens that one of the arms presents and sticks out, the positioning of the instrument requires particular care so that the child is not injured. First, every effort should be made to push the arm back, and if this cannot be achieved, the speculum should be opened enough to hold just the arm. Then the arm should be drawn into it

137. The old unit of measurement of a '*doigt*' is equivalent to about 1.85 cm, making the beak approx. 22 cm (or 8 inches) in length.
138. I.e. the cervix.

without causing any injury, and in such a way that it can be pushed back into the womb, and the child then turned to a suitable position.

If it happens that the child is dead, which will be apparent from the blackness and gangrene of the presenting part, there is no need to proceed so carefully. Instead, as described above, the arm should be cut off so that the speculum can be inserted more easily if the operation cannot be conducted in any other way.

LOUIS DE SERRES

*Treatise on the Nature, Causes, Signs and
Remedies concerning Failures to Conceive,
and Sterility among Women*
(1625)

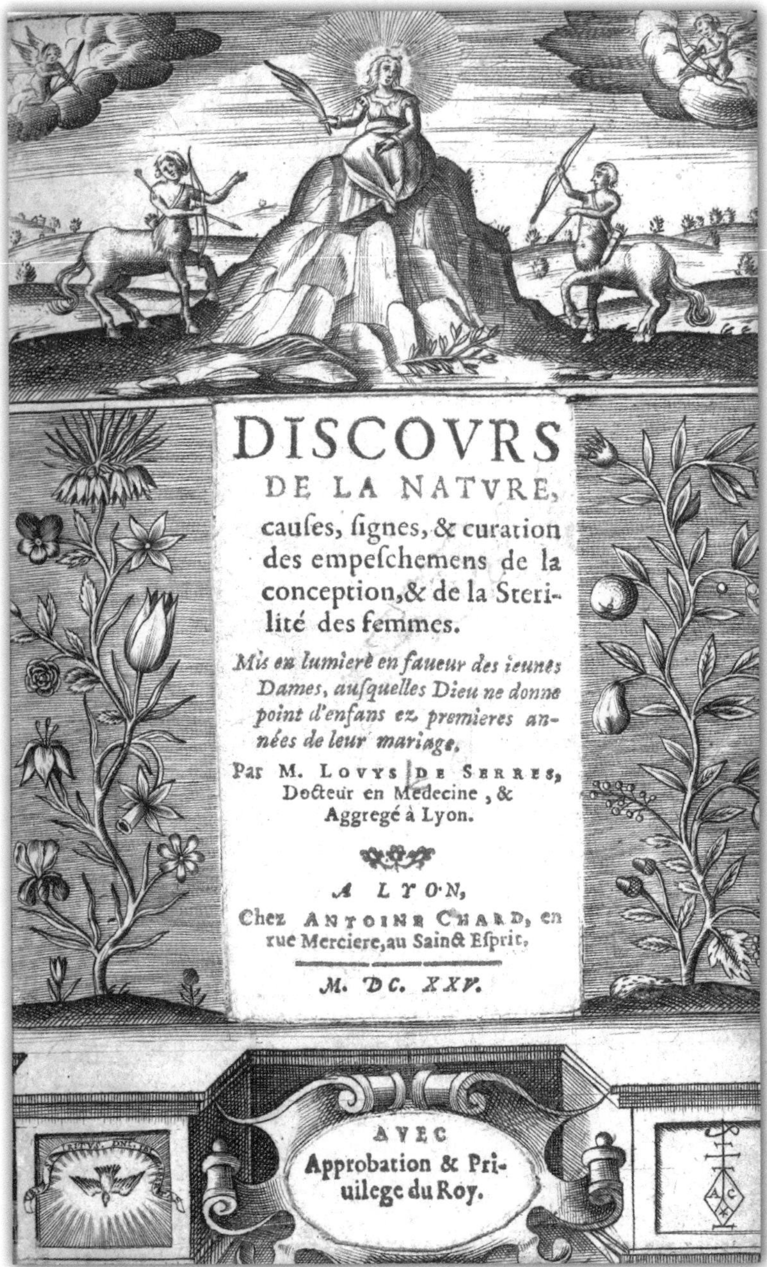

24) Title page: Louis de Serres, *Discours de la sterilité des femmes*, Lyons, 1625

(Library of Royal College of Obstetricians and Gynaecologists, London)

INTRODUCTION

TRANSLATION OF EXCERPTS FROM
TREATISE ON STERILITY AMONG WOMEN (1625)

Preliminary texts:

Main chapters:

INTRODUCTION

Like Rousset, de Serres composes a lengthy treatise to discuss his views on one aspect of pregnancy and childbirth that particularly interests him, namely the problems of women who are childless. Although to a modern reader the title of the work would suggest that he is concerned only with women unable to conceive, his definition of 'sterility' includes women who conceive but suffer repeated miscarriages. Hence, the work also encompasses recommendations for sustaining a healthy pregnancy. Other early modern French medical writers, including Joubert,[1] Liebault[2] and Bourgeois,[3] had treated infertility and miscarriages in the context of general reviews of women's reproductive health,[4] but de Serres is unique in making it the central focus of a whole treatise.[5] His evident compassion for those women unable to bear a child is striking.

Life and Works of Louis de Serres

We have little detail on the life of Louis de Serres (1588–1656), beyond what is revealed by the prefaces to his published works and some archival records in Lyons.[6] It is known that he came from a

---

1. Book II, chapter 11 of *Popular Errors* considers female sterility, while several other chapters of Book II also consider male sterility or limited fertility.

2. Chapters 2–10 of Book II of Liebault's *Three Books on the Health, Fertility and Illnesses of Women* (1582) are devoted to infertility (male and female).

3. Despite entitling her work *Diverse Observations on Sterility, Miscarriage, Fertility, Childbirth, and the Diseases of Women and Newborn Children*, Bourgeois confines her treatment of sterility to the first two chapters of Book I (on inability to conceive and repeated miscarriages, respectively). Unlike de Serres, she starts by postulating that women's failure to conceive is more often the woman's than the man's fault: *Diverse Observations*, I. 1.

4. In contrast, Guillemeau, writing as a surgeon, does not specifically treat infertility, although chapter 20 ('The way to treat women who do not carry their child to its term') of Book I of *On the Safe Delivery of Women* offers advice for women suffering from repeated miscarriages. Neither Rousset nor Duval specifically treats sterility, although both discuss fertility and conception at some length.

5. In this he typifies a resurgence of the later medieval preoccupation with fertility/ sterility, which is evidenced in a number of treatises specifically on sterility emanating from Montpellier (in Latin) in the fourteenth century. For discussion of these treatises and the broader context of later medieval medical discussions of fertility and sterility, see M. Green, *Making Women's Medicine Masculine*, 85–91.

6. See the website on French Huguenots: http://huguenots-france.org/france/lyon/, which cites the archival record (Rhone ER: 1322 R 719).

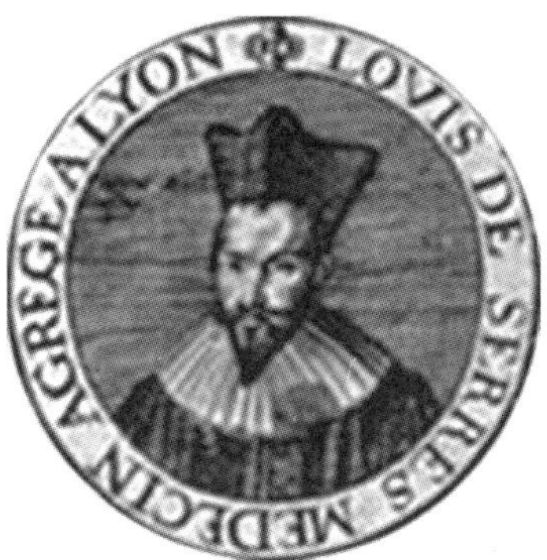

25) Portrait of Louis de Serres

Inset from title page of Jean de Renou, *Les Œuvres pharmaceutiques*, Lyons, 1626
(Centre d'Etudes supérieures de la Renaissance,Tours)

Protestant family, which had its roots in Dauphiné, a province under
the Protestant leadership of Lesdiguières.[7] He is recorded as having
studied medicine at Lyons, where he married another Protestant,
Anne Pellissari, and at least seven children were born to them between
1621 and 1637. Thus, by the time he composed his *Treatise on Sterility
among Women,* he wrote as both an experienced physician and a
father several times over.

This was his first published work, followed a year later, in 1626,
by a translation into French of the substantial *Pharmaceutical Works
[Les Œuvres pharmaceutiques]* of Jean de Renou (1560–1615), a doctor
from Coutances, the Latin text of which had appeared in 1608. Like the
Treatise on Sterility among Women, the pharmaceutical volume was
a scholarly work of vulgarization, undertaken to allow apothecaries
without a good reading knowledge of Latin to benefit from Renou's
work; it enjoyed enough success to be reprinted in 1637.

Circulation and Afterlife of the 'Treatise on Sterility among Women'

The only know edition of the *Treatise on Sterility among Women* is that
of 1625, of which a number of copies have survived, held in a range
of public libraries. Like Duval's *On Hermaphrodites,* de Serres's work

7. De Serres dedicated his treatise to the daughter of Lesdiguières. See 304.

was not translated into any other languages, but enjoyed a certain currency in its own day. We may assume that, once again, the absence of powerful patrons[8] and of any connections with Paris medical circles limited the circulation of de Serres's treatise. In addition, the subject of sterility, as he himself is the first to remark, might have made 'this gift a little distressing and displeasing on account of its subject matter'.

Structure of the 'Treatise on Sterility among Women' and Selection of Chapters for Translation

De Serres refers extensively to classical as well as contemporary medical works on sterility, notable amongst which was, of course, Hippocrates's *On Sterile Women*.[9] However, while drawing much of his material from earlier writers, he is concerned to recast it independently with the aim of adapting it for his intended readership, namely married women who have yet to conceive and give birth to an heir.[10] Hence, both the structure and style of his treatise are quite different from those of more scholarly works, dealing first and at length (chapters I-XI) with the reasons for sterility, and only subsequently (chapters XII-XV) with the solutions or remedies. He explains openly to his female readers that he seeks to gratify their curiosity and win their sympathy by adopting an engaging style in the first part, which he trusts will render them more receptive when he makes some necessarily harsh recommendations in the second part.[11] The use of questions in the titles of a number of the first eleven chapters sets the tone de Serres seeks to achieve, which is at once conversational and informative. Through the interrogative structure, he also indicates that he will question and nuance preconceived opinions before delivering his own advice For example: 'Whether women are more prone to

8. Although the work is dedicated to Françoise de Bonne-de-Lesdiguières, there is no indication that de Serres held a position in her household.

9. The treatise, the third in Hippocrates's *Diseases of Women*, deals primarily with sterility, but also contains sections on signs of pregnancy and the most favorable times for conception.

10. 'I thought I should give my work a new, aprochable form, so that it should be more deserving of being read by infertile ladies.' (313)

11. 'and will develop, as well as I am able, some interesting, pleasant questions I have identified relating to this subject, in order to draw the ladies, without their realizing it, into reading the second part, which is a little uninviting and bitter at the start.' (Ibid.)

sterility than men are to infertility, or the contrary?' — chapter I — or 'Whether women who are sterile are more lustful than those who bear children?' — chapter VI.[12]

My selection of chapters for translation demonstrates de Serres's initial defence of women in chapter I, and the forthright manner of its development, in chapter III, in support of the argument that women who bear only daughters are not to be considered sterile. Both of these chapters show how impressively de Serres tackles traditional misogynistic assumptions surrounding sterility. I then take the example of a pair of chapters, the first presenting a medical problem, the second de Serres's proposed solution: chapter X examines the causes of short-term sterility, and chapter XIV the cures for this affliction. Finally, I translate the closing section of the last chapter, XV, in which de Serres reaffirms his religious faith, before expressing his dutiful wishes for the birth of an heir to the French throne.

De Serres's Arguments and Style

Since de Serres reiterates at several points in the treatise that he is writing for a lay audience, primarily a female one, the reader does not expect this treatise to break new ground nor to offer a full scholarly account of sterility.[13] Yet his apparent modesty is belied by his acknowledgment in the Preface that physicians are also likely to read it, and his care throughout to cite his sources, sometimes giving precise references, including on occasions discussing Greek and even Hebrew as well as Latin terms.[14] While most of his material is based on classical sources, especially Hippocrates's *On Sterile Women*, he is quite prepared to add some recommendations and observations of his own,[15] and also on occasion silently to amend classical sources to

12. His approach may owe something to Laurent Joubert's highly successful *Popular Errors* (first published in 1578, and reprinted some 20 times in French, up to 1608).

13. 'I wish, in addition, to add a word of caution for the physicians and ladies who will read my book. To the former: let them not consider that this small work merits their criticism or further attention, for everything in it is lowly and for women.' (Preface by Author)

14. See 314.

15. E.g. nuancing the classical view that women cannot conceive unless they have menses by affirming that he had known several cases in Lyons of women who conceived without menstruating: *Treatise on Sterility among Women* [*Discours de la sterilité des femmes*, 108].

reflect early-seventeenth-century practice.[16] Nonetheless, with his lay, female audience in mind, he sometimes cuts discussion short, refusing to engage in 'obscure, hypothetical debate' of subjects such as the *reasons* for a womb not being suited for conception and pregnancy.[17] His avowed purpose, advising women suffering from sterility on how to overcome their condition, thus keeps the focus primarily on practical rather than theoretical issues.

There are, however, two major differences between the approach of de Serres and that of classical or indeed of most other early modern authorities. First, de Serres is guided throughout by his religious faith, according to which the physician is the servant of God, and fertility the gift of God.[18] Hence, his ultimate recommendation in chapter XIV for overcoming temporary sterility, if there are no obvious medical impediments, is to trust in God:

> … let [these women] seek the almighty hand of the ruler who cuts, shapes and decides the temperament, health, illness, sterility, life and death of men as seems good to Him.[19]

De Serres displays something perhaps close to a Calvinist acceptance of predestination: the physician and the woman should do what they are able to, but the fate of nations, families, individuals lies in the hands of God.[20] In this light, it is entirely logical that he should conclude his treatise with several quotations from the Old Testament, asserting that fertility is God's reward to his people when they have kept his

---

16. E.g. Hippocrates recommends that the woman should touch her own cervix to establish if she suffers from what would now be termed an over-wide cervix, unable to retain an embryo (*On Sterile Women*, 213). However, de Serres recommends the internal examination be conducted by a midwife: 'but the best thing is the touch of a midwife' (*Treatise on Sterility*, 385).

17. *Treatise on Sterility*, 301.

18. See the opening paragraphs of the Preface (307).

19. See 348.

20. He avoids any discussion of his Protestantism within the treatise, but it is likely that it underpins his thinking, and explains his frequent choice of examples from the Old Testament, which demonstrate God rewarding his people for keeping his covenant. However, while the work is dedicated to a leading Huguenot family (304, n. 31), it closes with formal good wishes for a much-awaited Catholic heir to the throne.

commandments, and — in a politically intelligent gesture — extending his prayers for fertility to Louis XIII and his Queen.

Secondly, in comparison with other medical writers on this topic, de Serres is singularly outspoken in his defence of women, especially of those suffering from sterility. As we have seen in the general introduction, his contribution to seventeenth-century echoes of the *Querelle des Femmes* is noteworthy.[21] Indeed, in the first chapter he declares himself 'in public to be the champion and father [of infertile ladies]'.[22] This metaphor of the knight in shining armor sets the tone for a treatise in which de Serres periodically returns to the image of undertaking combat on behalf of such women. The defence is necessitated by traditional beliefs that sterility might be either a punishment from God for women's pride or disobedience,[23] or the specific consequence of an individual woman's immoral way of life. On the latter point, de Serres achieves a delicate balance, castigating roundly the kinds of excess which jeopardize conception or lead to miscarriages, such as excessive dancing, drunkenness or promiscuity,[24] but showing a very genuine sympathy for the plight of chaste wives who cannot conceive or bear an heir.

His dedication to Françoise de Bonne-de-Lesdiguières is typical of the courteous, encouraging tone he adopts when addressing such female readers. Moreover, his defence of women goes beyond the issue of their infertility. After staging a debate between women and men in chapter I, with each side putting forward their case for holding the other more responsible for sterility, de Serres ventures his own opinion: 'I dare to claim that, in my view, men and women are equally subject to sterility.'[25] What is most interesting is the rational basis of this claim: his assertion that the bodies, souls and passions of men and women were both formed by God from the same mould, and that ancient medical writers also place them almost 'on the same level, in parallel' (albeit giving a slight advantage to man). Effectively,

21. See xiii-xxiv.

22. See 313.

23. De Serres allows men to put forward this argument against women in chapter I (317), but refrains from endorsing it himself.

24. See 336, n. 140.

25. See 318.

de Serres is arguing for quasi-equality of mind and body between the two sexes, a debate that he pursues with even greater vigour in chapter III when denouncing the common prejudice that women who bear only daughters suffer from a form of sterility.[26] He is in many ways a forerunner of Poulain de la Barre, but basing his beliefs on his Christian understanding, fully expounded in this chapter, that God's creation and redemption was common to men and to women.[27]

It is this underlying, conceptual framework of women as innately intelligent, and thus able to appreciate reasoned explanations, yet culturally unaccustomed to reading learned medical treatises, that accounts for de Serres's particular style. To a modern reader, some of his comments on the wish to avoid boring women with detailed explanations, or the need to include anecdotes in order to keep their attention, may seem patronizing, but his approach can be better understood as that of a professional seeking to engage a lay readership on a subject which he fears might appear forbidding. He uses a number of techniques, familiar from other writers in this volume: anecdotes and *exempla* are drawn from antiquity and his own experience; he cites a wide range of medical writers, but he also uses historians and even poets both to support his argument and to appeal to the reader's general curiosity;[28] some clever comparisons between medical principles and the natural world also allow the lay reader to grasp unfamiliar ideas.[29] Finally, we need to remember that de Serres is not always a serious mentor. While on occasion he can be both a fervent advocate and a harsh critic, he also relishes lighter tones, and his homage in the Preface to Rabelais, the 'French Democritus', is far from gratuitous. We sense that he would like his female reader to lay aside her worries about her fertility and smile from time to time when reading this work that is written primarily in her honor.[30]

26. In the course of this chapter, de Serres sides with physicians who believe the female seed contributes fully to the conception of the child.

27. *Treatise on Sterility*, 61–68. There is a neoplatonic idealization of woman's civilizing role in de Serres's comment on the creation of woman: 'God, the Creator of the female as well as of the male sex, foresaw that the beauty and excellence of the world would have been but chaos and unrelenting confusion without woman.' (323).

28. See 319-20 for an example of de Serres's judicious combination of a range of sources.

29. See for example 337.

30. See for example the humorous comparison to the farrier's bellows (341).

TITLE PAGE [1625]

TREATISE ON THE NATURE,
causes, signs and remedies
concerning failures to conceive,
and sterility among women.

*Published for the sake of young women
to whom God does not grant children in
the first years of their marriage.*

By Monsieur LOUYS DE SERRES, doctor
of medicine, registered in Lyons.

IN LYONS,

From the press of ANTOINE CHARD,
in the rue Merciere,
at the sign of the Holy Spirit.

M.DC.XXV.

WITH the King's Approval and Privilege.

TO THE MOST ESTEEMED AND REVERED LADY, FRANÇOISE DE BONNE-DE-LESDIGUIÈRES, MARESCHALE[31] DE CRÉQUY, ETC.

Madam,

Since your natural goodness generously and freely welcomes all those who appreciate your qualities, and who recognize the greatness of your illustrious house, I venture (counting myself among this number) to lay at your feet this small treatise in which sterility, the first monster of Nature, is vigorously attacked and defeated, so that henceforth and forever it may be banished from your distinguished family, and so that you may furnish the noble and ever victorious line of Créquy[32] with abundant children and grandchildren, who will be heroes and heroines.

I know well that at first you will find this gift a little distressing and displeasing on account of its subject matter, but when you have taken the time to look more closely at it, as a pleasant distraction, you will realize that I have not dedicated it to a lady of whom I think so ill that I would consider her to be sterile (such a thought never occurred to me), but rather to a heroine whom the power of procreation and fertility have kept waiting for a while, but delaying only the better then to spring forwards. I am confident that, with an open mind, you will judge my choice freely and favorably, and that you will come to confess that your most illustrious name alone, printed on the frontispiece of my book, will ever act as a shining beacon to its nascent reputation.

Please accept, therefore, Madam, this small gift of mine in the same good spirit as that in which it is offered to you, and trust that although it may be small in size, it is very large in the good wishes it holds; although sterile in its outward appearance, most fertile within. For not only will you find in it some fine balms to console you during the long wait you must patiently endure while unable to give birth as

31. Title denoting the wife of a Marshall of France (a senior military office). Françoise de Bonne-de-Lesdiguières was the second wife of Charles de Blanchefort de Créquy (or Crequi or Créquy-Blanchefort, c. 1575–1638). There is no record of her bearing any children, or at least none whose survival is recorded.

32. From the early Middle Ages, the Créquy family had enjoyed a distinguished reputation as military leaders and patrons.

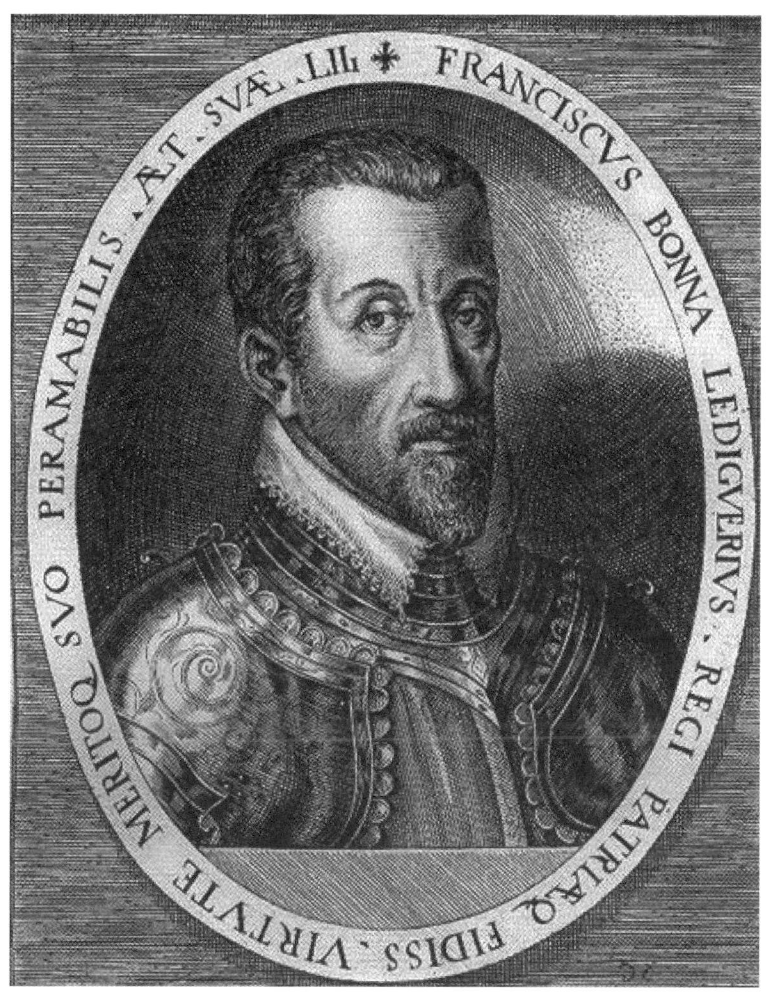

26) Nineteenth-century portrait of François de Bonne,
Seigneur de Lesdiguières (1543–1626)

by Joseph Nicolas Robert-Fleury
(Musée national des châteaux de Versailles et de Trianon)

soon as you would wish to a little lieutenant of the King, but it will also permit you to sample some excellent advice which will refresh your memory as to the rules you must closely observe in pregnancy when it shall please God to grant this to you.

May Heaven permit that in not too many months I may speak of you as the mother of a son who will be the living image of those two incomparable heroes, FRANÇOIS DE BONNE[33] and CHARLES DE CREQUY, his grandfather and father; a son who will truly imitate their heroism and be the ornament of the Dauphiné,[34] of France and of the whole world. May the Heavens also grant that I may see the greatness, prosperity and laurels of your two august families, the Lesdiguières and the de Créquy, increase. And that after having wished you fertility as great as that of the Emperor Albert[35] and of Anne of Carinthia,[36] I may ever, as now, be proud to call myself

Your most humble and most obedient servant,

Louys de Serres

Of the Dauphiné, Doctor of Medicine, and registered in Lyons.

33. François de Bonne (1543–1626), Seigneur de Lesdiguières et du Glaizil, then Duke de Lesdiguières and Marshall and Constable of France; father of Françoise de Bonne-de-Lesdiguières. A strong Protestant leader of Dauphiné in the later period of the civil wars (1575–1590), Lesdiguières took Grenoble back from the Catholic League, and became leader of the province, and then Lieutenant General from 1597 until his death in 1626.

34. The province of Dauphiné, previously an independent state, had been fully integrated into France in 1457.

35. Probably a reference to Albert I of Habsburg (1255–1308), whose wife Elisabeth bore him 12 children.

36. Anne of Hungary (1503–1547) gave birth to 15 children.

PREFACE BY THE AUTHOR

To the Ladies

Just as physicians are created by God only to serve the sick, so this book is written only for those ladies who are by way of becoming infertile, or others who are entirely so. Although its subject matter is most sterile since it deals only with sterility, I am nonetheless convinced that the latter group will find in it substantial matter to console them in their unhappiness,[37] and the former will discover advice and many good precepts to guide them to the end they desire, provided only that for their part they try to shake off the vexatious yoke of this monster of nature,[38] and work with me to recover their own freedom. For as it is not possible for the edicts of sovereign princes alone to check their subjects, unless the subjects themselves strive to take particular care to overcome their own nature and to submit to the rule which is imposed upon them, so too it is most difficult for women who are infertile to become fertile simply by reading my book, unless at the outset those who are ailing agree to subject themselves to the cures that I recommend, and those who are tainted with vices to rid themselves of those faults which are the product of their infertility.

This is why I make a general appeal to all women desirous of looking after themselves well, and particularly those who know within themselves that they are given to drunkenness, lechery, immoderate gambling, greed, or some other such vice, the least of which is capable of rendering them more sterile, to renounce and banish for ever more such evil tendencies, and to remember the promise of fertility which God gives, in the person of several women of Israel,[39] to those who are sterile yet fear to displease him. For then I can guarantee that, if they read and follow the advice and precepts that I shall give them, they will become as fertile as hares and doves, and indeed just the shadow of my book, like that of the bell towers of our French Democritus,[40] will make them produce as many fine offspring as the shoots produced by a vigorous olive tree.

37. Cf. ch. V in which, rather surprisingly, de Serres seeks to console infertile wives by listing the advantages of not bearing and bringing up children.

38. Cf. 304.

39. The Old Testament provides many examples of women who believed they were condemned to sterility only to be surprised by the gift of a child: such as Sarah, wife of Abraham, who bore Isaac in her old age (Genesis 18:1–5, 21:1–8).

40. Bell towers, given their phallic shape, were a widespread symbol of fertility in popular

I wish, in addition, to add a word of caution for the physicians and ladies who will read my book. To the former: let them not consider that this small work merits their criticism or further attention, for everything in it is lowly and for women; had I wished to produce something fit for the attention of physicians, I should have needed the lamp of Epictetus,[41] or to have spent years leafing through Hippocrates and Galen. Let the ladies, on the other hand, not consider me a misogynist like Aristarchus,[42] nor, even less, a courtly flatterer, for I do indeed have pity for those who are sterile through illness or misfortune, rather than through vices and excesses. Thus, without apology, I present the immoral behavior of some other women, so that they may be chastened by this, and that they may learn, at their own cost, to flee this horrible monster of nature, which creeps in everywhere, notably in great families. The readers may rest assured that I shall speak of their faults with as much discretion as my natural restraint and my profession bid me to. And if, as they cast their eyes upon this treatise, they should encounter a passage which is sterile in its vulgarity, or vulgar in its sterility, I ask them to remember that, according to Celsus,[43] it is impossible to discuss procreation, impotence and sterility, whether affecting men or women, without employing some vulgar expressions, like a sauce for such poor meat; and moreover medical advice on this subject cannot use such austerely decent language as would be required from, and is closely observed by, our theologians. Let him who has ears hear, and let him who can do better try his hand.

Zoilus, who laughs freely at our little pages,

If you have something better, show it, or bring your proof.[44]

---

culture. The 'French Democritus' is an allusion to the satirical comment made in François Rabelais's *Gargantua* (1534) by the monk, Friar John, to the hapless pilgrims whose wives are at home and prey to lascivious monks: 'May I catch the pox if you don't find them all big-bellied when you get home, for the mere shadow of the bell-tower of an abbey is fecund' (Rabelais, *Gargantua and Pantagruel*, trans. M. A. Screech, Penguin Classics, 43, 344). I am grateful to Hugh Roberts for identifying this humorous borrowing by de Serres.

41. Eminent Stoic philosopher of 1st century AD. After his death, his lamp was purchased for a great price by an admirer.

42. Aristarchus of Samos, philosopher of third century BC.

43. Aulus Cornelius Celsus's treatise *On Medicine* (c. 30 AD) was widely read during the Renaissance.

44. The two lines of verse are in Latin in de Serres's original text. Zoilus was a Cynic philosopher (c. 400–320 BC), whose reputedly harsh criticisms of Homer led to his name being associated, as here, with ungenerous literary criticism.

APPROVAL BY PHYSICIANS[45]

We the undersigned Doctors in medicine hereby certify that we have seen and read the Book entitled *Treatise on the failures to conceive, and on sterility among women*, composed by Monsieur Louys de Serres, doctor of medicine, and a registered member of our profession; in it we have found nothing which is not worthy to be read and published, containing as it does sound learning and various appropriate remedies, drawn up with care for the good and wellbeing of infertile women. In proof of which we have appended our signatures below.

At Lyons on this 4th December 1624.

Fournier.
Sarazin.
Du Bost.

---

45. Following a decree of the Paris Parlement, issued on 3 May 1535, the Faculty of Medicine had the right to judge every work published in Paris in the field of medical science. There was no Parlement in Lyons, but the city's physicians still issued Approvals.

EXTRACT FROM THE KING'S PRIVILEGE

By the grace and privilege of the King,[46] permission is granted to Antoine Chard, bookseller in Lyons, to print or have printed, and sell and distribute, as many times and in whatever format and typeface he wishes, a book entitled *Treatise on the failures to conceive, and on sterility among women*, composed by Monsieur LOUYS DE SERRES, Doctor of Medicine. With a prohibition to all other printers and booksellers throughout the kingdoms, countries and lands under the dominion of His Majesty, to publish or have published, sell or distribute, exchange or trade within or without these kingdoms, any copies of this book, or part of the same, except those which have been printed by order of Chard, on pain of a fine of 1500 Tours pounds,[47] half of which shall be paid to His Majesty and the other half to the said petitioner, with no reduction, and of all the expenses, damages and interest, and of confiscation of all the copies which shall be found to have been printed and sold in contravention of the present Privilege. And this for the term of five years,[48] starting from the day and date on which printing of the said book shall have been completed, with the obligation that two copies of the book shall be deposited in our library,[49] without which the present Privilege will be invalid, as is more fully stated in the letters of patent from His Majesty.

Issued in Paris on 27th December 1624 and in the fifteenth year of our reign. By the King in his Council

Renouard.

And sealed with the great seal in yellow wax.

Printing completed on 25th January 1625.

46. Louis XIII.

47. One of the standard units of currency in France in the early modern period.

48. Length of privileges for medical works varied, but five years is relatively short; printers of this period would more commonly seek six to ten years.

49. The decree of François I, of 28 December 1537, had imposed a legal obligation on printers and booksellers to deposit a copy of each of their publications in the King's library. In addition, by a decree of 1614, printers and booksellers in Paris were required to submit to the booksellers' guild a copy of any book deposited in the royal library.

TABLE OF THE CHAPTERS
CONTAINED IN THIS BOOK

Ch. I   Whether women are more prone to sterility than men are to infertility, or the contrary?

Ch. II   Whether it is probable that sterility more often affects beautiful women than those who are ugly and unattractive?

Ch. III   Whether women who bear only daughters should be called sterile?

Ch. IV   That women who remain childless after several years of marriage should not be judged to be sterile, even less, fit to be set aside, provided only that they show some indication and trace of fertility.

Ch. V   That women who are truly sterile are in some way fortunate in their misfortune.

Ch. VI   Whether women who are sterile are more lustful than those who bear children?

Ch. VII   On female sterility, its nature and different forms.

Ch. VIII   On the constitutional causes of female sterility.

Ch. IX   On the causes of female sterility only with respect to the present husband.

Ch. X   Of the causes of the last kind of female sterility, called temporary sterility.

Ch. XI   On the signs of female sterility.

Ch. XII   On curing constitutional female sterility.

And first on excessive coldness.

On excessive heat.

On excessive moistness.

On excessive dryness.

On windiness and rumblings of the womb.

On the toughness of the inner mouth of the womb.[50]

On the over-wide opening of the womb.

On the malpositioning or twisting of the womb.

50. I.e. cervix.

51. Like other physicians of the time, de Serres uses the word 'abortion' ('*avortement*') to signify miscarriage or spontaneous abortion.

52. The common term for leukorrhea.

TREATISE ON THE NATURE, CAUSES, SIGNS AND REMEDIES CONCERNING FAILURES TO CONCEIVE, AND STERILITY AMONG WOMEN

Chapter I: Whether Women Are More Prone to Sterility Than Men Are to Infertility, or the Contrary?

Having decided to take up arms against female sterility, I have drawn up this small treatise. I thought I should give my work a new, approachable form, so that it should be more deserving of being read by infertile ladies, of whom I declare myself in public to be the champion and father. I also wanted to distinguish it from the writings of a number of great people who have discoursed on this subject in learned detail. This is why I have taken a new path and resolved to treat it in two ways, expounding first the problems and then the solutions,[53] and thus I have divided my whole work into two parts. The first will provide the foundations for the second, and will develop, as well as I am able, some interesting, pleasant questions I have identified relating to this subject, in order to draw the ladies, without their realizing it, into reading the second part, which is a little uninviting and bitter at the start, yet promises them a most agreeable sequel and conclusion, lightened with various anecdotes, and augmented with all the best cures which my limited skill and experience could select and gather from various sources for their particular gratification.

I am well aware that I am tackling a subject which is sterile, tough and difficult, and which has often been tossed around and served up anew by very many great people who have forgotten more than I shall ever know about it in my whole life. Moreover, those of the inclination of Timon of Athens,[54] or Democritus[55] or Aristarchus,[56] who find nothing good unless they have done it themselves, will have sufficient cause to vomit bile and give vent to their calumnies at the expense of my new writings. But so be it; I shall emerge from it as best I can, and

---

53. Chs. I-XI treat the problems or causes, chs. XII-XV the solutions or remedies.

54. A citizen of Athens in the fifth century BC whose reputation for misanthropy was legendary.

55. A pre-Socratic philosopher who found mankind risible.

56. See 308, n. 42.

care not a fig for the critics. For my aim is not to please them, since I have set out only to satisfy those ladies who are in danger of becoming infertile and who will take the trouble to read my book.

As to the question which forms the title of this first chapter, I find that it is not greatly deserving of debate yet is much disputed by each side. For first, women claim vehemently that men are generally more dissolute and liable to follow their desires than women.[57] They claim that the course of men's nature tends more towards bad than good, towards vice rather than virtue, and to infertility because of their debauched lifestyle. For there is nothing which more easily causes this evil than the excessive use of unnatural things, as we shall see hereafter. Thus we read that Alexander the Great was '*de frigidis et maleficiatis*'[58] for loving wine too well; Henry VIII, King of England, for having indulged in excessive sexual debauchery; the Scythians for riding their horses too often without stirrups; and still others for having given themselves over to all kinds of excesses.

The Hebrews say that the word אִישׁ which means man also means fire, and is derived from the verb אֵשׁ which literally means to come from the nature of fire.

Secondly, they say that men are too hot and too ardent in their lovemaking, and that as a result they are more prone to become impotent than women are to become sterile. In what follows, we shall show that according to the arguments of Aristotle, Hippocrates and Galen, intemperance and excessive heat of seed are no less weighty as causes of sterility than the excessive coldness of women.[59] Now women demonstrate that men are excessively hot in two ways. First they refer to Hebrew, in which language the word 'man' means precisely fire, and to be a man is to have the nature of fire. And next, they cite the incontrovertible authority of a number of physicians, and notably Hippocrates in his book *On Regimen*,[60] and Galen in various places in his work, and Aristotle in the IVth book of *On the Generation*

---

57. In *On Sterile Women*, Hippocrates gives only brief space to ways in which men may contribute to infertility, but he does list excessive drinking as something they should avoid (Littré, *Hippocrate. Œuvres complètes*, vol. VIII, section 218).

58. The Latin expression used in the set legal phrase '*de frigidis et maleficiatis, et impotentia coeundi*' to denote impotence.

59. The references to (male) heat and (female) coldness reflect the traditional medical belief, within the humoral theory of the body, that while men are prone to the former, women to the latter, either extreme may harm the balance of humors or temperament.

60. The reference to *On Regimen* is hard to account for, and may be an error, since in this work, unlike some others in the Hippocratic corpus, there is not an explicit distinction between male and female humors and temperaments.

of Animals,[61] as well as a number of learned lawyers, including Jean Faber in his *Commentaries on the Institutes of Justinian* [*Justinianas institutiones Commentarii*[62]] and Giovanni d'Andrea in his *On Betrothals* [*De Sponsalibus*[63]] and various others who write that the coldest man in the world is a great deal warmer than the warmest woman that nature has created. From which they can argue from the least to the greatest, saying that if the coldest men are hotter than the hottest women, those men who are very hot for their sex must be endowed with a temperament and genital matter quite inappropriate for begetting children, as is quite evident given that fertility resides only in bodies which are moderately hot and moist.

Thirdly, they claim a great advantage over men by virtue of being exempt from the flaw in question. For since they are purged regularly by their menstrual flow they claim to be almost exempt from it, as well as from a number of other illnesses, such as gout, gravel and other such things, as can be gathered from the pronouncements of Hippocrates in his *Aphorisms*, and from Galen's *Commentaries* on these. The reason is that the monthly bleeding purges them of a great many superfluous humors which build up daily in the human body and which greatly weaken the natural heat, the radical balm, and thus the power to procreate whenever these humors are retained.[64] Men cannot benefit from such an advantage since they are not of the necessary nature, as is quite evident. And if hemorrhoids (to which women are also doubly subject) protect most of those suffering from them against quartan fever, epilepsy and sordid avarice, according to the same Hippocrates in Book VI of his *Epidemics*,[65] should women who have regular menses not hope that they may be exempt from sterility? Certainly I find there is nothing more able to sweep away the obstacles to procreation than this purging, provided it is well

---

61. *On the Generation of Animals*, IV. 1.

62. The commentaries on Justinian's *Institutes* by Jean Febre, a fourteenth-century French lawyer, were regularly reprinted in France in the Renaissance.

63. Giovanni d'Andrea (1275–1348), a celebrated Italian expert in canon law, whose works included the treatise *On Betrothals and on Matrimony* [*De Sponsalibus et Matrimonio*].

64. Renaissance physicians, like their classical forebears, for this reason always considered the retention of the menses to be dangerous, except in pregnancy.

65. *Epidemics* VI.3.23.

regulated, for women who are thus purged live healthy, happy and joyful lives.

On the other hand, men, relying on the precedence, perfection and excellence enjoyed by their sex, maintain most firmly that it would be an outrage against common sense, and a contradiction of the majesty of Nature, to believe that it could have intended to make man imperfect — he who is Nature's only dearest child and the be-all-and-end-all of all the most precious things it has created, the comforter and companion of women in the illnesses and sufferings which commonly afflict their sex. Sufferings (I say) which are numerous, and of which sterility is proven to be the most extreme.

Furthermore, they know that the principles of medicine (which are drawn from Nature) are entirely on their side; for just as their temperament is moderately warm and moist, women's is most cold and prone to discharges, as is recognized by both sexes, and unanimously confirmed by all the philosophers and physicians. They say that just as the first temperament is favorable to procreation, so the second truly encourages infertility.

Although women alleged above that the male sex is comparable to fire in its heat, and that the coldest of men is far warmer than the warmest of women, nonetheless this has to be understood sensibly and as a comparison. It is certain that although men are far hotter than women, nonetheless their heat remains moderate, otherwise it would be more likely to burn than to encourage fertility, as can be seen in various passages of Aristotle. And we know from Hippocrates that overly hot seed and a womb of the same temperature are incapable of procreation and conception.[66]

Thirdly, they prove by reference to the word of God and pagan historians that sterility is really women's affair, and that there are very few men in recorded history who were infertile, whereas there were countless women of all stations. For we read in the Holy Bible that Esther

---

66. Hence Hippocrates's recommendation, in *On Sterile Women,* that men should avoid hot baths before intercourse (Littré, *Hippocrate. Œuvres complètes,* vol. VIII, s. 218) and wash in cold water (*ibid.* section 220), and the various cooling fumigations recommended throughout the treatise.

the wife of Assuerus,[67] Judith,[68] Rachel[69] and various other honorable women were sterile. Modern history teaches us that Stratonice, wife of Deiotarus King of Galatia,[70] and Joan, the only daughter of Raymond V the Count of Toulouse and wife of Alphonse Count of Poitiers,[71] and Eleanor, daughter of William [X] Duke of Aquitaine and wife of Louis the Younger, King of France,[72] and Elizabeth, the most recent Queen of England,[73] and countless other princesses were entirely infertile. And this is leaving aside thousands of other lowly-born women who are entirely sterile, and whose names are not recorded in history. Thus it seems that God particularly wished to subject women to this kind of affliction in order to crush their pride, and that they might see that they are far less perfect than men.

Here are the arguments put forward by each side in attack and in defence of their case, and to uphold the honor of their sex. For my part, I shall refrain from making any judgment to decide the issue, for fear of offending one or other sex. Moreover, I should have had to consult Nature herself, or she would have had to whisper in my ear how to cut through the knot of the debate, a knot that is indeed more difficult to slice than that which Alexander cleft with his sword.[74] Thus, without showing myself to be in support of one or other side, but instead remaining neutral and objective, I shall simply give my opinion in a manner designed to be discursive rather than conclusive (although drawing on the established teachings of medicine) so that those who are possessed of finer judgment than myself may be left plenty of freedom to pronounce upon this topic.

67. In the *Old Testament*, Esther is not reported to have borne children.

68. In the Apocryphal *Book of Judith*, she is a pious and childless widow. Esther and Judith are often associated, in their purity and devotion to God, as forerunners of Mary.

69. Wife of Jacob: *Genesis* 30.

70. See Plutarch, *On the Bravery of Women*, ch. XXI.

71. Their marriage (from 1237 to 1271) remained childless.

72. Eleanor of Aquitaine and Louis VII of France (*Louis Le Jeune* / Louis the Younger) were married in 1137; but the marriage remained childless until 1145. Since de Serres gives her father as William V of Aquitaine (he was in fact William X), he may possibly be citing her name in error among women who were completely sterile.

73. Elizabeth I had died in 1603.

74. Reference to the legend of Alexander slicing the Gordian Knot. See also the use made of this by Rousset (17).

In short, I declare that men and women are a single species; the creation of their bodies was fashioned by the hands of a single craftsman, God Himself, and from the same basic matter; their souls were created from the same mould and the passions of their souls are inseparable. On this basis, I dare to claim that, in my view, men and women are equally subject to sterility, just as much as to the other illnesses that number some four or five hundred, according to the views of some writers,[75] notwithstanding the arguments put forward to the contrary by both sides. For when the good Job says that man born of woman lives for but a short time, and full of worries, that as long as his skin covers him, he is subject to grief;[76] when Hippocrates writes that the whole of man is subject to all illnesses;[77] when Aristotle says that man is the epitome of weakness, the cast-off of time, the plaything of fortune, the image of inconstancy, the balance of envy and calamity, and that for the rest he is nothing but phlegm and choler,[78] we must believe that such authorities do not exclude either of the two reasonable sexes, but they place both of them on the same level, in parallel, albeit that men can claim to have an advantage over women by virtue of some natural prerogatives, but these are very slight and of little consequence.

Chapter III: Whether Women Who Bear Only Daughters Should be Called Sterile?

The women and unmarried girls who take the trouble to read this chapter will at first think that I deliberately set out to attack and strike them from all sides, and they will consider me to be another arch-misogynist or sworn enemy of their sex. However, I would fervently beg them not to judge my methods unfavorably before they have read the whole chapter. For just as I undertook in this short book to uphold the particular cause of those women who are wrongly accused of

75. Classical physicians had sought to define all the kinds of illness, arriving at a list of this number.

76. Job 14: 1.

77. See, for example, *On Affections*, I. 1, where Hippocrates attributes all human illnesses to an excess of bile or phlegm.

78. This comes from a work no longer usually attributed to Aristotle: see *Aristoteles Pseudepigraphus*, ed. Valentin Rose (Leipzig, 1863) (*Stob.* p. 610: 20). I am grateful to Mike Inwood for locating this reference for me.

being sterile and infertile, so in this present chapter I have determined to be the public father, or indeed the official defender, of their sex in respect of the question under debate.

So that they should not think I have proposed this subject simply to develop my views without a good basis, I want them to realize that their sex is held in such poor repute by the majority of men of all stations, and notably by married men, that it would seem (from the men's account) that God did them a disservice by subjecting them to the company of women,[79] and uniting them in the thorny bonds of matrimony. Indeed, they consider it to be a great shame and disgrace to have daughters, even legitimate, wise, beautiful, well-born ones. Now the hatred that such men have for women arises not so much from their natural feelings (for who ever wished to hate another being like himself?), but from bad imitation and bad lessons drawn from the writings of those who once displayed all their imperfections for the world to see. They include Socrates, Plato, Aristotle, Diogenes,[80] Montaigne,[81] André Tiraqueau, the famous lawyer who furiously tore women's imperfections apart in his book on the *Laws of Marriage*, and on the rights of husbands.[82] And even more so, a certain nameless modern poet who left us his 'Six-line verses' which are a summary and epitome of all the insults and curses (O come Lord, come!) against women which can be imagined. Here they are:[83]

> Woman is like the great waves
> Which ceaselessly toss the sailors
> In some storm:
> The most experienced pilot
> Is likely to drown
> Over such moving sands.

79. Genesis 2:18–22.

80. Diogenes the Cynic, a controversial Greek philosopher (c. 412–323 BC).

81. Michel de Montaigne (1533–1592), French humanist and thinker, author of the *Essays* (first French edn, 1580).

82. Tiraqueau (1488–1558) published a lengthy Latin treatise in 1513 on the laws of marriage.

83. I have translated the meaning, but not imitated the French meter or the rhyme scheme of this '*sizain*' (aabcbc).

> She is a snake covered with flowers,
> Laughter accompanies her tears,
> All is pretence and deceit.
> What crime have men committed
> To deserve such torture,
> Except to have loved their enemies?

However, if we leave aside our search for such foolish, ill-substantiated examples of animosity, together with the authors who composed them, we need to discover if there is anyone armed with good reasons to induce people to believe the statement in the title to this chapter.

Aristotle, speaking of the generation of man in various places in his works, and especially in his book *On the Generation of Animals*, says expressly that woman contributes nothing to the conception of man; indeed he asserts that she is the first monster of nature.[84]

Galen, in chapters 6 and 7 of Book XIV of his *Usefulness of the Parts of the Body*, writes that woman is an imperfect animal, the product of hasty chance.

Plato, in his *Theaetetus*,[85] and in his books on the *Laws*, really does not know what kind of animal woman should be classified under, for first he puts her among the reasoning and then among the unreasoning.

St Jerome, or the person who wrote to a certain Oceanus on the life of clerics,[86] says that woman is the door to the devil, the path to all iniquity, the bite of a scorpion, and in all ways a harmful animal.

St Epiphanius, in his first book of *Heresies*, writes that the Severian heretics believed that women were a masterpiece of the devil.[87]

When the philosopher Simonides was questioned and asked to say what he thought about womankind, he answered that she was nothing but a deadly asp, a decorated bitch, the ruin of men, a cause

84. *Generation of Animals*, I. 17–20.

85. Dialogue in which Socrates draws a lengthy comparison between the work of a midwife delivering a child and that of a philosopher delivering souls.

86. See Jerome's letter of 397 (letter LXIX in *The Principal Works of St Jerome*) to Oceanus, a Roman nobleman, in the context of a dispute over the remarriage of the Spanish bishop Carterius.

87. Epiphanius (c. 320–403), Bishop of Salamis and Metropolitan of Cyprus, waged war against heretics, compiling a large compendium of some 80 heresies, including those of the Severians, a gnostic sect that believed that the devil created woman and the lower half of man.

of disquiet, a domestic wild animal, the vessel of adultery, the storm of a household, an unbearable burden, a lifetime's imprisonment, and a necessary evil.[88]

St Augustine and St Jerome write that Origen[89] resolutely held that women will not be resurrected in their present sex, and that they will cease to be women on the Last Day.

Moreover, our experts in matters of statecraft declare firmly that those monarchies and sovereign states that do not allow women to inherit the throne have always considered themselves unfortunate when they have been ruled by kings whose wives have been unlucky enough to bear only daughters. For they have left their states without heirs, torn apart and rife with factions, as has often been seen in the reign of a number of princes, and in this kingdom particularly in the reign of Philippe of Valois,[90] who was accorded the crown by the Estates-General in Paris against the claim of Edward King of England,[91] son of Isabella, daughter of Philippe the Handsome,[92] excluding the daughter of Charles the Handsome,[93] to whom Charles claimed to be the legitimate heir and thus successor to the crown of France, as first cousin of the deceased lady. For although the salic law was upheld, the daughter of Charles refused any hope of the succession, Edward's claim dismissed by the Estates, and the whole kingdom reunited under its rightful king, nonetheless history records that this kingdom suffered strange persecutions and atrocities perpetrated by Edward. This would not have happened had King Charles left a male child.

If, therefore, we are to agree with Aristotle that women bring nothing to the conception of a child, and that they are monsters of nature; with Galen that they are imperfect in all ways, and the product of chance; with Plato that they should be classed as unreasoning rather than reasoning creatures; with St Jerome that they are the door to the

88. Simonides of Amorgos, seventh-century BC poet who wrote a *Pedigree of Women* in which different kinds of women were compared unflatteringly to animals.

89. Early Church Father (c. 185–254) who argued that the body would be resurrected in a pure, spiritual state (or '*eidos*').

90. I.e. during the first phase of the Hundred Years' War (1337–1453) between England and France.

91. Edward III of England (1312–1377), son of Edward II and Isabella of France.

92. Philippe IV of France, known as *Philippe le Bel* (1268–1314).

93. Charles IV, known as *Charles le Bel* (1294–1328), who left only a daughter at his death.

devil and the path of all iniquity; with the Severians that they are a masterpiece of the devil; with Simonides that they are a deadly asp and decorated bitches; with Origen that they will not be resurrected in their present sex at the Last Day; and finally with all good experts on statecraft who live under monarchies, as we do, that they are not capable of inheriting the crown from their fathers, then it would seem that those who argue in favor of this assertion are correct in saying that women who bear only daughters should be compared alongside and considered to suffer from the same degree of sterility as those women who bear neither males or females. For (they add), just as the wild fig trees[94] and the apple trees of Sodom[95] are considered no less barren than the weeping-willow or poplar in that they appear to produce good fruits, yet these fruits are useless, so women who bear only daughters should not be considered any better than those who are entirely sterile. For they produce only fruits which appear beautiful and pleasing to behold, but are in truth thorny, wild, full of bitterness, and indeed the abortive products of nature. And, moreover, what a cause of heartache it must be for so many good people to see their houses full of animals without tails,[96] which have no natural ability or activity, which are very difficult and dangerous to look after, and which very often bring into disrepute and ruin those who brought them up, just as ivy ruins the wall which has supported it for so long.

Certainly, we should not be surprised if the majority of husbands who have daughters and no sons fall into a state of frenzy for a few days after their wives are delivered. For they find themselves in the same situation as those who come into a small inheritance which brings in its wake a dozen heavy lawsuits, or those who have sown good, fine grain yet reap only the chaff. 'For my part', says one of these men, 'I knew a distinguished lord whose wife had borne him a fourth daughter but no sons, and he felt as though he could have thrown away his house and his wife, such was his rage and fury seeing

94. Cf. the parable of the barren fig tree in Matthew 21:19, Mark 11:13, Luke 13: 6–9. De Serres is probably referring to uncultivated fig trees, bearing a crop of small figs, which do not ripen.

95. A form of crab apple.

96. In French 'sans queue' ('without tail') is also a pun on the popular meaning of 'queue' ('penis'). Women are thus both imperfect animals (lacking a tail) and imperfect males (lacking a penis).

himself old, near to death, with no hope of a true male inheritor to whom he would leave his responsibilities and incomes, which were not insignificant'.

Nevertheless, all these reasons are more injurious than acceptable, more full of bitterness than of truth, and cannot shake the steadfastness of those who concentrate on the pure truth of the question at issue, taking the side of God and of nature against the false claims of the large number of infirm minds which exist only to resist the works of the Lord. Let me explain myself by saying that although the arguments I have rehearsed above against the dignity and merits of the female sex seem to leave no place for any defence or response, and to be intrinsically robust and male, yet we hope that our responses, which are drawn from the well of Democritus,[97] that is to say from the center of truth, will remove their attraction for ever.

And so that they do not think we are lacking in good, compelling arguments to defend our position, which they attack from all sides, they should indeed know that God, the Creator of the female as well as of the male sex, foresaw that the beauty and excellence of the world would have been but chaos and unrelenting confusion without woman.[98] Further, He preordained from all eternity that the salvation of His children would have been incomplete and imperfect unless He united their souls, true rays of the divine, with bodies made of elementary matter and molded with the admirable efforts of the procreative matter of both sexes, as we shall see more fully later in this treatise. And that it would also have been incomplete unless later, after the Fall of Man, he had deigned through His great, overwhelming mercy to send His own son, our only Redeemer, to take on human flesh in the womb of the Blessed Virgin. This may be so, someone will object, but Aristotle, Plato, Socrates, Diogenes and a whole array of other pagan writers who write about the brazenness of women, both in procreation and in other matters, did not know these two great, incomprehensible mysteries of the creation and the redemption of man. Thus, it would seem more appropriate to counter them through

97. An image commonly associated with the Greek philosopher Democritus (c. 460–370 BC).
98. In the following passage, de Serres is using a series of neoplatonic ideas and images which share similarities with those used by Pena in his revisions and extension of Liebault (see 71-74).

natural reason than by reference to the sacred writings in which they never believed. I would reply that it is as easy for me to undermine them with natural reasons as by reference to religious authority. However, since these two mysteries, and especially the latter, are the two cornerstones of our salvation, which it would scarcely appear they ever shared, I determined to use them as an impenetrable rampart that withstands all attacks without regard for person or manner. And it is of little significance to us how we attack them given we have dismissed their insults. Thus, we prefer to take on those who are called Christians, yet unfortunately profess impious and profane ideas, and cling tenaciously to the belief that woman plays no role at all in procreation, and cannot be reckoned among reasoning creatures.

If they had taken the trouble to search out the truth by reading good books, notably holy scriptures, they would first have found that the divinely inspired prophet David acknowledges that his mother conceived him in sin,[99] and that she contributed to his conception; for the natural conception of a human never occurs without the contribution of male and female genital matter, as all our physicians unanimously agree.[100] Next, if this divine, irrefutable authority does not satisfy them, they should inform themselves fully about natural history which speaks of the generation of man: this would teach them that woman contributes as much, or more, than man in the act of generation. For what, if not generation, is the purpose of the preparatory and ejaculatory vessels, the testicles, with which Nature has furnished her just as much as it has man?[101] Or of the womb, of the menstrual blood which is intended to nourish the foetus during pregnancy, and of all the other natural parts, which are so wonderfully designed? Would they be so presumptuous as to accuse the Maker of Nature of having created what they see as so many useless parts?

In addition, do they know that lawyers claim that the mother is always certain, the father uncertain, which shows that the female contributes much more than the male to procreation? If, according to all the most learned physicians, she contributes more, why should

99. Psalms 51:5, 'Behold, I was shapen in iniquity; and in sin did my mother conceive me.'
100. An important indication that by the 1620s the one-seed argument had all but vanished.
101. De Serres is following the tradition of likening the woman's fallopian tubes and ovaries to the man's *vas deferens* and testicles.

a woman who bears only daughters be held to be sterile, since daughters are blessed with the same immortal soul as males, and the contribution of the seminal matter of both man and woman is just as necessary for the generation of daughters as of males? Moreover, have they ever paid attention to the fact that there are as many, or more, male and female children whose facial shape resembles their mother's more than it does their father's? They must indeed acknowledge that these individual resemblances (as our doctors call them) can come only from the procreational strength, which is in the seed of both father and mother, and in the strong imagination of the mother.[102] She imprints first on the mind and spirit (which are summoned in such a noble act), then also at the appropriate moment on the living seed, the form, character, nature and idea which she imagined during the heated struggles of the loving battle.[103] This could not be so if the woman did not do half the work and did not contribute half the matter to make such a noble male or female construction.

Finally, can they deny the daily experience that shows us that women suffering from gout, manias, epilepsy, pleurisy or some other similar illness, produce children subject to the same ailments, even if their husbands and relatives are well? Now this would not happen if they contributed nothing of their own to the conception and development of the child throughout the pregnancy. All these reasons are most powerful to strengthen the case of Nature and also of women, whose side we are also taking. So I do not think it necessary to advance other major arguments to prove that those who hold the opposite view are in error and motivated by hostility.

Thus, it remains only to reply in detail to each one of the arguments, or rather calumnies and outrageous insults, proposed by the authors mentioned above. For our views would be of little importance and very poorly received by the women we support if we did not demolish the case of those who try to undermine our position.

102. De Serres is citing the conventional belief that the pregnant woman's imagination may influence the physical development of the child as an argument for the mother contributing even more than the father to procreation. For other examples in this volume of accounts where the mother's imagination is held responsible for the foetus's form, see 175, n. 76.

103. I retain de Serres's metaphors likening the sexual act to a fight. They echo his use of the metaphor of a battle when referring to his defence of women.

First, therefore, we say in reply to Aristotle that he does great wrong to himself and to women with regard to this question he raises, for he does not remember that he wrote the opposite of what he said above concerning women's inability to contribute to conception. This is seen when he speaks eloquently in Book X of the *History of Animals* and in various other places in his work, saying that it is necessary for the male and female to contribute their share of seed for conception, which must take place in the woman's womb.[104] Moreover, in this he must have followed the opinion of many great men who lived some centuries before him, notably our divine Hippocrates, who was a much better physician and anatomist than Aristotle, and who wrote in his book *On Generation* and in his books on *Regimen* that not only does woman contribute her share to the generation of mankind, but also that she has a double seed, like men.[105] The first kind is the material cause either of less vigorous males or of strong women, dare I say Amazons, when the woman's seed is hotter, more plentiful and stronger than the man's; the other kind serves only for the generation of a weak little woman, because it has little heat, assuming the man's seed is proportionate in nature.

So Aristotle needs to admit one of two things: either he was daydreaming when he wrote such clearly contradictory statements,[106] or he was never a good doctor since he wrote things that directly contradict the principles of medicine and nature. Similarly, he must honestly acknowledge that he was misled and insulting when he wrote that woman is a monster of Nature, given that he himself well knew what all the best natural historians after him have known. That is to say, that among animals a monster in the true sense is simply an offspring born from any animal which is either of a different species or greatly unlike it both in appearance and in the number, proportion and position of its limbs. Now if one applies all these things to woman, is it not to criticize openly the Author of Nature and to wage war on commonsense? For everyone knows that women are of the same

---

104. See X. 2 of the *History of Animals*, in which the author considers how women's semen is projected so that it meets men's.

105. See *On Generation*, 6. 1–2 and *Regimen*, ch. 28.

106. De Serres does not allow for the possibility that some of these works may be erroneously attributed to Aristotle.

species as men, according even to Aristotle himself who says in Book X of his *Metaphysics* that man and woman differ only in their sex, which is an accidental rather than a fundamental difference.[107] Thus it would have been more acceptable if he had said that truly those women are real monsters of Nature who form monstrous ideas in their brains when they are carried away by imaginary jealousy against their husbands, or those who conceive and carry out monstrous plans to satisfy their desire for revenge or their lust, or finally those who couple monstrously with animals, like Pasiphae[108] and others of her kind.

Let us come now to Galen, and let us reply to him with what he himself taught us following Aristotle: it is true that woman is an imperfect creature in comparison with man, but nonetheless within her own sex she is as perfect as man is within his. For Nature, having anticipated that it was necessary to have two sexes for the accomplishment of the generation of all animals, and especially that of man, her dearest child and the unique epitome of all her wonders, did not wish to give the woman less perfection than the man, in as much as one of them is destined to procreate within the other, and the other within her own body, as all our doctors unanimously agree. Had she done otherwise, she would have made us like a great number of plants which do not have any female form; but it would be irreverent to think this of such a good mother.

As regards what he said about woman being produced by mere chance, we would say either that he is indulging in an attack on woman by writing this, or that he made an enormous mistake. The reason is that the intention of Nature was to produce females as well as males because of the procreation to which these two sexes need to contribute equally, as we have already said. For, because of this it follows that Nature would cause its own destruction if it ceased to produce females, as everyone knows. And there is no point in citing the vices and faults of their sex in order to add weight to this argument, for moral vices are different from bodily imperfections. The majority of women are born morally flawed, as are men, but almost all are born

107. *Metaphysics*, X. 9.

108. The figure in Greek mythology, daughter of the sun-god and wife of King Minos of Crete, who fell in love with a bull and conceived the monster of the Minotaur.

perfect in their bodily and sexual form, and are duly equipped with all the parts required for life and procreation.

As for the abusive arguments against women proposed by Plato, St Jerome and the Severian heretics, we shall answer in few words, that either Plato wanted to show posterity that he was possessed of more stupidity than learning, or he was taking account of the flaws of the female mind, like St Jerome, and not of the miraculous body which it inhabits, for it is most certain that females generally have a much weaker mind than men in all good things, despite the fact that their body is just as naturally perfect in all ways as that of males. So that it must be thought that he spoke as he did to provoke and goad the women of his day, rather than to be unfair to the whole sex. For I cannot imagine that such a great person (I mean Plato) would have wished to err on this fine subject by overlooking the difference between species, excluding women from the category of reasoning creatures, unless he intended himself eventually to admit that he was the natural, legitimate son of an animal.

What shall we say to the Severian heretics who go beyond the worst insults, professing stubbornly that woman is a masterpiece of the devil? We must indeed reply to them in few words, saying that they are possessed by a fanatical and pernicious spirit, which is completely diabolical, since they attribute to the devil the creation of the noblest of all creatures. What effrontery and prodigious madness! That men born, like others, of women, and created, like others, by God, should boldly deny their divine origin, and claim to be children of he who could not even create a midge, nor produce the slightest thing in the world without the permission of God! Moreover, we shall tell them that their insults and lies are out of order, since they act as both prosecutor and judge. For writing about their errors, amongst other things, St Jerome, Sophronius and Epiphanius tell us that they hate women to their very bones, and they forbad all of their disciples to marry. So that it is not because of them that the world has not returned to the state it was in immediately after the flood, that is to say deserted, unpopulated and without offspring; or that women have not been condemned to endure perpetual enforced virginity, which today would be more unbearable to most women than the heaviest breastplate.

Let us leave the rest aside, but not fail to voice the necessary response to Simonides' disrespectful speech on women. Let us tell him that if he were still alive, he would deserve to be delivered naked into the hands and power of women, since he was not ashamed to call them mortal asps, decorated bitches, etc., and moreover to be struck from the rank of men since he denies and angrily scorns half of himself by deriding the sex which contributed in part to his reasoning being, made in the image of God. Should he not be classed among animals, rather than among famous philosophers?

Moreover, let us respond to Origen that his opinion about the resurrection of the sexes is quite wrong and heretical, and was criticized by St Augustine, St Jerome, St Epiphanius, and almost all the early Church Fathers who are in unanimous agreement in their belief that woman will be resurrected in her present sex, just as man will in his. This can be proved by reference to various authorities and arguments. First, in Book IV of *The Orthodox Faith*, Damascene says clearly that after the resurrection we shall keep the same face, the same bodily form and the same characteristics which distinguish us from one another in this life.[109] From this, I would argue that if the same characteristics, the same face, the same limbs and the same body endure after the resurrection, it then follows that women's bodies will endure, since women's bodies have their individual characteristics, their faces and their forms just like those of men. Now, it is so evidently clear that women's bodies have all these things that it does not need to be proved; and even the most ignorant know that although there is a great degree of conformity between the bodies of men and women, nevertheless, as far as the parts for generation are concerned, they cannot and must not be taken to be one and the same. Therefore, if man is resurrected in his sex, why should woman not also be in hers?

Secondly, in chapter 17 of Book XXII of *The City of God*, St Augustine plainly states that He who created both sexes in this life will resurrect the same in the next life. And although Jesus Christ replied to the Sadducees that there would be no marriage in the Kingdom of His Father,[110] he did not tell them that woman would not exist; for He

109. St John Damascene, a Syrian monk and priest (c. 676–749), author of *An Exact Exposition of the Orthodox Faith*.
110. Matthew 22:23–33.

Himself knew that God His Father had created woman from the side of the first man, saying, 'It is not good that the man should be alone, I shall make him a helpmate like himself.'[111] From St Augustine's words, I deduce the following brief argument. He who created man and woman in His image and likeness did not create them to keep His said likeness and image in only one of them; otherwise, we would accuse Him of being powerless, which would be a blasphemous claim. Rather, He created them both using the same strength and power, as all true Christians believe, and as it says at the beginning of Genesis. Thus, it follows that He will always retain His said image and likeness in both sexes, since they are equally destined to receive eternal life after the resurrection, in which St Thomas, in the third part of his *Summa Theologica*,[112] declares that the same substance, the same flesh, the same hair will be retained, not only through a specific identity (as he calls it), but also an individual and incommunicable one. Moreover, would Origen and his followers dare to deny that the Blessed Virgin is eternally blessed in her sex? And that the same is true for many others, since this sex is inseparable from their female nature?

Finally, if condemned women are damned in their present sex, why should those who are chosen for all eternity not be truly blessed in theirs, by the argument of opposites? This view of Origen's is indeed so repellent and contrary to our Christian belief that it should never be put forward without regretting the wretched condition of the man who lent it currency.

As for the succession to the crown: the first leaders and the founders of monarchic states, which do not allow women to inherit, have deprived married and unmarried women of this for ever. I maintain that this does not in any way undermine the perfection and merits of their sex, given that God furnished them with souls equally, if not more excellent and capable of assuming leadership than those of many men, even though their bodies may be weaker, frailer and less fit to withstand the tribulations which commonly accompany those who wear the diadem. In any case, we know that these rigorous laws do not apply throughout the whole world, for Spain had its

111. Genesis 2:18.

112. St Thomas Aquinas wrote his great work on the Christian faith in 1265–1274; the third part, treating the incarnation and the sacraments, was left incomplete at his death.

Isabella,[113] England its Elizabeth,[114] Assyria its Semiramis,[115] Scythia its Penthesilea[116] and Amazons, all sovereign princesses who have overshadowed the achievements of very many great princes with their prudence, bravery and greatness of spirit.

In our present age, Flanders rejoices that it is under the sweet, yet solemn authority of the great Isabella Clara Eugenia,[117] sole female star of the house of Austria (as her niece, our most generous and munificent Queen[118] is of the house of France), and she is the true refuge of chastity, gentleness, prudence and wisdom. Furthermore, if we leaf through the history of this kingdom, we shall discover that it would have been in a desperate state more than 170 years ago but for the sword and invincible courage of Joan of Arc to whom Charles VII (whom the English had previously in jest named the King of Bourges) owed the return of his crown, and to whom France owes her greatness and power.[119] Although the Salic law entirely excludes our French women from the succession to the throne, it does not prevent them from holding the Regency, which is a second form of royalty. This shows that in all ages and in almost all kingdoms, the female sex has taken its turn, sooner or later, in commanding, and indeed often with such success, discretion and good conduct that it has put to shame the

113. In listing each of these names in French, de Serres uses the plural form of the female name, although there is only one recent example in each case, the first being Isabella I of Spain (1451–1504), Queen of Castile and Leon in her own right from 1474, and, after her husband Ferdinand acceded to the throne of Aragon in 1579, joint monarch of the united kingdom of Spain.

114. Elizabeth I of England (1533–1603), queen from 1558.

115. The name of Semiramis was often attributed to the mythical queen of Assyria (ninth century BC), married to Nimrod, and noted for her wisdom and beauty.

116. In Greek mythology, Penthesilea, queen of the Amazons, fought heroically with the Trojans at the Battle of Troy before being killed by Achilles.

117. Isabella Clara Eugenia (1566–1633), archduchess of Austria, was the eldest daughter of Philip II of Spain and of his French wife, Elisabeth of Valois. She was married to Albert of Habsburg in 1599, with whom she jointly ruled the Spanish Netherlands until his death in 1621. Since Isabella's three children had all died in infancy, the Spanish Netherlands reverted to the crown of Spain, but Isabella acted as Governor (for her nephew Philip IV) until her death in 1633, while also devoting herself to acts of charity and wearing the habit of a nun in the order of the poor Clares.

118. Anne of Austria, daughter of Philip III of Spain and Margaret of Austria.

119. Joan of Arc (c. 1412–1431), claiming she was inspired by visions from God, led the French army to a series of victories in the Hundred Years' War, before being captured and burned at the stake by the English. Charles had been marooned south of the Loire, near the town of Bourges, hence the pejorative nickname given to him by the English.

reigns of various of our kings, who are as spineless and effeminate as any Heliogabalus.[120] Thus, without looking any further, the regency of the Sun of Italy and of France, Marie de Medici,[121] was so happy and successful that it deserves to be ranked alongside that of Blanche of Castile,[122] or the reign of a number of our oldest and greatest kings, and much more highly praised than that of Charles VI[123] or those of John son of Philippe of Valois,[124] of Charles the Fat,[125] of Theodoric,[126] of Childeric,[127] of Clotaire I[128] and of others who similarly were kings in no more than name.

Thus, since it is an unchallengeable and sacred truth that God created woman to serve as a companion and helpmate to man, and particularly for the purpose of procreation, as was indeed asserted by St Thomas in question 91 of the first part of his *Summa Theologica*, by Daneau in his commentaries on St Augustine's *Manual*,[129] and by various other famous theologians, we must recognize and accept as a matter of proven fact that women who bear only daughters are equally as fertile as those who bear only males, and that the procreation of

120. Heliogabalus (or Varius Avitus Bassianus, or Elagabalus) was Roman Emperor 218–222; he became a byword for irreligion and sexual debauchery, on account of which he was assassinated in 222, aged 18, by some of the Praetorian Guards.

121. De Serres's positive portrayal of Marie de Medici (who acted as regent for the young Louis XIII from the death of Henri IV in 1610) is controversial. Many other contemporaries depict her as weak and an easy prey to the different Catholic factions.

122. Blanche of Castile (1188–1252), widow of Louis VIII of France, acted as regent when her son, the young Louis IX (later known as St Louis), came to the throne in 1226. She was generally celebrated as a strong ruler who held France together against external threats.

123. Charles VI (reigned 1380–1422), called the Beloved (*le Bien-Aimé*) and the Mad (*le Fol or le Fou*); his periods of madness led to instability among powerful nobles.

124. Philippe of Valois reigned 1328–1350, and was succeeded by his son John II (*Jean Le Bon*, or John the Good) who reigned 1350–1364. He was taken prisoner by the English at the Battle of Poitiers, and to the dismay of the French went voluntarily into captivity in England after being shamed by the escape of his son, who had been acting as a hostage.

125. *Charles le Gros*, or Charles the Fat (839–888), was king of East Francia from 882 and of West Francia from 884, but was deposed in 887.

126. Theodoric or Thierry III (652–691), King of all the Franks from 679, was accused of being merely a puppet king, real power lying with the mayor of the palace.

127. Childeric I (440–481), King of the Salian Franks from 457, was then expelled by the Franks.

128. Clotaire I (c. 497–561), King of Soissons, Orleans and France; the end of his reign was troubled by internal strife.

129. Lambert Daneau (1530–1595), a disciple in Geneva of de Bèze, wrote a commentary on St Augustine's *Enchridion* (or *Manual*).

the female sex is as necessary as that of males for the continuation of the human race and for the replacement of the number of souls which were lost by the rebellion of the bad angels,[130] notwithstanding that woman's faults and imperfections are great. Indeed, I would venture to say that without women, in this world men would be like a lamp with no light; a well without a rope; a bell with no clapper; a body without a soul; a sky without stars and a fire without warmth. And it is wrong to assert that their sex is not worthy to exist because of its imperfections, given that St Augustine, in the passage cited above, learnedly and concisely refutes those who advance such a weak and feeble argument, saying that the female sex is not a vice, but rather is human or female nature. By this he wishes to imply that the flaws and imperfections are inseparably bound up simply with human nature, and not with the sex; and that consequently men are equally or more deficient than women, since their nature is equal in everything, and that it is based on the same creation, and the same elementary principles.

Were it not that I wish to preserve the honor of my masculine sex (for fear lest women, who are already naturally quite ambitious enough, might venture to assert superiority over men at the demand of some new Guillaume Postel,[131] and seek to shake off the yoke of their lords and masters, as the ancient Amazons did), I could demonstrate through reasoning and authorities that the education of males is commonly far more painful and less fruitful than that of girls. The latter are capable of fully observing good discipline, indeed comporting themselves very well, provided that from the cradle they are brought up according to the pedagogy of good people, fearing God, and nourished on the milk of piety, wisdom, sweetness and chastity.

But I prefer to stop here, and to allow someone better placed than myself to take up this purpose, for I undertook in this chapter only to defend the female sex in respect of procreation, in the fulfilment of which men must admit that women have better mistresses than men, as we have shown above.

130. Reference to the War in Heaven (Revelations 12:7–9) in which the bad angels (and the dragon) are cast out by St Michael.

131. A polymath (1510–1581), whose sanity was questioned by the Inquistion, which disapproved of several of his works. *The Most Miraculous Victories of the Women of the New World* (*Les Très Merveilleuses Victoires des femmes du nouveau monde*, 1553) argued that women should rule the world.

Chapter X: Of the Causes of the Last Kind of Female Sterility, Called Temporary Sterility[132]

In this chapter we shall go carefully through the causes of the kind of sterility from which the majority of infertile women believe they are suffering, thinking that they will not die before sooner or later seeing an heir delivered from their womb. But in order to achieve our aim more easily, we must first recall that our authorities[133] distinguish two different forms of this kind of sterility. The first is that which affects only women who are too young, by which I mean those who marry before they are 12 or 14, when they are in their first year of fertility according to the majority of natural philosophers.[134] The second is the kind into which many women fall, some through their own fault, and others through the violence and duration of various illnesses or other natural infirmities.

As far as the first kind is concerned, I think we have sufficiently discussed its causes already at the beginning of chapter VIII, so that I do not consider it necessary to say anything further, for fear of lapsing into tiresome repetitions that could only be displeasing and wearisome to those ladies who deign to look through this book.[135]

Thus we shall content ourselves with declaring that there are various causes that bring about and maintain the second kind of sterility. For first, as everyone knows, frequent injuries or miscarriages are the very essence of it, as we have shown earlier with reference to the authority

132. This chapter discusses the causes of temporary sterility; ch. XIV will discuss the possible remedies. Since I do not include a translation of the later chapter in its entirety, I summarize the main points from ch. XIV in the footnotes to this chapter.

133. I.e. the classical authors on whom de Serres draws throughout, notably Hippocrates, Galen and Aristotle.

134. Renaissance physicians (and moralists) hotly debated the youngest age at which a girl could become pregnant. Joubert, for example, was criticized for having treated the subject in the *Popular Errors* where he cited the exceptional case of a girl who conceived her first child at the age of nine (*Erreurs populaires*, Bordeaux, 1578, Book II, Ch. 2, 149–156).

135. Similarly, in Ch. XIV de Serres advises that women who married before the age of 14 should simply wait until they are older before being concerned about possible infertility.

of Hippocrates,[136] Mercatus,[137] da Veiga[138] and some others. Yet, we see today that various pregnant women willingly expose themselves to this evil when they imprudently exert themselves in all kinds of dances and other violent movements, which threaten the life of the children they carry. They would have Nature believe that she was quite wrong in wishing them to abstain from these dances, from riding in carriages and other such immoderate exercises during their pregnancies. I do not, however, deny that there are some women who are sufficiently robust that they can easily partake in such exercises without coming to any harm, but I maintain that both groups do a great wrong to both Nature and themselves in undermining their health, especially those who are more fragile and easily subject to injury. For Hippocrates, in his third book on common diseases, asserts that such women are subject to any number of diseases and live rather pitifully.[139]

Nonetheless, I do not doubt that various wise and moderate women may often suffer an injury which may even make them infertile not as a result of excesses and incontinence, as with the previous group, but rather because of their inner disposition, or because of an unexpected fall, or through stumbling. But I would say that these women must think of themselves just as the first group must, and seek a timely remedy so that their wombs do not become accustomed to shuddering and then expelling their fruit at a premature stage. For I have said and will repeat that, just as in some people Nature becomes accustomed to vomiting when it has once been allowed to become established, so also it can adopt the habit of expelling the child from the womb before its full term when it has often been driven to do so by some violent force. We may be certain that Nature acts not rationally or knowingly, but by instinct, as physicians say, following the same pattern when it is once inculcated, whether for good or bad, and it does not know

136. For Hippocrates's remarks on the causes of repeated early miscarriages and the treatment of them, see Littré, *Hippocrate. Œuvres complètes*, vol. VIII, sections 237–240.

137. Luis de Mercado, author of On *the Common Diseases of Women* [*De mulierum affectionibus*, Valladolid: D. Fernandez, 1579].

138. Tomas Rodrigues da Veiga (1513–1579), a Portuguese physician who edited and commented on the works of Galen.

139. This seems to be an erroneous reference. De Serres may be half-remembering another Hippocratic text, *On the Diseases of Women,* which states (I.1) that women who have not yet born children are likely to be more afflicted by menstrual disorders than those who have already carried a pregnancy to term.

how to restrain itself in the face of such actions and movements, like persons running headlong down a steep path.[140]

In addition, our authors, both ancient and modern, write that white discharges[141] often cause this form of sterility in women, yet Hippocrates asserted the opposite in Book IV *Of Common Diseases* and Book II of the *Diseases of Women*, as then did Aretaeus,[142] Montanus[143] and various other well-known doctors. Furthermore, experience shows us every day that these discharges do not prevent women from bearing a number of children, as we have said earlier, in chapter IV. On such subjects, we must treat the differing opinions of both sides in a friendly manner, so that the truth may be established, and people will no longer believe that medicine is a science full of quarrels and pointless disputes; and the difficulties in it are of the same nature as the Gordian Knot which Alexander sliced with his sword when he could not untie it.[144]

We need to recognize, therefore, that this unhealthy white discharge (otherwise known as 'white flowers') can occur in any women, whether married, unmarried, relatively young or old, fertile or infertile. The reason for this is that since women have a cold, mucousy temperament, and are thus incapable of digesting and consuming the great multitude of excrements which gather and stagnate in their bodies, Nature decided to provide the womb for them, the first and main role of which concerns the conception, gestation and birth of man; its other role is the elimination and expulsion of such unpleasant

140. In ch. XIV, de Serres provides advice on avoiding early miscarriage by care before and after conception. He counsels women to consult their ordinary physicians before conceiving so that humors and temperament may be corrected (by bleeding, purges, appropriate foods). Once pregnant, they should follow all the standard advice: seek out temperate conditions (avoiding excessive heat or cold), avoid over-vigorous exercises (notably dancing and horse-riding), and keep an even temper (avoiding quarrels with their husbands), since it was believed that anger might provoke a miscarriage. A number of gentle 'tonics' and calming poultices are recommended, but in conclusion de Serres reminds the women to consult their physician in case of any problem; his general advice is never meant to replace the specific care of the regular physician.

141. The medical condition of leukorrhea.

142. Physician contemporary to Galen, c. 150 AD.

143. Johannes Baptista Montanus (1498–1551) — or Giovanni Baptista da Monte — was professor of medical practice at Padua and a friend of Vesalius.

144. See 317.

excrements. This is why our authors say that the womb is like the sewer of women's bodies.[145]

Now these foul substances are either red or white or yellow or blackish, and all of these can be either hot or cold. The red ones are the most common and are also the least dangerous; indeed I would say they are very healthy provided they occur once a month, according to the pattern Nature admirably set. The yellow and blackish ones are less common but the most painful, according to Hippocrates in the second book of the *Diseases of Women*.[146] And Aetius says in chapter 63 of his fourth book that as the yellow ones come from a warm, bilious and bitter humor and are the colour of the yolk of an egg, and as the blackish ones betoken a dried-out, black, melancholic and corrosive humor, both can only be disagreeable and troublesome for women. As for the white ones, which are the main subject under discussion here, I would comment that whether Nature sends them from the whole body to the womb, whence they are expelled to protect the body from them, or whether they gather in this organ as a result of its own weakness, it is clear that they are either liquid, or serous like milk, or like an ass's urine, as Hippocrates says,[147] or dirty, foul-smelling and fetid like the discharge from an ulcer, or cold and runny like water, or finally they may be sticky, warm, prone to ulceration, like the discharge from clap.[148]

Now it happens that those which are too cold and runny may cause infertility by leaving the mark of their excess in the womb; so, too, those which are exceptionally hot, bitter, bilious and prone to ulceration may produce the same effect by dissipating the natural heat of this organ, destroying women's ability to bear children, even making them become wasted and dried out like wood.[149] But when

---

145. A commonplace among various authorities, including notably Avicenna, but disputed by other writers who argue for the positive qualities of uterine or menstrual blood. See H. King, *Midwifery, Obstetrics and the Rise of Gynaecology* (Aldershot: Ashgate Publishing Limited, 2008), 55.

146. *Diseases of Women*, II. 117.

147. *Diseases of Women*, II. 116.

148. De Serres uses the common colloquial term *'chaude-pisse'* (literally 'hot piss') to denote blennorrhea.

149. In ch. XIV, de Serres recommends treating problematic cases of leukorrhea primarily through diet, poultices and baths, and pharmacy (e.g. a pessary of sorrel leaves), according to the nature of the humoral imbalance in the patient. Since he believes that all parts of the

a woman's nature is healthy, and the white discharges (even though they occur at all times, without any rule) do not in themselves have an excess of any quality such that they might corrupt and perturb the temperature of the womb in which they often linger for a certain time, it is clear that in such cases they do not harm her fertility. Nor will they do so if, running down the whole length of the spine, they simply pass down the neck of the womb, being expelled to relieve Nature, that was troubled by them. Thus, when our authors write that the white discharges cause female sterility in themselves, I would affirm that their opinion has to be understood with reference to the first group, that is to say those women who are too cold or too hot and prone to ulcers. When Hippocrates writes that they occur primarily in women who have had, or are having, many children, his view should be taken as referring to those who have no undesirable quality in themselves but simply have a mucousy, rather cold and serous humor, which Nature expels in order to rid itself of a general surfeit. This is what I think we should understand in respect of this question, and how we should reconcile the differing opinions on the subject.

Similarly, when women have too much fat or are over-thin, this is not the least cause of this kind of sterility.[150] For, first, our authors declare that where there is an excessive amount of fat in either men or women, there is correspondingly little prolific seed, since both come from the same matter, the blood, so that a decrease in one is related to an increase in the other. Not that I would wish to conclude that all fat or fleshy bodies are sterile; and this the more so because of what Hippocrates wrote in the fifth book of his *Aphorisms*.[151] For, on the contrary, I consider that men and women who are moderately fat, regularly proportioned, that is to say who are born plump and usually

---

body can produce the excessive humors which pool in the womb and must be expelled in the menses or the leukorrhea, his treatments are designed to cure the whole body.

150. See for example various of Hippocrates's aphorisms, including: 'Women who are very lean, have miscarriages when they prove with child, until they get into better condition', and 'When unnaturally fat women cannot conceive, it is because the fat presses the mouth of the womb, and conception is impossible until they grow thinner' (*Aphorisms*, V. 44, 46). The latter is also cited by Rousset (56). Extreme thinness and fatness are also discussed as causes of infertility in Hippocrates's *On Sterile Women* (see Littré, *Hippocrate. Œuvres complètes*, vol. VIII, sections 229 and 237), and in Aristotle, *Generation of Animals* (II. 7).

151. Hippocrates does not directly state this in Book V of the *Aphorisms*, but does express more concern about conception and pregnancy in over-thin than in over-fat women.

stocky (we must assume that Hippocrates is talking about such women as this in his *Aphorisms*), are very fertile, as experience generally proves to us, and in accordance with the remarks of Hippocrates in his book *On Superfetation*.[152]

But I want to point out that those men and women who were born thin and emaciated but later become excessively fat are usually infertile for various reasons. The first is that most and the best part of their blood is converted into fat, which means that these women do not have enough blood to sustain themselves and any fruit of their womb. The second is that their menses are very slight, which indicates a deficiency of the blood — without which they cannot conceive, as is quite evident. And indeed Hippocrates (whom we have already cited on this subject), in examining the causes of sterility among Scythian women, puts this as one of the first and main ones, and claims that such a deficiency of the blood resulted only from the lack of exercise that they took, and on account of their over-pampered and cosseted lifestyle, whereas their female servants who were brought up in austerity and poverty, with constant physical exercise, were all overflowing with blood, and as fertile as mice.[153] The third reason is that this fat so compresses the womb by virtue of the epiploon that the womb can neither receive nor keep the seed as it needs to. And even if it does receive it, it can certainly not hold the child for the necessary term because of the limited space.

As for thinness, we must consider two types, as we have already said above. One is natural and appropriate, and we shall not speak of it for two reasons. First, it is often associated with fertility, unless there is some other problem. Secondly, it cannot be dissociated from sterility if it is extreme and indeed incurable. The other type is that which is called 'foreign', and which may be cured and corrected in both men and women, provided one does not delay until it has given way to extreme consumption of the fleshy parts of the body. Now

152. *On Superfetation*, 21.

153. Most of de Serres's advice in Chapter XIV calls for a degree of asceticism. He asks over-plump women to abstain from foods that induce weight-gain or flatulence, and to adopt a tough lifestyle, seeking colder air, plentiful exercise and less sleep. He considers the mind and body to be equally affected by the excess fat, recommending that women wishing to lose weight may sometimes be advised to give way to sadness, jealousy and anger, since the emotional outbursts will consume their excess fat.

it is quite evident and widely acknowledged that this thinness is an impediment to female fertility, first because it attacks all the natural parts, especially the abdomen, according to Aristotle in Book V of his *Problems*, from which I cite the following argument: 'that since it destroys the fleshiness of natural parts such as the muscles of the lower abdomen, the epiploon, the womb, the veins, the seed-bearing vessels,[154] and other such things, in the radical balm of which lies the natural heat without which procreation, the noblest of all natural functions, cannot take place, it is, in consequence, the cause of female sterility'.[155] I would add, further, that sterility is normally caused by an over hot and dry temperament, which is a direct enemy of conception, as everyone knows; so it is not surprising if it brings with it infertility.

To all these we can add these four other causes which are no less important: the natural weakness of women, and particularly of their womb; painful, difficult and dangerous births; infection caused by a child which has remained in the womb for a long time after its death; and finally a mole or mass of flesh which a woman has carried for some years.[156]

As to the first, it is quite commonly observed that, just as we find some weak, thin and rather feeble men who carry but one child within them, even though they desire their wives who are naturally and fully fertile, so too there are some women who are so delicate and of such a weak constitution, both with respect to their general health and to their womb in particular, that they can bear only one child and will spend the rest of their lives sterile and infertile. This is natural in their case, according to Hippocrates in his book *On Sterile Women*.[157] In this, they are quite the opposite of some others who are like farriers'

---

154. I.e. what are now know as the fallopian tubes.

155. Unsurprisingly, de Serres's remedies in ch. XIV for excessive thinness are essentially mirror images of those for excessive fatness. The thin woman should seek warmer air, eat foods that fortify the blood (including not only ass's milk, but the milk of the strong lactating mother of a son!), and avoid too much exercise, or causes of emotional distress, while taking every opportunity to sleep.

156. For Hippocrates's comment on these causes of sterility in *On Sterile Women*, see Littré, *Hippocrate. Œuvres complètes*, vol. VIII, sections 227 (on an unhealthy womb), 228 (on a womb damaged after miscarriage or birth), 233 (on moles).

157. This seems to be an erroneous reference. Hippocrates does, however, consider the cases of women whose constitution is weak and who habitually miscarry after two months (*On Sterile Women*, 238).

bellows, that is to say no sooner empty than full again, no sooner full than empty.

The second kind (painful, difficult and dangerous births) certainly deserves recognition, for our physicians and midwives observe every day that those women who undergo such births suffer an enormous number of difficulties, of which the least is often quite sufficient to make them infertile for ever. Thus if it happens that the neck of the their womb loses its normal shape, and instead of being straight, is now at an angle and bent in a curve, they are unable to receive the seed as they need to. Nor can they if the womb, dislodged from its rightful place, falls and comes out with the child (which happens most often because of the brutality and ignorance of the midwives, who take it for the placenta).[158] Or if, finally, the ligaments which keep it in place stretch so that they cannot resume their former state or hold the womb as they did before, hereafter the womb will definitely not be able to hold the foetus in future pregnancies.

As to the third kind (infection caused by a child which has remained in the womb for a long time after its death), I consider that just as the vapors from muddy waters or a privy tarnish bronze and copper, making them quite dull, so the strange putrefaction which arises when a dead child has rotted in the womb for a long time can corrupt and blight the nature of this vessel which contains the fruits of procreation, so that hereafter it will no longer be capable of a new pregnancy.

Finally, the last kind (a mole or mass of flesh which a woman has carried for some years) is no less destructive. This is because when any mole (which, according to Galen, is simply a piece of excess flesh, unable to move, shapeless, incompletely formed and inanimate) lingers too long in the womb, not only does it waste and dry out the woman because of the great amount of blood it drains, but also when it comes out — an action which cannot be accomplished without great force — it will often break and shatter the womb because of its heavy weight. As it leaves the body, it brings in its wake guaranteed sterility, especially if the woman is particularly fragile and of a delicate constitution.[159]

158. Various writers, including Duval (274), caution against causing uterine prolapse.
159. See 340.

I shall leave aside several other causes of this affliction, such as blockages or obstructions, the absence of the menses, and such like.[160] The reason for this is that I did not intend to write a complete work on women's health,[161] but rather to treat briefly the most common and frequent causes of sterility among women. This is why I shall stop here, to pass on to how to recognize the condition in question.

Chapter XIV: On Curing the Last Kind of Female Sterility, Called Temporary Sterility

The women whom God afflicts with this kind of sterility have good cause to be consoled by the fact that even though it is burdensome to them for a time, it will finish much sooner than they might think, provided only that they arm themselves with prayer and patience, following the examples of Leah,[162] of the mother of Samuel,[163] of Saint Elizabeth,[164] and of many other such women; and they should also behave as is necessary and as we shall explain in what follows.

[De Serres then divides the chapter into five subsections, corresponding to the causes of sterility identified in chapter X:

> And first on miscarriage or injury.
> On white flowers.[165]
> On excessive fat or unnecessary plumpness.
> On abnormal thinness.
> On bad deliveries and other remaining causes.

I have summarized in the footnotes to the relevant sections of chapter X the lengthy advice and cures he offers on the first four topics. I resume the translation with the last section, which directly concerns childbirth.]

160. These conditions are discussed by Hippocrates in *On Sterile Women*.

161. De Serres uses the French term '*un Gynaecée*', a Latinism coined from '*gynaeceum*' (of / about women). This is one of the earliest attested uses of the word in the vernacular.

162. Wife of Jacob, who conceived one last child after she thought herself no longer fertile (Genesis 29:31–35; 30:9–21).

163. Hannah had previously been childless (1 Samuel 1:11–20).

164. Mother of John the Baptist, and cousin of the Virgin; she had been sterile for many years before conceiving her son (Luke, 1:5–66).

165. I.e. leukorrhea.

On bad deliveries and other remaining causes

Whenever women remain sterile after bad deliveries, we must believe that this happens for two main reasons. Either the womb is too small, and, in contrast, the child too large and most vigorous, and thus during its delivery the child breaks and shatters some great vessel or the inner mouth of the womb;[166] or, which is worse, it dislodges the womb from its rightful place, as a result of which the womb can neither retain the seed it receives nor carry to term any child conceived in subsequent pregnancies. This is because of both the obvious disturbance it has endured and the abnormal relaxation of the ligaments which previously held it in place. Or, alternatively, if the child chances to die and rot in the womb, not only does it affect the noble parts with the ghastly vapors which emanate from its body, but it also so alters the temperature of the shelter in which it dwells that in the future the womb cannot return to its former state, and so is unable to retain seed, conceive and then, in due course, give birth to what it took in. Thus we shall try to overcome these obstacles as best we can.

As far as the first problem is concerned, there is no doubt that, if the small size of the womb reflects its natural shape, it is very difficult, if not impossible, to change it, as everyone knows. But, if it happens that the problem derives wholly from the child being too large, swollen and full of liquid from the mother, as is often the case, then it is necessary to take good care of the womb, and give it plenty of rest, and then return to the section above which deals with treating abnormal openings of the womb, where I have given all the appropriate remedies which should be used in this situation. And it should not be believed that this problem is as great as some women who suffer from it might think. For in such a case their private parts are like stagnant water into which a great stone is thrown: it breaks the surface sharply, but when the stone sinks to the bottom, the surface of the water becomes as smooth and even as before, so that no trace is left of the disruption. Similarly, after the painful and violent birth of such children, the womb returns to its former state, provided it is given good care, rest, and the remedies listed above. In a very short time, the women are fully restored to the same health they enjoyed before, except in those cases where the problem was so great that neither the skill of physicians, nor the work of midwives could avail.

166. I.e. the cervix.

However, when they are entirely recovered and before they become pregnant once more, it is necessary to treat these women so that they do not suffer such a problem again, that is to say so that the fruits of subsequent pregnancies do not become as swollen as the earlier ones. This can be done by the use of remedies to purge, change and dry the body both internally and externally, and also by attention to diet. For it is likely that their temperament, which is nothing if not over-cold and damp, provides not good, noble blood which can feed children, but rather moisture and other such humors which are unable to feed them well, and of which there is sometimes such a great abundance that they suffocate the fruit of the womb. Midwives observe this daily, and as a result the child becomes quite swollen and excessively fat, and thus during its birth is capable of causing all the problems of which we have just spoken.

Now the cures for this imbalance of temperament have already been so fully described that I do not intend to repeat them here.

If it happens that the sterility is caused by an infection resulting from one or several children dying in the womb, first it is important to remember to provide a good diet, and then to use cordials which will stimulate internally and externally. Finally, baths should be used, or injections, perfumes, poultices and other such remedies which have the power not only to dull, but even to eliminate entirely the noxious effect on the womb of the rotten and cadaverous vapors from the dead children. As for bathing, I believe the following prescription might be appropriate:

Take roots of galingale, round buckwheat, blue ginger, angelica, lichen, clove, three ounces of each; leaves of citronella, artemisia, matricaria, devil's bit, borage, sorrel, soapwort, Roman wormwood, catnip, four good handfuls of each; laurel and juniper berries, Ethiopian cumin, mace, an ounce and a half of each; seeds of flax, aniseed, fennel, one ounce of each; flowers of small centaurea, water lilies, borage, violets, roses of Provins, three pinches of each of these; let them be infused in a container suitable for a bath or a half-bath, as they wish.

The woman should bathe in this twice a day, morning and evening, remaining in it for an hour or two on each occasion if she feels able to. This bath, or half-bath, will suitably and profitably change the womb.

She should herself inject the infusion into the womb when she is in the tub, and it will consume entirely all the poisons which may still be in it. It will strengthen the woman's whole constitution, and provide a strong encouragement to Nature to favor conception.

Each time she comes out of the bath, the following tablets should be burned so that the fumes may pass into her womb:

Take powdered birds from Cyprus, powdered violet, one ounce of each; weeping storax, mace, juniper seeds, mastic, incense, laudanum, one dram of each; powder of alipta moscata, two small pinches, which may be powdered. This should be mixed with sufficient quantity of turpentine to make tablets weighing half a dram, which you must use as described.

Finally, to fortify and delight the womb, she can place the following poultice on the navel:

Take pure laudanum, half an ounce; mastic, incense, myrrh, nutmeg, a dram of each; half a dram of castoreum; grind to a powder those ingredients which should be mixed with good Venetian turpentine;[167] then reduce it to the consistency of a poultice, adding yellow wax as necessary.

This poultice should be round in shape, and renewed every week, and each time it is applied to the navel, a couple of grains of musk must be put into the cavity, and the poultice then applied on top.

Further, if this problem results from a large mole,[168] either remaining in the womb or protruding from it, particular care must be taken. For it must at all costs be extracted if it has been stagnating there for too long. This can easily be achieved through potions to purge or cause abortion or expulsion; or through blood-letting, perfumes, frictions, cuppings, medicines to induce sneezing, and other such cures of which thousands can be found in the writings of those who have dealt fully with the diseases of women, like Mercado,[169] Varanda[170] and such like, and about which I shall say no more for the present in order to avoid verbosity.

167. A form of natural resin.

168. See 340.

169. See 335, n. 137.

170. Jean Varanda (1563/4–1617) was Professor of Medicine at Montpellier; his work *On the Diseases and Afflictions of Women* [*De morbis ei affectibus mulierum*] appeared posthumously in 1619.

If the expulsion of the mole causes a large constant hemorrhage or loss of blood, as it breaks and shatters most of the great vessels of the womb, care must be taken to nourish these women on good foods which are not too hot, but rather astringent and glutinous such as gruel, broths made with foot of veal or sheep or beef, which are excellent in such cases, rice, vermicelli, wheatcakes, jellied quinces and such like. They should avoid all strong wines, drinking only those that are not heavy, and are dark red, and they should drink only a small quantity diluted with water. They should also keep to their bed, avoid any anger, sadness, sneezing and other such violent movement of either the body or the mind; they should keep their stomach empty, and sleep moderately and regularly. As for treatments, revulsions[171] and purgatives should certainly be applied in such cases in order to divert Nature from this unnatural growth. Similarly, potions, injections, perfumes, poultices, cataplasms and other such remedies, which are astringent and strengthening, should also be applied. You will find descriptions of all these cures in the authors mentioned above.

In short, if the natural weakness of their body in general, or of their womb in particular, is the only cause of their sterility, let these women not seek the medicine of those men who with all their vain and confused learning have nothing to change the nature or constitution of those men or women they undertake to relieve of their illnesses; but rather let them seek the almighty hand of the ruler who cuts, shapes and decides the temperament, health, illness, sterility, life and death of men as seems good to Him. For Hippocrates, Aristotle, Galen, Plutarch and various other such authors teach us that the natural indispositions of the mother's womb, which are associated with the noble, solid parts of the body, are totally incurable. And physicians who would undertake to cure them would be no less rash than those who would make so bold as to attempt to transform the nature of the four elements, from the combination of which the human body has been wondrously created.

---

171. The practice of applying a strong substance (e.g. mustard) to an area of the body at some distance from the affected area, to draw away blood.

Chapter XV: On Specific Foods and Remedies against Female Sterility

[De Serres concludes his work with a chapter on some generic remedies for female sterility, although at the start he severely cautions the reader not to assume that his remedies will be a panacea. The recommendations cover a standard range of foods to nourish the blood, medicines and herbs to take internally, and treatments to apply externally. I translate the conclusion to the chapter, interesting both for its reassertion of de Serres's faith in God, and for the reference to the continued childlessness of Anne of Austria, Queen of France.]

And this indeed is what God's Spirit said to the women of Israel, and through them to all gentlewomen, about the final, true cures for sterility. 'If you hear my voice,' he said, 'and if you serve me, I who am your Eternal God, there will be none who miscarries or is barren in your country.' (Exodus 23:26). And also, 'If you follow my commandments, you will be blessed above all peoples, and there will be no man or woman among you who is sterile, nor among your animals' (Deuteronomy 7:14).

This work on female sterility has reached its conclusion to coincide precisely with the year that we safely left a few days ago.[172] Thus, at the start of the year, we must renew our good wishes and prayers to the King of Kings for our invincible LOUIS, and his chaste wife ANNE OF AUSTRIA,[173] the Queen of Princesses, and the Princess of Queens, who (if my wishes are prophetic) will in this year or shortly afterwards give birth to the finest, most perfect young *'fleur de lis'*[174] ever seen in France since the thirteenth century, and this child will cause the noble line of Saint Louis to multiply,[175] and give to the French Empire a King, to the King a Dauphin, and to the Universe a Monarch, whose conquests will far outstrip those of various other Kings, and who in his

---

172. The printing privilege was granted on 27 December 1624; the *imprimatur* is dated 25 January 1625.

173. The marriage of Anne of Austria and Louis XIV had been consummated in 1615 when both were only 14. (See de Serres's earlier comments on marriages which remain sterile in the early years if the bride is too young: 334.) To the concern of many in France, the Queen remained childless for 23 years, until the birth of Louis *'Dieudonné'* (God-given), the future Louis XIV, in 1638.

174. The lily flower was the heraldic symbol of the French monarchy.

175. St Louis (Louis XI) reigned from 1226 to 1270.

time will show that France can achieve all it wants so that it becomes the very center and circumference of the world. Amen.

Sterilitas Galliam foecundabit.[176]

176. 'Sterility shall make France fertile.' (The Latin phrase, suggesting that de Serres's treatise will allow childless women to conceive, reads like a motto beneath an emblem.)

GLOSSARIES

The glossaries are intended to provide readers with a quick reference tool for: 1) names of medical practitioners and writers, 2) common medical terms, and 3) common herbs and medicinal remedies cited in the texts in this volume. The entries are necessarily brief, and readers wishing for further information should consult standard works of reference.

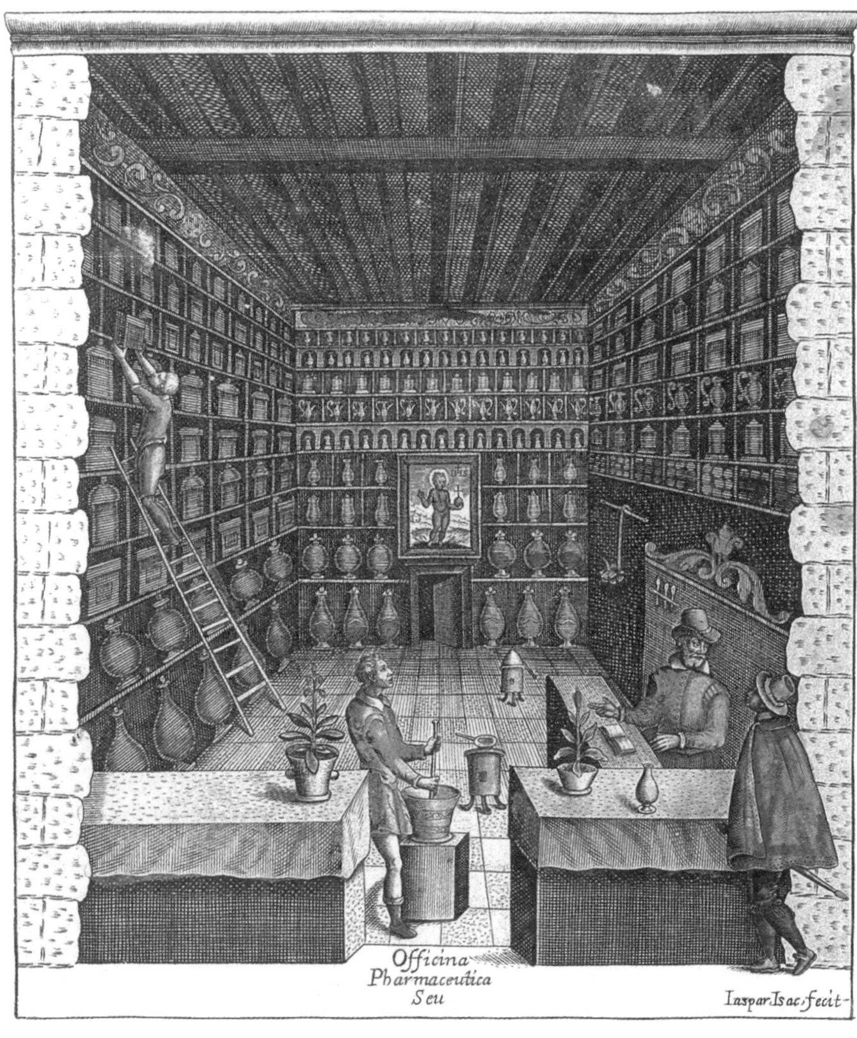

27) Apothecary's shop

Jean de Renou, *Institutionum pharmaceuticarum, libri quinque*, Paris, 1608
(Wellcome Library, London)

MEDICAL AUTHORITIES FROM CLASSICAL
TO EARLY MODERN TIMES

Aegineta	*See* Paulus Aegineta.
Aesculapus (or Asclepius)	God of medicine in Greek mythology, son of Apollo.
Aetius of Amida	(late–5th or early–6th centuries) Byzantine physician and author of *Books on Medicine* [*Tetrabiblus*], compiled from ancient sources — especially from Galen and Oribasus.
Ailleboust (or Aliboux), Jean	(?1518–1594) Physician at Autun and then at Sens; first physician to Henri III. Author of a Latin epistle (*The Monstrous Stone-Child* [*Portentosum lithopaedion*, 1582]) describing the discovery of a calcified foetus that had remained in the mother's womb for 28 years.
Albertus Magnus	(?1193–1280) German biologist, author of a widely read Latin treatise on *The Secrets of Women and Men* [*Secreta mulierum et virorum*].
Albucasis	(c. 936–1013) Personal physician to Calif of Cordoba; author of a highly respected medical encylopedia [*Al-Tasrif*].
Alpharabius (Al-Farabi)	(c. 872–950) Muslim polymath, philosopher and scientist.
Aretaeus (of Cappadocia)	(1st century) Greek physician.

Aristotle	(384–322 BC) Greek philosopher and natural scientist, pupil of Plato. Author of scientific works, including *On the Generation of Animals.*
Asclepiades (of Bithynia)	(c. 124–40 BC) Settled in Rome and established a new theory of atomic or corpuscular medicine, opposed to Hippocratic humoral medicine.
Avenzoar (Ibn Zuhr)	(1091–1161) Muslim physician and surgeon; introduced methods of human dissection and anatomy.
Avicenna	(c. 980–1037) Arab philosopher and physician whose works remained highly influential throughout the Renaissance.
Bourgeois (or Boursier), Louise	(?1563–1636) Midwife to French Queen, Marie de Medici. Author of three volumes of *Diverse Observations* on deliveries (1609, 1617, 1626).
Caelius Aurelianus	(5th century) Roman physician and writer; translated Soranus' work from Greek to Latin.
Cardano, Gerolamo	(1501–1576) Italian physician and author of various scientific works, including *On the Subtlety of Things* [*De subtilitate rerum*, 1550].
Celsus, Aulus Cornelius	(c. 25 BC–50 AD) Roman medical writer; author of *On Medicine* [*De re medicina*].
Cornax, Mathias	(born c. 1520) Physician in Vienna; one of the first to perform a cesarean on a living woman (in 1545).

Daleschamps, Jacques	(1513–1588) Physician and botanist in Lyons; author of several medical works, including *French Surgery* [*Chirurgie françoise*, 1570].
Dioscorides	(c. 40–90) Greek physician and botanist: author of a five-volume treatise on herbal medicine.
Du Laurens, André	(1559–1609) Professor of Medicine, then Chancellor at Montpellier, physician to Henri IV and Marie de Medici. His *Works on Anatomy* [*Opera anatomica*] were published in 1593.
Ebreo, Leone (or Abravanel, Judah Leon)	(c. 1465–1523) Jewish Portuguese physician and philosopher; influential proponent of neoplatonism.
Erasistratus (of Ioulis)	(c. 325–250 BC) Instrumental in foundation of medical school of Alexandria; short fragments of his works were preserved by Galen.
Estienne, Charles	(1504–1564) French anatomist, medical writer and printer; father-in-law of Jean Liebault.
Falloppio, Gabriele	(1523–1562) Italian physician and leading anatomist; famous for his work on the head and the reproductive organs.
Fernel, Jean	(1497–1558) First physician to Henri II (accredited with curing the king's sterility). Author of various scientific treatises in Latin.

Galen	(129-?227) Roman physician, surgeon and philosopher, of Greek extraction. His major works included commentaries on Hippocrates' aphorisms, *Book on the Natural Faculties, On the Usefulness of Parts.*
Gelée, Théophile	(1566-?1650) Physician in Dieppe; trained under Du Laurens; published a report (1622) of a successful cesarean on a living woman in which a retained, calcified foetus was extracted.
Girault, Jean	(late–16th-early–17th centuries) Surgeon in Paris; revised and extended Daleschamps's work on surgery, including (in 1610) additional notes on obstetric practice in Paris.
Gorris, Jean	(1505–1577) Physician in Paris.
Guillemeau, Jacques	(1549-?1613) Surgeon who trained under Ambroise Paré, and served four successive French kings. Author of works in French on childbirth, care of newborn child and ophthalmic disorders.
Héroard, Jean	(1551–1628) First Physician to the young Louis XIII; specialist in paediatrics.
Herophilus (of Chalcedon)	(c. 335–280 BC) Greek physician instrumental in founding the medical school of Alexandria, one of the first anatomists to dissect corpses. His works are now lost, but his treatise on midwifery was cited by Galen.

Hippocrates	(c. 460–370 BC) Greek physician often hailed as 'Father of Western medicine'. Among the texts known to the Renaissance in the Hippocratic corpus (i.e. attributed to Hippocrates) were: *Aphorisms, Animadversions, Epidemics, On the Nature of Woman, On the Diseases of Virgins, On the Diseases of Women,* and *On Sterile Women.*
Honoré	(late–16th, early–17th centuries) Surgeon in Paris with outstanding reputation for conducting difficult deliveries.
Houllier, Jacob	(1500–1562) Regent of the Faculty of Medicine in Paris from 1546 to 1548.
Joubert, Laurent	(1529–1582) Physician and Chancellor of Faculty of Medicine of Montpellier; author of Latin and French works on medicine, including *Popular Errors* [*Erreurs populaires*, 1578].
Lemnius, Levinus (or Lemne, Levin)	(1505–1568?) Dutch physician, author of widely read Latin work *On the Secret Miracles of Nature* [*De miraculis occultis naturae*, 1559].
Marchand, Jacques	(later–16th-earlier–17th centuries) Surgeon with expertise in deliveries, son-in-law of Jacques Guillemeau; composed two tracts in Latin against the use of cesareans on living women (1590).
Marinelli, Giovanni	(16th-century) Italian physician from Formia: author of two manuals on women's health and beauty, which were adapted in French by Jean Liebault.

Mercado, Luis de (or Mercatus)	(?1525–1611) Physician to Philip II and Philip III of Spain: author of a Latin treatise *On the Diseases of Women* (*De mulierum affectionibus*, 1579).
Montanus (or da Monte, Giovanni Baptista)	(1498–1551) Friend of Vesalius and Professor of Medicine at Padua; promoted revival of Greek medical texts in Italy.
Paré, Ambroise	(c. 1510–1590) Royal surgeon and celebrated anatomist; author of various French treatises on surgery.
Paulus Aegineta (or Paul of Aegina)	(625–690) Surgeon and famous compiler of medical works in Greek.
Pineau, Séverin	(c. 1550–1609) Surgeon and anatomist in Paris; author of controversial treatise in Latin on signs of virginity (1597).
Plato	(c. 428/7–348/7 BC) Greek philosopher, mentor of Socrates and teacher of Aristotle; author of philosophical dialogues, including *Symposium, Timaeus, Theatatus*.
Pliny (the elder)	(23–79) Latin naturalist and author of an encyclopedic *Natural History*.
Plutarch	(c. 45–125) Greek historian, essayist and philosopher; his extensive *Moral Writings* were regularly cited by Renaissance physicians.
Provanchières, Simon de	(1540-?1617) Physician in Sens; published a report in French on the extraction of a calcified foetus that the mother had carried for 28 years.

Quintus Severus Sammonicus	(2nd century) Physician and author of Latin poem on *The Precepts of Medicine*.
Rhazes (or Rasis)	(865–925) Persian physician and philosopher; his extensive writings became an essential part of the Western canon.
Roderigo de Castro	(c. 1550–1627) Portuguese physician; served king of Denmark. Author of a work in Latin on *The Universal Medicine of Women*.
Rodrigues da Veiga, Tomas	(1513–1579) Portuguese physician; edited and commented on the works of Galen.
Rondelet, Guillaume	(1507–1566) Physician and Chancellor of Faculty of Medicine of Montpellier; author of a general textbook in Latin on curing diseases.
Ronsseus, Baldvinus (or Ronsse, Baudouin)	(d. 1596) Flemish physician; vol. II of his *Medical Treatises* [*Opuscula medica*], was *On the Diseases of Women* [*De morbis mulieribus*].
Rösslin, Eucharius	(1470-?1526) German physician and author of best-selling German midwifery treatise *A Rosegarden for Pregnant Women and Midwives* [*Der Swangern Frawen und Hebammen Roszgarten*, 1513].
Rousset, François	(1535–1590?) Student of Houllier and Rondelet, then personal physician to Duke of Nemours. Author of a treatise defending use of cesareans on living women (published 1581 in French).

Soranus of Ephesus	(93–138) Greek physician; author of important lost treatise on gynecology, known to the Renaissance via various fragmentary translations and epitomes.
Varanda, Jean	(1563/4–1617) Professor of Medicine at Montpellier: author of work in Latin *On the Diseases and Afflictions of Women* [*De morbis et affectibus mulierum*, posthum. 1619].
Villeneuve (or Villeneufve), Nicolas de	(16th century) Physician in Valréas (Provence).

MEDICAL TERMS

Allantois	One of the four extra-embryonic membranes.
Amnion	Thin, innermost membrane of the sack containing the foetus.
Blennorrhea	Excessive discharge of mucous from urethra or vagina.
Breech presentation	Baby entering the birth canal with buttocks or feet presenting.
Cachexia	Weight loss and deterioration of physical condition.
Calculus	Stone within the body (e.g. in womb or urinary tract).
Cataplasm (or poultice)	Soft moist mass, often heated and medicated, spread on cloth over the skin to treat aches or inflammation.
Caul	Thin, fatty membrane lining abdominal cavity.
Cautery	White-hot irons applied to cauterize site on body.
Cephalic presentation	(Normal) presentation whereby baby enters the birth canal with its head first.
Cervix	Lower, narrow portion of the uterus which joins the vagina; usually called the 'neck of the womb' in early modern usage.
Chorion	Outermost membrane of the sack containing the foetus.
Chyle	Milky fluid, consisting of lymph and containing absorbed food materials.

Clavicle	Collar bone.
Coccyx	Final segment of the spine, also known as the tailbone.
Condyloma	Genital wart.
Cotyledon	Placental cotyledons were considered by early modern physicians to be ligaments binding the foetus to the uterus.
Crowning	Stage in the delivery when the widest part of the baby's head (the crown) is emerging.
Cupping	Therapy involving application of glass cups to the skin in order to draw the blood to them.
Electuary	Drug mixed into a paste for administration.
Emollient	Substance used to soften the skin or passage.
Enema	Introduction of liquids into the rectum and colon, via the anus, causing the colon to be emptied.
Epigaster	Part of upper abdomen, immediately over stomach.
Epiploon	Also known as the greater omentum; a fold of the peritoneum, from the stomach to abdominal organs.
Erisypelas	Red soreness of the skin (now considered to be caused by bacterial infection).
Fistula	Abnormal connection, passageway or hole between two parts.
Fomentation	Substance applied as warm, moist medicinal compress.

Fumigation	Use of vapours to treat infections or medical problems.
Fundus	Top, or highest, portion of the womb.
Gastrotomy	Surgical incision of abdominal wall.
Hymen	Membrane surrounding, or partially covering, external vaginal opening in a woman who is a virgin.
Hypogastrium	Part of abdomen situated below navel.
Iliac bones	The two upper and largest bones of the pelvis, either side of the sacrum.
Labia minora	Inner lips of the vulva.
Leukorrhea	Excessive, or offensive, white discharge from vagina (known in the early modern period as 'white flowers').
Lochia	Post-partum vaginal discharge, containing blood, mucus and placental tissue.
Mole	Hydatidiform mole is an abnormal development of placental tissue in absence of a viable foetus.
Nymphae	Renaissance term for the labia minora of the clitoris.
Oedema	Fluid retention in the body, producing swelling.
Omphalotomy	Cutting of umbilical cord.
Paracentesis	Drainage of fluid from the peritoneal cavity by a catheter or needle.
Peritoneum	Membranes lining pelvic and abdominal cavities.

Pessary	Small, soluble block inserted into vagina to treat infection OR rigid device inserted into vagina to support uterus.
Petrous bone	Hard portion of the temporal bone, forming a protective case for the inner ear.
Phimosis	Constriction preventing the male foreskin from being fully retracted, OR in women an adhesion affecting vaginal labia.
Phthisis	Wasting or atrophy of all, or part, of the body.
Pica	Appetite for abnormal, non-nutritive substances (especially in early pregnancy).
Poultice (or cataplasm)	Soft, moist mass, often heated and medicated, spread on cloth over the skin to treat aches or inflammation.
Prolapse	An organ (e.g. uterus) falling down or slipping out of place.
Quarter fever	Intermittent fever, markedly raised temperature appearing after about two days.
Revulsion	Medical therapy involving application of a strong substance (e.g. mustard) to an area at some distance from the affected area, in order to draw blood.
Rhagades	Fissures, lesions, linear scars.
Sacrum	Large, triangular bone situated at base of spine and in upper and back of pelvic cavity, between the two hip bones.
Scarification	Scratching or superficial cutting of body.
Schirrus	Type of hard tumor.

Speculum	Instrument inserted into vagina to dilate it so physician can view the womb.
Suffocation of womb	Phenomenon believed in the early modern period to result from upward movement of the womb into the upper abdomen, causing stiff breathing ('suffocation') and sharp pains.
Superfetation	Conception of another pregnancy after a first is already established.
Suppository	Medical tablet inserted into rectum, vagina or urethra.
Trachea	Windpipe.
Trepanation	Cutting a hole in the skull to relieve pain.
Uterus	Womb (term comprises both cervix and body of womb).

EARLY MODERN HERBAL REMEDIES
AND MEDICINES

I list the ingredients cited in the translations in this volume, with a summary indication of the common uses in the early modern period most relevant to these texts. (Note: some of the ingredients would now be viewed as extremely dangerous, e.g. hellebore or hemlock. None of the comments on their uses in the early modern period should be taken as any endorsement for modern usage.)

I am indebted for a number of my definitions to the 'Medical glossary' at the end of Elaine Hobby's edition of Thomas Reynalde's *The Birth of Mankind*; I indicate these by [EH]. Readers will also find it useful to refer to the detailed Medical Glossary provided by Alison Klairmont Lingo at the end of the edition and translation in this series (by herself and Stephanie O'Hara) of Louise Bourgeois's *Observations*: this provides full definitions and recipes for many early modern remedies, and cites the best known classical and early modern printed sources referring to them.

Agarwood / lignum aloes	Fragrant resinous heartwood forming as a result of mould in aquilaria trees of Southeast Asia; used for incense and essential oil to relax muscles.
Alchermes (confection of)	Dark red syrup, made from spices, flowers and kermes colouring (produced from insects), thought to promote longevity.
Alipta moscata	Apothecary's remedy containing storax, calamint, lignum aloes, myrrh, amber [EH].
Aloes (aloe vera)	For constipation, suppressed menstruation, and for healing the skin [EH].
Althea / rose-of-sharon	Emollient, used for digestive disorders.

Angelica	For chest congestion, fevers, to promote menstrual flow; avoided in pregnancy.
Aniseed	For catarrh, cough, colic [EH].
Aristolochia (heartwort)	Stimulant of uterus.
Artemisia	Family of bitter plants — including mugwort, tarragon and wormwood — generally used for dyspepsia, or to promote labor.
Balm / lemonbalm	For anxiety, depression, dyspepsia, mild fever, menstrual problems [EH].
Bedellium	Aromatic gum, similar properties to myrrh [EH].
Belladonna (deadly nightshade)	To ease pain and inflammation.
Benedicta	Laxative, containing turbith, spurge roots, cloves, spikenard and other ingredients [EH].
Blessed thistle water (carduus benedictus)	Made by distilling thistles and herbs, to purge thick, slimy humors, cure pleurisy and strengthen the heart; an antidote to venomous bites.
Borage	For premenstrual symptoms and for external skin complaints [EH].
Buckwheat	For hemorrhage, to suppress menstruation.
Bugloss	Plant close to borage, used similarly.
Camomile	For menstrual pain, morning sickness, digestive disorders, headaches; applied to sore skin [EH]; sometimes avoided in pregnancy since likely to promote menstruation.

Cassia	Aromatic bark similar to cinnamon, used as mild purgative and tonic.
Castoreum	Dried scent glands of a beaver, used to treat a range of ailments.
Catholicon	Common panacea containing many ingredients, usually including senna, rhubarb, cassia and tamarinds.
Catnip	For colic, cramps and 'suffocation' of the womb; to relieve insomnia and tension.
Centaurea / centaury	For indigestion, liver complaints, fever; avoided in pregnancy [EH].
Cinnamon	Stimulant, sometimes avoided in pregnancy, or used to promote labor.
Citronella / lemongrass	To relieve fever, flatulence and painful menstruation.
Clove	An astringent, used for digestive problems; also to prime the womb for childbirth [EH].
Clover / sweet clover	To prevent miscarriage.
Colocynth / bitter apple	(Part of gourd family) strong purgative and abortifacient.
Coriander	To treat digestive disorders and diarrhea.
Cumin	For indigestion, coughs and colds [EH].
Cyclamen	Roots used as a powerful purgative [EH].
Devil's bit	Plant of the scabious family with anti-pyrexic and cleansing properties.

Diacassia	Mixture with laxative properties, containing cassia and manna.
Dictaminus / dittany	Stimulant — avoided in pregnancy.
Euphorbia	Plant with peppery smell, used for respiratory disorders, diarrhea and to promote lactation.
Fennel	Used to promote lactation; for mucous membrane inflammations [EH].
Fenugreek	Powerful stimulant of uterus, to promote lactation.
Flax seed / linseed	To draw boils, for bronchitis and constipation [EH].
Galingale	(From the ginger family) digestive stimulant, mild laxative and used after childbirth.
Gentian	To stimulate appetite and improve digestion.
Ginger	To treat dyspepsia, constipation, colic — a stimulant.
Ground-ivy	For rheumatic pains, bronchitis, skin eruptions, swollen tissues [EH].
Hellebore	Strong stimulant of menses, abortifacient.
Hemlock	For mastitis and hemorrhoids.
Henbane	To induce sleep and relieve pain.
Hippocras	Cordial made from wine mixed with spices, including cinnamon.
Hydromel	Common drink made from water and fermented honey.

Hypericum	*See* St John's wort.
Hyssop	For bronchitis, fever and exhaustion.
Juniper	Berries used for cystitis, gout, joint pain, colic, flatulence; abortifacient [EH].
Labdanum	Sticky brown resin from cistus shrubs, used as expectorant.
Laudanum	Stimulant and expectorant [EH].
Laurel / bay leaves	Ointment for painful joints; gentle stimulant.
Lichen	For lung diseases and rabies.
Lily (oil of)	For burned or dry skin.
Mace / bitter oleander	(Unlike modern mace this is the bark of *holarrhena antidysenttierca* [EH]). Used for diarrhea and skin diseases.
Madder / rubia	Used to make red dye, to bring on the menses and for problems of the liver or spleen.
Maidenhair fern	For catarrh, coughs; a diuretic.
Mallow / marshmallow	Emollients with laxative properties, also used for 'suffocation' of the womb.
Manna	Sugary syrup secreted by certain species of ash tree, with laxative properties.
Mastic	Used externally for boils, bronchitis, muscular stiffness [EH].

Matricaria	(Or feverfew, from the camomile family) Used for flatulence and inflammation.
Mauve	(Species of the mallow family) Emollient and laxative properties, used for 'suffocation' of the womb.
Mercurialis / herb mercury	Diuretic and purgative [EH].
Motherwort	For dysmenorrhea, false labor pains, nervous tension; avoided in pregnancy [EH].
Mucilage	Thick gummy substance produced by plants such as mallows.
Mugwort	*See* Artemisia.
Myrrh	For indigestion, menstrual and circulatory problems, locally for minor wounds; avoided in pregnancy [EH].
Nutmeg	For dyspepsia, colic, inflammatory diseases of gut — sometimes avoided in pregnancy [EH].
Panax	Kind of ginseng.
Patience / impatiens	Diuretic.
Pellitory	Diuretic, also used for 'sufffocation' of the womb and for bronchial infections.
Pennyroyal	For menstrual pain, but avoided in pregnancy [EH].
Periwinkle	For inflammation and congestion.

Polygonon / sanguinalis herba	Kind of buckwheat (*see above*).
Purslane	Astringent, used for inflammation and problems of digestive and urinary tracts.
Rhubarb	Purgative and stimulant.
Roses of Provins (rosa gallica officinalis)	For digestive problems, to cleanse skin.
Rue	For bronchitis, absence of menses, abortifacient [EH].
Saffron	For headache, depression, to stimulate the menses [EH]; sometimes avoided in pregnancy.
Sage	Evergreen herb with widespread healing properties, including as a diuretic and stimulant, and for 'suffocation' of the womb.
St John's wort / hypericum	For burns, and to 'drive out the inner devil'.
Savory	For digestive and menstrual disorders, bronchial congestion [EH].
Scammony	(Of the bindweed family) Gum resin acting as strong purgative.
Senna	Common purgative and laxative.
Soapwort	Mild diuretic, expectorant and tonic.
Sorrel	For fevers, locally for boils [EH].

Spikenard / nard	The oil used as a perfume and a sedative, including for difficult births.
Storax / weeping storax	Complex resin used in medicines and perfumes; for mucous membrane inflammation; an ingredient in proprietary lung medicines [EH].
Tamarind	(Fruit of the tree) Mild laxative and purgative.
Theriac	Commonly used medicinal compound of up to 64 drugs, antidote to poisons.
Turbith	Obtained from roots of convolvulus turpethum, strong purgative.
Venetian turpentine	Form of natural resin.
Verjus	Acidic liquid from the juice of green grapes, used in cooking and as an astringent for treating stomach and liver disorders.
Violet	For congested lungs, cancer pain [EH].
Water lily	To reduce sexual excitement; for diarrhea, bronchitis, uterine infections [EH],
Wormwood	For dyspepsia, to promote menstruation, externally for bruises [EH].

BIBLIOGRAPHY

This Bibliography comprises works directly cited or discussed in the translations or in the introductions, and some key general studies on early modern medicine. For items mentioned in passing and which are not included here, full bibliographical details have been given in the footnotes.

For works originally published in languages other than English, if the English title is well known in its own right (e.g. the works of Aristotle, Galen, etc.), or has been published in a modern edition, this is the form used here. In other cases, I give first my own English translation of the title and then, in square brackets, the title in the original language and the date of the published edition I have used.

With regard to spelling and capitalization, I have followed in the Bibliography the same principles as in the rest of this volume (see xiii).

Where sixteenth- and seventeenth-century works have particularly lengthy titles, I have shortened them appropriately.

PRIMARY BIBLIOGRAPHY

Aetius of Amida, *Tetrabiblus in XVI volumes* [*Aetii contractae ex veteribus medicinae tetrabiblos, id est sermones XVI, per Ianum Cornarium Latine conscripti*, Lyons: ex officina Godefridi et Marcelli Beringorum, 1549].

Agrippa, Henricus, *Declamation on the Preeminence and Nobility of the Female Sex*, trans. and ed. A. Rabil (Chicago: University of Chicago Press, 1996).

Ailleboust, Jean d', *The Monstrous Stone-Child, or the Putrefied Embryo of the Town of Sens* [*Portentosum lithopaedion, sive embryon putrefactum urbis Senonensis*, Sens: Jean Savine, 1582].

[pseudo-] Albertus Magnus, *Women's Secrets. A Translation of pseudo-Albertus Magnus's 'De Secretis Mulierum' with commentaries*, trans. H. Rodnite Lemay (Albany: State University of New York Press, 1992).

Aristotle, *On the Generation of Animals*, trans. A. L. Peck (London: Heinemann, 1953).

______. *On Generation and Corruption*, trans. J. Stock (Forgotten Books, 2007).

______. *The History of Animals*, ed. and trans. D. M. Balme (Cambridge–MA: Harvard University Press, 1991).

______. *Politics*, ed. and trans. H. Rackham (Cambridge–MA: Loeb Classical Library, 1959).

Avicenna, *The General Principles of Avicenna's Canon of Medicine*, trans. M. H. Shah (Karaki: Naveed Clinic, 1966).

Bauhin, Caspar, ed. *Books on the Diseases of Women* [in the *Gynaeciorum libri*], 2nd and enlarged edition (Basel: Conrad Waldkirch 1586–1588); original edn ed. Hans Kaspar Wolf (Basel: Thomas Guarinus, 1566).

Bourgeois, Louise, *True History of the Births of the Royal Children of France*, in *Observations*, 1617 [*Récit véritable de la naissance de messeigneurs et dames les enfans de France*, ed. F. Rouget and C. Winn, Geneva: Droz, 2000].

______. *Diverse Observations on Sterility, Miscarriage, Fertility, Childbirth and the Diseases of Women and of Newborn Children* [*Observations diverses sur la sterilité, perte de fruits, foecondité, accouchements et maladies des femmes et enfants nouveaux naiz*, vol. I, Paris: A. Saugrain, 1609; vols. I and II, Paris: A. Saugrain, 1617; vols I, II and III, Paris: Melchior Mondiere, 1626].

______. *Diverse Observations on Sterility, Miscarriage, Fertility, Childbirth, and the Diseases of Women and Newborn Children (1626)*, trans. Stephanie O'Hara; ed. Alison Klairmont Lingo (Toronto: Toronto University Press, forthcoming).

Cardano, Gerolamo, *On the Subtlety of Things* [*De subtilitate rerum*, Nuremberg: Johannes Petreius, 1550].

Celsus, Aulus Cornelius, *On Medicine* [*De re medicina*], trans. G. F. Collier (London: 1840).

Cheselden, William, *A Treatise on the High Operation of the Stone* (London: John Osborn, 1723).

Cornax, Mathias, *Two Memorable Histories* [*Historiae duae memorabiles*, Augsburg: Johannes Zimmerman, 1555].

Daleschamps, Jacques, *French Surgery* [*Chirurgie françoise recueillie par M. Jacques Dalechamps*, rev. and ext edition Jean Girault, Paris: Olivier de Varennes, 1610 (original ed. 1569)].

Dioscorides, Pedanius, *De materia medica: being an herbal with many other medicinal materials*, trans. T. Osbaldeston (Johannesburg: Ibidis Press, 2000).

Duval, Jacques, *On Hermaphrodites, Deliveries of Women, and the Treatment which is required after Childbirth* [*Des Hermaphrodits, accouchemens des femmes, et traitement qui est requis pour les relever en santé, et bien élever leurs enfans*, Rouen: David Geuffroy, 1612].

______. *Response to the Discourse by Monsieur Riolan on the Tale of the Hermaphrodite of Rouen* [*Responce au discours fait par le sieur Riolan contre l'histoire de l'hermaphrodit de Rouen*, Rouen: Julien Courant, 1615].

Estienne, Charles, *Maison rustique, or The Countrie Farm*, trans. Richard Surflet, London: E. Bollifant for B. Norton, 1600 [*Praedium rusticum*, Paris: C. Stephanus, 1554; *Agriculture et maison rustique de M. Charles Estienne*, trans. Jean Liebault, Lyons: 1564].

Galen, *Book on the Natural Faculties*, trans. A. Brock, 1916 (cited from the Directory of Classic Literature, www.greektexts.com).

______. *On the Usefulness of the Parts of the Body*, trans. M. Tallmadge May (2 vols.), (Ithaca: Cornell University Press, 1968).

Gelée, Théophile, *The Rare, Marvelous but True Tale of a Woman from the Village of Neufville near Dieppe* [*Histoire rare et merveilleuse, mais veritable d'une femme du village de Neufville aupres de Dieppe*, Dieppe: Nicolas Acher, 1622].

Guillemeau, Jacques, *On the Safe Delivery of Women* [*De l'heureux accouchement des femmes*, Paris: Nicolas Buon, 1609].

______. *On the Care and Upbringing of Children from the Very Time of their Birth* [*De la nourriture et gouvernement des enfans, des le commencement de leur naissance*, Paris: Nicolas Buon, 1609].

______. *Child-birth or, The Happy Deliverie of Women* [...] *To which is added, a treatise of the diseases of infants, and young children: with the cure of them*, trans. anon. (London: A. Hatfield, 1612).

Hippocrates, *Aphorisms*, in *Hippocrates, with an English translation*, trans. W. H. S. Jones, vol. IV (Cambridge–MA: Loeb Classical Library, 1931).

______. *Œuvres complètes. Traduction nouvelle avec le texte grec en regard*, ed. and French trans. E. Littré (10 vols.), (Paris: 1839–1861).

______. *On the Nature of the Child*, in *Hippocratic Writings*, ed. G.E.R. Lloyd, trans. J. Chadwick (Hardmondsworth: Penguin, 1983; original edition, 1950).

Horace, *The Art of Poetry*, in *Horace: Satires, Epistles and Ars Poetica*, trans. H. Fairclough (Cambridge–MA: Loeb Classical Library, 1926).

Joubert, Laurent, *Popular Errors*, trans. G. de Rocher (Alabama: University of Alabama Press, 1989) [*Erreurs populaires*, Bordeaux: Simon Millanges, 1578].

La Croix Du Maine, François de, *Les Bibliothèques françoises de La Croix Du Maine et de Du Verdier, sieur de Vauprivas* (6 vols.), ed. M. Rigoley de Juvigny (Paris: Taillant and Nyons, 1772; first edn. 1584).

Lemne, Levin, *On the Secret Miracles of Nature* [*Occulta naturae miracula*, Antwerp: apud G. Simonem, 1559; *Les Secrets Miracles de nature et divers enseignemens de plusieurs choses, par raison probable et artiste conjecture expliquez en deux livres*, French trans. Lyons: Jean Frellon, 1566].

Leone, Ebreo, *Dialogues of Love* [*Dialoghi d'amore*, posthum. Rome: Antonio Blado d'Assola, 1535; French trans. Pontus de Tyard, Lyons: Jean de Tournes, 1551].

L'Estoile, Pierre de, *Memoirs-Papers* [*Mémoires-Journaux*, ed. P. Bonnefon, Paris: A. Lemerre, 1888–96].

Liebault, Jean, *Three Books dealing with the Infirmities and Illnesses of Women* [*Trois livres appartenant aux infirmitez et maladies des femmes*, Paris: Jacques Dupuis, 1582].

______. *Three Books on the Embellishment and Adornment of the Human Body* [*Trois livres de l'embellissement et ornement du corps humain*, Paris: Jacques Dupuis, 1582].

Liebault, Nicole, 'The Sufferings of the Married Woman' ['Les Misères de la femme mariée', c. 1587].

Marchand, Jacques, *Declamation against François Rousset's Apologia* [*In Fr. Rosseti apologiam, declamatio*, Paris: Nicolaus Delouvain, 1598].

Marinella, Lucrezia, *The Nobility and Excellence of Women and the Defects and Vices of Men* [*Nobiltà e Eccellenza delle donne, coi difetti et mancamenti degli uomoni*, Venice: 1600], trans. and ed. A. Dunhill, intro. L. Panizza (Chicago: Chicago University Press, 1999).

Marinelli, Giovanni, *The Ornaments of Women* [*Gli ornamenti delle donne*, Venice: Francesco de Franceschi, 1562; 2nd extd edn Venice: Giovanni Valgrisio, 1574].

______. *Medicine pertaining to Women's Diseases* [*Le Medicine partenenti alle infermità delle donne*, Venice: G. Bonadio for Francesco de Franceschi, 1563; 2nd extd edn. Venice: Giovanni Valgrisio, 1574].

Mauriceau, François, *Diseases of Women with Child, and in Childbed*, trans. Hugh Chamberlen, 2nd edn. London: John Darby, 1683 [*Maladies des femmes grosses et accouchées*, Paris: Charles Coignard for the author, Jean d'Houry and Robert de Ninville, 1668].

Mercado, Luis de, On *the Diseases of Women* [*De mulierum affectionibus*, Valladolid: D. Fernandez, 1579].

Mercurio, Scipione, *The Midwife* [*La Commare o raccoglitrice*, Venice: G. B. Ciotti, 1601].

Meyssonnier, Louis, *The Care of Newly Delivered Women* [*Le Regime des femmes accouchées*, Lyons: J. Du Creux, 1646].

Paul of Aegina, *The Medical Works of Paulus Aegineta, the Greek Physician*, ed. and trans. Francis Adams (London: J. Welsh, 1834).

Pineau, Séverin, *Physiological and Anatomical Treatise* [*Opusculum physiologum et anatomicum*, Paris: S. Prevosteau, 1597]; republished as *On the Signs of Intact and Despoiled Virgins* [*De integritatis et corruptionis virginum notis*, Lyons: 1639].

Plato, *Timaeus*, ed. and trans. R. Bury (Cambridge–MA: Loeb Classical Library, 1960).

______. *Symposium*, trans. W. Lamb (Cambridge–MA: Loeb Classical Library, 1925).

______. *Republic*, trans. P. Shorey (Cambridge–MA: Loeb Classical Library, 1930).

______. *Theaetetus*, trans. H. Fowler (Cambridge–MA: Loeb Classical Library, 1921).

Pliny the Elder, *Natural History*, trans. H. Rackham (Cambridge–MA: Loeb Classical Library, 1950).

Plutarch, *The Moralia* (14 vols.), (Cambridge–MA: Loeb Classical Library, 1927).

Provanchières, Simon de, *The Monstrous Stone-Child, or the Putrified Embryo of the Town of Sens* [*Portentosum lithopaedion, sive embryon putrefactum urbis Senonensis*, Sens: Jean Savine, 1582].

Rabelais, François, *Gargantua and Pantagruel*, trans. M. A. Screech, Penguin Classics [*Pantagruel*, Lyons: Claude Nourry, 1532; *Gargantua*, Lyons: François Juste, 1534].

Reynalde, Thomas, *The Birth of Mankind: otherwise named, The Woman's Book*, ed. Elaine Hobby (Farnham-Burlington USA: Ashgate Press, 2009; orig. edn. 1540).

Riolan, Jean (the younger), *Discourse on Hermaphrodites* [*Discours sur les hermaphrodits*, Paris: Pierre Ramier, 1614].

Rondelet, Guillaume, *The Method of Curing all Diseases of the Human Body* [*Methodus curandorum omnium morborum corporis humani*, Paris: apud Jacobum Maceum, 1570].

Rösslin, Eucharius, *A Rosegarden for Pregnant Women and Midwives* [*Der Swangern Frawen und Hebammen Roszgarten*, Hagenau: H. Gran, 1513].

______. *Eucharius Rösslin: when midwifery became the male physician's province*, ed. and trans. W. Arons (Jefferson NC and London: McFarland, 1994).

Rousset, François, *New Treatise on Hysterotomotoky* [*Traitté nouveau de l'hysterotomotokie, ou enfantement cæsarien*, Paris: Denis Duval, 1581].

______. *Caesarean Birth. The work of François Rousset in Renaissance France. A new treatise on hysterotomotokie or caesarien childbirth*, ed. and trans. R. Cyr and T. Baskett (London: RCOG Press, 2010).

______. *Hysterotomotoky, that is a Historological Defence of Caesarean Delivery* [*Hysterotomotokias, id est Caesarei partus assertio historologica*, Paris: Denis Duval, 1590].

______. *Dialogue in Defence of Caesarean Delivery* [*Dialogus apologeticus pro caesareo partu*, Paris: Denis Duval, 1590].

______. *Response to the Declamation of Jacques Marchant* [*Responsio ad Jacobi Marchant declamationem*, Paris: n.d.?1590].

Serres, Louis de, *Treatise on the Nature, Causes, Signs and Remedies concerning Failures to Conceive, and Sterility among Women*, [*Discours de la Nature, causes, signes, et curation des empeschemens de la conception, et de la sterilité des femmes*, Lyons: Antoine Chard, 1625].

Soranus, *Gynaecology*, trans. O. Temkin (Baltimore: John Hopkins University Press, 1956).

The Trotula: a medieval compendium of women's medicine, ed. and trans. M. H. Green (Philadelphia: University of Pennsylvania Press, 2001).

Varanda, Jean, *On the Diseases and Afflictions of Women* [*De morbis et affectibus mulierum*, published posthumously, Lyons: B. Vincent, 1619].

SECONDARY BIBLIOGRAPHY

Albaric, K., *Un Médecin ébroïcien, Jacques Duval. Son traité des hermaphrodites (1555?–1615?)*, (Paris: Librairie Le François, 1934).

Bates, A., *Emblematic Monsters. Unnatural conceptions and deformed births in early modern Europe* (Amsterdam-New York: Rodopi, 2005).

Benedict, P., *The Huguenot Population of France: the demographic fate and customs of a religious minority* (Philadelphia: American Philosophical Society, 1991).

Berriot-Salvadore, E., *Un corps, un destin: la femme dans la médecine de la Renaissance* (Paris: Champion, 1993).

Blumenfeld-Kosinski, R., *Not of Woman Born. Representations of caesarean birth in medieval and Renaissance culture* (Ithaca and London: Cornell University Press, 1990).

Bracke, W. and Deumens, H., ed., *Medical Latin from the Late Middle Ages to the Eighteenth Century* (Brussels: 2000).

Brockliss, L. and Jones, C., *The Medical World of Early Modern France* (Oxford: Clarendon Press, 1997).

Broomhall, S., *Women's Medical Work in Early Modern France* (Manchester: Manchester University Press, 2004).

Daston, L. and Lunbeck, E., eds., *Histories of Scientific Observation* (Chicago and London: The University of Chicago Press, 2011).

Doe, J., *A Bibliography of the Works of Ambroise Paré* (Chicago: University of Chicago Press, 1957).

Dubard, P., *La vie et l'œuvre de Jacques Guillemeau* [no place], 2006.

Flemming, R., 'Women, Writing and Medicine in the Classical World, *Classical Quarterly* 57–1 (2007), 257–279.

Frère, E., *Manuel du bibliographe normand* (Rouen: A. Le Brument, 1858).

Gélis, J., *L'Arbre et le fruit: la naissance dans l'Occident moderne, XVIe-XIXe siècle* (Paris: Fayard, 1984).

______. *La Sage-femme ou le médecin. Une nouvelle conception de la vie* (Paris: Fayard, 1988).

Goldstein, C., *Print Culture in Early Modern France. Abraham Bosse and the purposes of print* (Cambridge: Cambridge University Press, 2012).

Green, M., *Women's Healthcare in the Medieval West: texts and contexts* (Aldershot: Ashgate Press, 2002).

______. *Making Woman's Medicine Masculine. The rise of male authority in pre-modern gynaecology* (Oxford: Oxford University Press, 2008).

______. 'The Sources of Eucharius Rösslin's "Rosegarden for Pregnant Women and Midwives"' (1513)', *Medical History*, 53–2 (April 2009), 167–192.

Harris, J., '"La force du tact": representing the taboo body in Jacques Duval's *Traité des hermaphrodits* (1612)', *French Studies* 57 (2003), 311–322.

King, H., *Hippocrates' Woman. Reading the female body in Ancient Greece* (London and New York: Routledge, 1998).

______. *Midwifery, Obstetrics and the Rise of Gynaecology. The uses of a sixteenth-century French compendium* (Aldershot: Ashgate, 2007).

Klairmont Lingo, A., 'The Fate of Popular Terms for Female Anatomy in the Age of Print', *French Historical Studies* 22–3 (1999), 335–349.

Laqueur, T., *Making Sex: body and gender from the Greeks to Freud* (Cambridge MA-London: Harvard University Press, 1990).

Long, K., 'Jacques Duval on Hermaphrodites' in *High Anxiety. Masculinity in crisis in early modern France*, ed. K. Long. (Kirksville, Missouri: Truman State University Press, 2002).

______. *Hermaphrodites in Renaissance Europe* (Aldershot: Ashgate, 2006).

Maclean, I., *Woman Triumphant: Feminism in French Literature, 1610–1652* (Oxford: Clarendon Press, 1977).

______. *The Renaissance Notion of Woman. A study in the fortunes of scholasticism and medical science in European intellectual life* (Cambridge: Cambridge University Press, 1980).

McTavish, L., *Childbirth and the Display of Authority in Early Modern France* (Aldershot: Ashgate, 2005).

Pantin, I., 'La traduction latine des *Œuvres* d'Ambroise Paré', in *Ambroise Paré (1510–1590). Pratique et écriture de la science à la Renaissance. Actes du Colloque de Pau (6–7 mai 1999)*, ed. E. Beriot-Salvadore and P. Mironneau (Paris: Honoré Champion, 2003).

Park, K., *The Secrets of Women. Gender, generation and the origins of human dissection* (New York: Zone Books, 2006).

Perkins, W., *Midwifery and Medicine in Early Modern France: Louise Bourgeois* (Exeter: University of Exeter Press, 1996).

Pomata, G., 'Sharing Cases: the *Observationes* in early Modern Medicine', *Early Science and Medicine* 15 (2010), 193–236.

Pomata, G. and Siraisi, N., ed., *Historia: Empiricism and erudition in early modern Europe* (Massachusetts: Massachusetts Institute of Technology, 2005).

Poulain, F., *La Vie et l'œuvre de deux chirurgiens: Jacques Guillemeau (1550–1613) et Charles Guillemeau (1588–1656)*, doctoral thesis, Montpellier, 1961.

Read, K., *Birthing Bodies in Early Modern France: Stories of Gender and Reproduction* (Farnham: Ashgate, 2011).

Renouard, P., *Imprimeurs et libraires parisiens du XVIe siècle* (Paris: Service des Travaux Historiques de la Ville de Paris, 1964.)

Reynolds-Cornell, R., '*Les Misères de la femme mariée*: another look at Nicole Liebault and a few questions about the woes of the married woman', *Bibliothèque d'Humanisme et Renaissance*, LXIV–1 (2002), 37–54.

Stone, H., 'The French Language in Renaissance Medicine', *Bibliothèque d'Humanisme et Renaissance* XV (1953), 315–343.

Tucker, H., *Pregnant Fictions: Childbirth and the Fairy Tale in Early Modern France* (Detroit: Wayne State University Press, 2003).

Wilson, A., *The Making of Man-Midwifery: childbirth in England 1660–1770* (London: UCL Press, 1995).

Worth-Stylianou, V., *Les Traités d'obstétrique en langue française au seuil de la modernité: bibliographie critique des 'Divers Travaulx d'Euchaire Rösslin' (1536) à l'Apologie De Louyse Bourgeois sage femme' (1627)*, (Geneva: Droz, 2007).

______. 'La théâtralisation de la naissance du dauphin (1601) chez Louise Bourgeois, sage-femme de Marie de Médicis', in *Le*

«Théâtral» de la France d'Ancien Régime, ed. S. Chaouche (Paris: Honoré Champion, 2010), 137–154.

______. 'The definition of obscene material 1570–1615: three medical treatises held to account', *EMF: Studies in Early Modern France*, 14 (2010), 148–167.

INDEX

INDEX OF PROPER NAMES

This Index comprises references to names of people from Antiquity through to the end of the seventeenth century. For authors of modern critical studies, the reader should consult the General Index or the Bibliography.

INDEX OF PLACES

This Index comprises the names of villages, towns, regions and countries referred to in the texts or in the discussions of them.

GENERAL INDEX